PEDIATRIC NURSING PROCEDURE MANUAL

PEDIATRIC NURSING PROCEDURE MANUAL

As per the Revised INC Syllabus for BSc Nursing (also useful for MSc students)

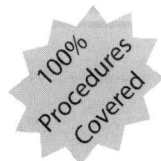

SECOND EDITION

A Padmaja MA (Psy) MSc (N) PhD
Professor (Retd)
College of Nursing
Sri Venkateswara Institute of Medical Sciences
Tirupati, Andhra Pradesh, India

Officer-Special Duty (OSD), Allied Health Science (AHS)
Sri Padmavathi Medical College for Women
Sri Venkateswara Institute of Medical Sciences
Tirupati, Andhra Pradesh, India

Forewords
Saradha Suresh
K Rajalakshmi

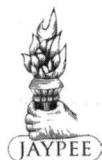

JAYPEE BROTHERS MEDICAL PUBLISHERS
The Health Sciences Publisher
New Delhi | London

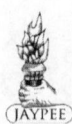 **Jaypee Brothers Medical Publishers (P) Ltd**

Headquarters
Jaypee Brothers Medical Publishers (P) Ltd
EMCA House
23/23-B, Ansari Road, Daryaganj
New Delhi 110 002, India
Landline: +91-11-23272143, +91-11-23272703
+91-11-23282021, +91-11-23245672
E-mail: jaypee@jaypeebrothers.com

Corporate Office
Jaypee Brothers Medical Publishers (P) Ltd.
4838/24, Ansari Road, Daryaganj
New Delhi 110 002, India
Phone: +91-11-43574357
Fax: +91-11-43574314
E-mail: jaypee@jaypeebrothers.com

Overseas Office
JP Medical Ltd.
83, Victoria Street, London
SW1H 0HW (UK)
Phone: +44-20 3170 8910
Fax: +44(0)20 3008 6180
E-mail: info@jpmedpub.com

Website: www.jaypeebrothers.com
Website: www.jaypeedigital.com
© 2022, Jaypee Brothers Medical Publishers

The views and opinions expressed in this book are solely those of the original contributor(s)/author(s) and do not necessarily represent those of editor(s) of the book.

All rights reserved by the author. No part of this publication may be reproduced, stored or transmitted in any form or by any means, electronic, mechanical, photocopying, recording or otherwise, without the prior permission in writing of the publishers.

All brand names and product names used in this book are trade names, service marks, trademarks or registered trademarks of their respective owners. The publisher is not associated with any product or vendor mentioned in this book.

Medical knowledge and practice change constantly. This book is designed to provide accurate, authoritative information about the subject matter in question. However, readers are advised to check the most current information available on procedures included and check information from the manufacturer of each product to be administered, to verify the recommended dose, formula, method and duration of administration, adverse effects and contraindications. It is the responsibility of the practitioner to take all appropriate safety precautions. Neither the publisher nor the author(s)/editor(s) assume any liability for any injury and/or damage to persons or property arising from or related to use of material in this book.

This book is sold on the understanding that the publisher is not engaged in providing professional medical services. If such advice or services are required, the services of a competent medical professional should be sought.

Every effort has been made where necessary to contact holders of copyright to obtain permission to reproduce copyright material. If any have been inadvertently overlooked, the publisher will be pleased to make the necessary arrangements at the first opportunity.

Inquiries for bulk sales may be solicited at: jaypee@jaypeebrothers.com

Pediatric Nursing Procedure Manual

First Edition: 2014
Second Edition: **2022**

ISBN: 978-93-5465-622-4

Printed at: Sterling Graphics Pvt. Ltd.

DEDICATED TO

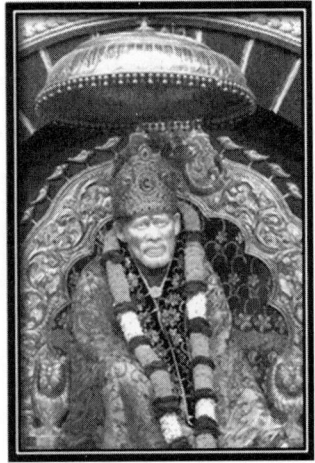

I am heartfully dedicating my work to "Sri Shiridi Sainath", who strengthens me by helping in each and every second in all my deeds by showering His blessings abundantly through various resources, which helped me in the accomplishment of all the tasks in my life.

This book is also dedicated to my incredible family, without whom I could never have accomplished this monumental task. In loving memory of my father, Late A Adinarayana, for his eternal blessings and my mother, Smt A Kausalyamma and my mother-in-law, Smt K Chengamma, for rendering emotional support. My husband, Dr K Munuswamy, SMO, Causality, Sri Venkateswara Institute of Medical Sciences (SVIMS), has unfailingly stood by my side, providing continuous positive affirmation and infinite support for this project. My brothers, S Somprakash, founder President of Viswadharma Peetam (Center for Universal Philosophy), A Venkata Ramanaiah, founder of Sri Shiridi Sai Industries, Avilala, for their motivation and moral support. My sister, A Nagaraja Kumari and my son, K Prabhat Kiran, for their patience and tireless efforts to help me in computer work.

DEDICATED TO

FOREWORD

The book *Pediatric Nursing Procedure Manual* is very valuable as it will help the nurse to prepare the patient and also the equipment required for that. As teachers we all know good books are hard to come by as it takes enormous effort to write one. I really congratulate Professor Dr A Padmaja, for her enthusiasm and hard work in writing and bringing out this book which I am sure will be found useful to each and every working nurse not to mention teachers and other medical faculties involved in teaching and care of sick children. It is with great pleasure and a sense of honor that I am writing the Foreword for this book and I am not hoping but am very sure that this book will go into several edition and prints as it readily deserves. Once again I express my appreciation to Dr A Padmaja and her Guru Professor Dr K Rajalakshmi who had been instrumental in inspiring her to write this book.

Saradha Suresh MD PhD FRCP (Glas)
Former Director and Superintendent
Institute of Child Health and Hospital for Children
Chennai, Tamil Nadu, India
Head
Department of Pediatrics
Madras Medical College
Chennai, Tamil Nadu, India

FOREWORD

It gives me immense pleasure to pen this Foreword to the *Pediatric Nursing Procedure Manual* written by Professor Dr A Padmaja. She is very enthusiastic, interested but calm and quite to contribute to education, practice, service, administration and research. She has published articles on Pediatric Nursing in India and presented papers in India and abroad. Since, there is no such well-written book available on procedures in child health, she has taken interest to bring out this procedure manual. It is very much useful to treat patients in hospital/community to provide high quality holistic care with competence and compassion. This book will give all the nursing as well as medical students and staff as a manual to do the procedure scientifically with rationale. It is a well-planned and hard work of the author in a simple, excellent material and easily understandable language to teach and learn on the procedure, start from the history taking, physical examination, newborn assessment, developmental assessment, methods of feeding, drugs administration, exchange transfusion, total parenteral nutrition, restrains, play needs, psychological support, and all the procedures in surgical and medical intervention including, thoracic drainage for tension pneumothorax, etc., are the outstanding features of this manual.

The author exhibits her vision and critical thinking in each section of this procedure book. It has great value and standardized one to treat to the satisfaction and requirement of the need of the child and it is useful for educators and students on this subject. I am happy and confident that this procedure book will be helpful for students and practitioners to provide health to improve the children's health status.

I am privileged to know Professor Dr A Padmaja as a best outgoing student as a graduate, postgraduate, doctoral scholar, as examiner for PhD program in different universities and educator. I know her aspirations through my personal close contact and correspondence.

K Rajalakshmi
RN, MN (PhD)
Professor, Pediatric(N) and Research Guide
CSI Jeyaraj Annapackiam College of Nursing
Madurai, Tamil Nadu, India

PREFACE TO THE SECOND EDITION

It gives me immense pleasure to present the second edition of this *Pediatric Nursing Procedure Manual* to the nursing students, educators and practitioners in the field of child health nursing.

A reasonable time has been spent in the revision of this book. The whole book is updated according to the current concepts of child health nursing procedures. Some of the topics have been added such as family assessment, nutritional assessment, assisting with common diagnostic procedures, monitoring of babies, pediatric drug calculation, oral rehydration therapy (ORT), empowering parents on prevention of malnutrition, empowering parents on immunization, ureterostomy and enterostomy care, insertion of suppositories, endotracheal tube suctioning, umbilical cord blood collection and analysis.

This book is my sincere effort to help BSc nursing and MSc nursing students prepare for child health nursing practical examination, and in turn helps in theory examination also, as the text covers complete child health nursing procedures as per the syllabus prescribed by Indian Nursing Council (INC), New Delhi. Each procedure was begin with practice competencies, and ends with points to note. Multiple choice questions (MCQs) were given at end of each chapter, will help the students to evaluate their understanding of the matter and ability to recall the information. This manual is definitely going to be a valuable companion to all nursing students and personnel.

I sincerely invite suggestions, constructive criticism and comments of the readers about this book so that acceptable changes can be made in the forthcoming edition. Kindly mail me at raajinaidu@rocketmail.com.

I wish all readers success in nursing career.

A Padmaja

PREFACE TO THE FIRST EDITION

I am very much delighted to present this book titled *Pediatric Nursing Procedure Manual*, to the nursing students in India. This textbook promotes nursing as an evolving art and science, directed to child health and well-being. The primary objective of this book is to prepare nurses who combine the highest level of scientific knowledge and technologic skills with responsible caring practice.

Since, it is prepared according to the syllabus of Indian Nursing Council, the undergraduate and postgraduate nursing students will find it as a textbook for their studies. The nursing educators will find it easy to teach their students and prepare them for the examinations.

This book will also bring a uniform standard of the nursing education in India. It also serves as a reference manual for the practicing nurse.

I will be much appreciated, if readers send their criticism, suggestions, corrections, if any for further improvement of this book.

A Padmaja

ACKNOWLEDGMENTS

I am most grateful to my teacher Professor Dr K Rajalakshmi and Professor Dr Saradha Suresh, who have kindly honored me by writing the forewords.

I would like to have the opportunity to thank Professor Dr B Vengamma (Director), Professor Dr D Rajasekhar (Head, Department of Cardiology and Dean), and Professor Dr PV Ramasubba Reddy (Registrar), Sri Venkateswara Institute of Medical Sciences (SVIMS) and other administrators, for permitting me to publish this book.

I extend my special thanks to Professor Dr Alladi Mohan (Head, Department of Medicine), SVIMS and all my colleagues, friends and well-wishers, who have cooperated directly or indirectly on completion of the task. I am thankful to all my past and present students, who have insisted me to accept this work, especially Ms J Samhitha, for drawing the figures.

A grateful acknowledgment is extended to Shri Jitendar P Vij (Group Chairman), Mr Ankit Vij (Managing Director), Mr MS Mani (Group President), Dr Madhu Choudhary (Publishing Head -Education), Ms Pooja Bhandari (Production Head), Ms Sunita Katla (Executive Assistant to Group Chairman and Publishing Manager), Mr Rajesh Sharma (Production Coordinator), Ms Seema Dogra (Cover Visualizer), Ms Geeta Barik (Proofreader), Ms Uma Adhikari (Typesetter), Mr Ratan Lal (Graphic Designer) and all the other staff of M/s Jaypee Brothers Medical Publishers (P) Ltd, New Delhi, India, especially Mr Venugopal (Branch Manager, Bengaluru), Mr Shanta Raj, for publishing this book.

During the revision of second edition of this manual, Ms S Anjali (Development Editor), who was working on this book had developed COVID-19. In spite of that, she worked from home during this crucial period and completed the task successfully. I express my gratitude from the bottom of my heart for her hard work with great patience and sincerity. I feel proud of our Jaypee Publications, especially Ms Samina Khan (Executive Assistant to Publishing Head–Education). I pray Lord Balaji to bless them with health, wealth and happiness.

CONTENTS

1. **Pediatric History Taking and Physical Examination**   1
   - Profile of the Child   2
   - Immunization History   2
   - Physical Examination   3
   - Case Presentation   6

2. **Family Assessment**   9
   - The Family History   9
   - Observation   11
   - Interviewing Technique   11
   - Phases of Interview   11
   - Family History   12

3. **Nutrition Assessment**   15
   - Nutrition Assessment   15
   - Physical Assessment   16
   - Anthropometric Measurements   16
   - Biochemical Indices   18

4. **Newborn Assessment**   20
   - Purposes and Precautions   20
   - Immediate Examination at Birth   21

5. **Anthropometry Measurements**   26
   - Definitions   27
   - Anthropometric Measurements   27

6. **Developmental Assessment**   36
   - Development   36
   - Assessment of Development   37
   - Development of Newborn   37
   - Reflexes of Newborn   37
   - Important Milestones at Glance   40
   - Language Development   40
   - Developmental Screening Test   41
   - Denver Development Examination   43

7. **Assisting with Common Diagnostic Procedures**   46
   - Definition   46
   - Throat Swab Specimen Collection   48
   - Sputum Specimen Collection   49
   - Stool Specimen Collection   50
   - Venepuncture   52
   - Blood Cultures   53

8. **Monitoring of Babies**   57
   - Aim   57
   - Observations and Monitoring   58
   - Management   61
   - Parent Engagement   62

9. **Kangaroo Mother Care**   64
   - Definition   64
   - Components of KMC   65

10. **Methods of Feeding**   70
    - Principles of Feeding Children   71
    - Breastfeeding   71
    - Bottle Feeding   72
    - Spoon/Paladi/Katori (Cup) Feeding   73
    - Gavage Feeding   73
    - Gastrostomy Feeding   76
    - Gastrojejunal Feeding   77

11. **Drug Administration**   79
    - Oral Administration of Medications to Children   79
    - Intramuscular Drug Administration   84
    - Fluid Calculation for IV Infusion   88
    - Exchange Transfusion   92
    - Total Parenteral Nutrition   99

12. **Pediatric Drug Calculation**   104
    - Metric Units   104
    - Dosage Calculations   105
    - Volume of Drug to Give   106
    - Percentage Calculations   107
    - Ratio Calculation   108

13. **Oral Rehydration Therapy**   112
    - Definition   112
    - Recommended Home Fluids   112
    - How to Prepare ORS?   113

14. Empowering Parents on Prevention of Malnutrition in Children — 117
- Teaching Mothers/Parents: Feeding and Weaning 118

15. Empowering Parents on Immunization — 121
- Do's and Don'ts during Immunization 121
- Immunization Schedule, Source—WHO 2013 122

16. Urine Specimen Collection — 124
- Definition 124
- General Principles 124
- In Elder Children 127
- In an Infant 127
- Nursing Responsibility 128

17. Restraints — 130
- Definition 130
- Types of Restraints 131
- Hazards of Restraints 134

18. Play Needs for Different Age Groups — 136
- Functions of Play 137
- Development Role of Play 138
- Types of Play According to Socialization 139
- Toy Safety 142
- Selection of Play Materials for Different Age Groups 143
- Therapeutic Play During Bedside Care 146

19. Care of Child with Phototherapy — 148

20. Care of the Child in Incubator — 152
- Thermoregulation 153
- The Neutral Thermal Environment 154

21. Care of the Child in Radiant Warmer — 159

22. Ostomy Care — 162
- Colostomy Care and Irrigation 162
- Urostomy Care 168
- Gastrostomy Care 169
- Ureterostomy and Enterostomy Care 172
- Enterostomy Care 175
- Documentation 177

23. Care of Surgical Wounds, Dressing and Suture Removal — 179
- Definition 179
- Purposes of Dressings 179
- Types of Dressings Used 179

24. Catheterization in Children — 184
- Procedure for Pediatric Urinary Catheterization General Guidelines 187

25. Insertion of Suppositories — 191
- Definition 191
- Ideal Suppository Measures 191
- Equipment 192
- Indications 192
- Contraindications 192
- Pre-procedure Guidelines 192
- Complications 194

26. Oxygen Administration in Children — 196
- Oxygen therapy 197
- Indications 197
- Methods of Oxygen Therapy 198

27. Cardiopulmonary Resuscitation — 205
- Objectives 205
- Purposes 206
- Indications 206
- Preparation for Resuscitation 206
- Equipment Required 206
- The TABC of Resuscitation 207
- Signs to Evaluate for Resuscitation 207
- Initial Steps of Resuscitation 207
- Positive Pressure Ventilation Bag and Mask 209
- Technique of Positive Pressure Ventilation 209
- Chest Compression 210
- Technique of Chest Compression 210

28. Endotracheal Intubation — 213
- Indications 213
- Technique of Intubation 213
- Procedure of Endotracheal Intubation 214
- Orotracheal Intubation 214
- Medications 215

29. Endotracheal Tube Suctioning — 217
- Definition 217

- Indications for Suctioning   217
- Essential Equipment   218
- Nurses Responsibilities   222

30. Care of Child on Ventilator   225
- Indications   225
- Definitions   226
- Types of Ventilatory Support   227
- Care of Infants on Ventilator   228
- Ventilator Sighs   229
- Endotracheal Tube Suction   229
- Complications During Ventilation   230
- Bradycardia During Ventilation   231
- Extubation   231

31. Intravenous Therapy   234
- Indications for IV Therapy   234
- Common IV Solutions   234
- Common IV Additives   235
- Equipment   235
- Preparations   235
- Hints for Prolonged IV Infusions   236

32. Blood-Drawing Technique in the Neonate   238
- Heel Puncture   238
- Blood-Drawing Techniques in the Neonate   239
- Complications   240
- Arterial Puncture   242

33. Central Venous Catheters and Long Lines   245
- Definitions   245
- Procedure if Intralipid is Used   247

34. Umbilical Arterial Catheterization   249
- Indications   249
- Complications   251

35. Umbilical Vein Catheterization   254
- Arterial/Venous Catheter Insertion: Umbilical   255
- Documentation   257

36. Umbilical Cord Blood Collection and Analysis   259
- At Birth   260
- Background Information   260
- Post-Birth Specimen Collection/Examination   260
- Normal Cord Blood Gas and pH (During and Post-Labor)   262

37. Thoracic Drainage for Tension Pneumothorax   264
- Indications   265
- The Nurse's Role in Managing Unplanned Chest Drain Events   268

Bibliography   271
Index   273

INC SYLLABUS

CHILD HEALTH NURSING - I & II CLINICAL
(3 Credits – 240 hours)

PLACEMENT: V and VI SEMESTER
PRACTICUM: Skill Laboratory: 1 Credit (40 hours)
CLINICAL: V SEMESTER—2 Credits (160 hours)
VI SEMESTER—1 Credit (80 hours)
PRACTICE COMPETENCIES: On completion of the course, the students will be able to:
- Perform assessment of children: Health, developmental and anthropometric.
- Provide nursing care to children with various medical disorders.
- Provide pre and postoperative care to children with common pediatric surgical conditions/malformation.
- Perform immunization as per NIS.
- Provide nursing care to critically ill children.
- Give health education/nutritional education to parents.
- Counsel parents according to identified counseling needs.

Skill Laboratory
- Use of manikins and simulators
- PLS, CPAP, endotracheal

Suction Pediatric Nursing Procedures
- Administration of medication: Oral, IM and IV
- Oxygen administration
- Application of restraints
- Specimen collection
- Urinary catheterization and drainage
- Ostomy care
- Feeding: NG, gastrostomy, jejunostomy
- Wound dressing
- Suture removal

CLINICAL POSTINGS
8 weeks × 30 hours per week (5 weeks + 3 weeks)

Clinical area/ unit	Duration (Weeks)	Learning outcomes	Procedural competencies/ clinical skills	Clinical requirements	Assessment methods

Pediatric Medical Ward	V sem – 2 weeks
	VI sem – 1 week
		Provide nursing care to children with various medical disorders	• Taking pediatric history
			• Physical examination and assessment of children
			• Administration of oral, IM and IV medicine/fluids
			• Calculation of fluid replacement
			• Preparation of different strengths of IV fluids
			• Application of restraints
			• Administration of O_2 inhalation by different methods
			• Baby bath/sponge bath
			• Feeding children by Katori spoon, Paladai cup
			• Collection of specimens for common investigations
			• Assisting with common diagnostic procedures
			• Teaching mothers/parents
			  » Malnutrition
			  » Oral rehydration therapy
			  » Feeding and Weaning
			  » Immunization schedule
			• Play therapy
				• Nursing care plan
				• Case study presentation – 1
				• Health talk – 1
					• Assess performance with rating scale
					• Assess each skill with checklist OSCE/OSPE
					• Evaluation of case study/presentation and health education session
					• Completion of activity record

Pediatric Surgical Ward	V sem – 2 weeks VI sem – 1 week	• Recognize different pediatric surgical conditions/malformations	• Calculation, preparation and administration of IV fluids • Bowel wash, insertion of suppositories	Nursing care plan – 1 Case study/presentation – 1	• Assess performance with rating scale • Assess each skill with checklist OSCE/OSPE

Clinical area/ unit	Duration (Weeks)	Learning outcomes	Procedural competencies/ clinical skills	Clinical requirements	Assessment methods
		• Provide pre and postoperative care to children with common pediatric surgical conditions/ malformation • Counsel and educate parents	• Care for ostomies: » Colostomy irrigation » Ureterostomy » Gastrostomy » Enterostomy • Urinary catheterization and drainage • Feeding » Nasogastric » Gastrostomy » Jejunostomy • Care of surgical wounds » Dressing » Suture removal		• Evaluation of case study/ presentation • Completion of activity record
Pediatric OPD/ immunization room	V sem – 1 week	• Perform assessment of children: health, developmental and anthropometric • Perform immunization • Give health education/ nutritional education	• Assessment of children » Health assessment » Developmental assessment » Anthropometric assessment » Nutritional assessment • Immunization • Health/nutritional education	• Growth and developmental study: » Infant – 1 » Toddler – 1 » Preschooler – 1 » Schooler – 1 » Adolescent – 1	• Assess performance with rating scale • Completion of activity record
NICU and PICU	VI sem – 1 week	Provide nursing care to critically ill children	• Care of a baby in incubator/warmer • Care of a child on ventilator, CPAP • Endotracheal suction • Chest physiotherapy • Administration of fluids with infusion pumps • Total parenteral nutrition • Phototherapy • Monitoring of babies • Recording and reporting • Cardiopulmonary resuscitation (PLS)	• Newborn assessment – 1 • Nursing care plan – 1	• Assess performance with rating scale • Evaluation of observation report • Completion of activity record

CHILD HEALTH NURSING- II- CLINICAL PRACTICUM (1 Credit- 80 hours)
Given under Child Health Nursing - I as I and II

CHAPTER 1

Pediatric History Taking and Physical Examination

PRACTICE COMPETENCIES

On completion of the chapter, the students will be able to:

- Demonstrate accurate knowledge of physical and psychological development changes in children
- Apply this knowledge for further examination and treatment.
- Demonstrate accurate referrals
- Provide good pediatric emergency care on the basis of high priority.
- Deliver high quality, timely and efficient pediatric care.

ABSTRACT

A number of factors distinguish the pediatric from adult history and physical examination. Depending on the age of the patient, the primary historian may be the patient and/or another person, usually the parent. Developmental factors are commonly considered. The differential diagnosis of a condition may vary depending on the age of the patient. Healthcare maintenance (e.g., immunization, and safety issues) and social issues play a major role in emergent and routine care. A non-threatening touch can facilitate a physical examination. In contrast to examining older patients, the pediatric examination should start with the organ systems requiring the greatest amount of cooperation. This may vary depending on the type of examination required. In the normal infant, this is usually the cardiovascular and pulmonary examination. The head and neck examination tends to be the most disturbing to the patient and should be deferred until the end of the examination. In older infants and toddlers most of the examination can be more successfully accomplished in the patients lap than on a cold examination table. Telling a story, examining a doll the patient brought to the clinic or engaging the patient in a conversation can significantly decrease the stress associated with the examination for both the patient and examiner, older children and adolescents should be addressed and treated as individuals. The present chapter designed for nursing students to perform the pediatric clerkship. It is designed to take a history and performing physical examination on children of varying ages and to plan nursing process.

Keywords: Developmental stage, family tree, body built, anthropometric measurements, reflexes, case presentation, nursing process, pedigree charts, consanguineous marriage.

Chapter 1: Pediatric History Taking and Physical Examination

■ PROFILE OF THE CHILD

Name of the child	:	Master or baby's name
Age	:	In months or years
Gender	:	
IP No.	:	
Ward	:	
Developmental stage	:	Whether infant or toddler or preschooler or school age child.
Name of the father	:	Occupation of father
Name of the mother	:	Occupation of mother
Income	:	
Address	:	
Introduction to child	:	A brief note about the child, siblings, family position of child in the family, religion, language, schooling and note about the first encounter with the child and the significant others.
Current complaints	:	Complaints at present
Past health history	:	History of any life threatening or chronic problem, which needed admission to hospital, treatment given, prognosis and follow up measures taken.
Birth history	:	
Antenatal	:	Whether the child's mother during pregnancy had taken folic acid tablets, TT injection, regular antenatal checkups, and any other medicine used by her.
Intranatal	:	The child delivered normally or by cesarean section, APGAR score of the child, any birth trauma, and anesthesia (if known), onset of respiration, first cry, kind of labor.
Postnatal	:	History of neonatal convulsion or jaundice, rashes, congenital abnormalities.
Family history	:	Describe any family health problems hereditary/communicable diseases.
Family tree	:	Mention the child's three degree generation
Sibling history	:	The siblings of the child, any illness, their relationship with each other to be mentioned.

■ IMMUNIZATION HISTORY

Name of the vaccine	Schedule time	Child's due	Inference

Chapter 1: Pediatric History Taking and Physical Examination | 3

Development milestones	:	The child's milestones attained up to three years of age.
Play history	:	The play activity of the child to be mentioned, which games the child likes to play and with the peer group.
Personal history	:	Child's relationship with siblings, peers and family members, child's communication skill.
Habits	:	Any habits of thumb sucking, nail biting, temper tantrum, head banging, pica, etc., to be mentioned.
Dietary history	:	Breastfeeding, weaning foods, vegetarian food, non-vegetarian food, likes and dislikes, number of meals taken to be mentioned.

■ PHYSICAL EXAMINATION

A. Head to Foot Assessment

Nourishment	:	
Body built	:	The child's body built whether mild, moderate or severe to be mentioned.
Activity	:	The child is dull, active or very active.
Mental status	:	Whether the child is in conscious, semi-conscious or unconscious stage to be mentioned.
Head	:	Size, shape, circumference, asymmetry, cephalohematoma, craniotabes, molding, fontanel (size, tension, number, abnormally late or early closure), sutures, dilated veins, scalp, hair (texture, distribution, parasites) face.
Face	:	Symmetry, paralysis, distance between nose and mouth, depth of nasolabial folds, bridge of nose, distribution of hair, size of mandible, swellings, hypertelorism, Chvostek's sign, tendernesss over sinuses.
Eyes	:	Photophobia, visual acuity, muscular control, nystagmus, epicanthic folds, lacrimation, discharge, lids, exophthalmos or enophthalmos, conjunctiva, papillary size, shape, reaction to light and accommodation, media (corneal opacities, cataracts), fundi, visual fields (in older children). At 2–4 weeks an infant will follow light. By 3–4 months, coordinated eye movements should be seen.
Nose	:	Exterior, shape, mucosa, patency, discharge, pressure over sinuses, flaring of nostrils, septum.
Mouth	:	Lips (thinness, down turning, fissures, color, cleft), teeth (number, position, caries, mottling, discoloration, notching, malocclusion or malignant), mucosa (color, redness of Stensen's duct, Epstein's pearls). Gum, palate, tongue, uvula, mouth, breathing.
Throat	:	Tonsils (size, inflammation, exudates, crypts, inflammation of the anterior pillars), mucosa, hypertonic lymphoid tissue, epiglottis, voice (hoarseness, stridor, grunting, type of cry, speech). The number and condition of the teeth should be recorded.
Ears	:	Pinnas (position, size), tympanic membranes (landmarks, mobility, perforation, inflammation, discharge). Mastoid tenderness and swelling, hearing (including hearing screen).

Neck	:	Position (torticollis, opisthotonus, inability to support head, mobility), swelling, thyroid (size, contour, bruit, isthmus, nodules, tenderness), lymph nodes, veins, position of trachea, sternocleidomastoid (swelling, shortening), webbing, edema, auscultation, movement, tonic neck reflex.
Thorax	:	Shape and symmetry, veins, retractions, and pulsations, beading, Harrison's groove, flaring of ribs, pigeon chest, funnel shape, size and position of nipples, breasts, length of sternum, intercostals and substernal retraction, asymmetry, clavicles.
Lungs	:	Type of breathing, dyspnea, prolongation of expiration, cough, expansion, fremitus, flatness or dullness to percussion, resonance, breath and voice sounds, rales, wheezing.
Heart	:	Location and intensity of apex beat, precordial bulging, pulsation of vessels, thrills, size, shape, auscultation (rate, rhythm, force, quality of sounds compare with pulse rate and rhythm friction rub) murmurs (location, intensity, position in cycle, pitch, effect of change of position, transmission, effect of exercise).
Abdomen	:	Size and contour, visible peristalsis, respiratory movements, veins (distension, direction of flow), umbilicus, hernia, musculature, tenderness, rigidity, tympany, shifting, dullness, tenderness, rebound tenderness, pulsation, palpable organs or messes (size, shape, position, mobility) fluid wave, femoral pulsations, bowel sounds.
Male genitalia	:	Circumcision, meatal opening, hypospadias, phimosis, adherent foreskin, size of testes, cryptorchidism, scrotum, hydrocele, hernia, pubertal changes.
Female genitalia	:	Vagina (imperforate, discharge, adhesions), hypertrophy of clitoris, pubertal changes.
Rectum and anus	:	Irritation, fissures, prolapsed, imperforated anus, rectal examination should be performed with the little finger (inserted slowly). Note the muscle tone, character of stool, masses, tenderness, sensation, examine stool on glove finger (gross, microscopic, culture) as indicated.
Extremities	:	Deformity, hemiatrophy, bowlegs (common in infancy), knock knees, paralysis, edema, coldness, posture, asymmetry, extra digits, gait, clubbing, curvature of little finger, deformity of nails, splinter hemorrhages, abnormalities of feet, dermatoglyphics, width of thumbs and big toes, syndactyly, dimpling of dorsa, temperature.
Spine and back	:	Posture, curvatures, rigidity, webbed neck, spine bifida, pilonidal dimple or cyst, tufts of hair, mobility, Mongolian spots, tenderness over spine, pelvis or kidneys.

B. Basic Physiological Data

Vitals	Normal value	Child's value	Inference
Temperature			
Pulse			
Respiration			

Anthropometric Measurements

Name of the measurement	Child's value	Normal value	Inference
Height			
Weight			
Head circumference			
Chest circumference			
Abdominal circumference			

Reflexes: Need to be assessed if the child is newborn or neonate.

C. Summary of Physical Examination

Investigations

Sl. No.	Name of the Investigation	Child's value	Normal value	Inference

Drug Regimen

Sl. No.	Drug name	Dose and route	Action	Indications	Contraindications	Side effects	Nursing implications

Time plan : Note: Time plan can be changed according to hospital policies, doctors' rounds and condition of the child.

List out Nursing Diagnoses: (As per NANDA)

1. ....
2. ....
3. ....
4. ....
5. ....
6. ....
7. ....
8. ....
9. ....
10. ....
11. ....

Chapter 1: Pediatric History Taking and Physical Examination

12. ....
13. ....
14. ....
15. ....
16. ....
17. ....
18. ....
19. ....
20. ....

Nursing Process: (As per priority)

Assessment	Nursing diagnosis	Goal	Planning	Implementation	Rationale	Evaluation
Subjective data						
Objective data						

Case Presentation

Apart from the above following need to be included,
Review of literature (detailed description of the disease)
- ❖ Definition
- ❖ Incidence
- ❖ Etiology
- ❖ Pathophysiology
- ❖ Clinical features

Book features	Child's features

- ❖ Complications
- ❖ Investigations

Book features	Child's features

- ❖ Treatment: Medical Management, Surgical Management, Nursing Management need to be mentioned

Book features	Child's features

Chapter 1: Pediatric History Taking and Physical Examination

Nursing process: As given above:

Brief summary of the care given with evaluation :
Conclusion and self-evaluation of care given :
Bibliography :

Note: Select a patient who is acute/subacute stage of illness. Continued care must be given for a minimum of 5 days. Nursing process for the first day should be submitted within 24 hours.

Family tree — **Pedigree charts**

Family tree	Pedigree charts
Male	☐
Female	○
Mating	☐—○
Parents and children 1 boy and 1 girl (In order of birth)	☐—○ with ☐ ○
Dizygotic twins	☐ ○ (separate lines)
Monozygotic twins	☐—○ (joined)
Sex unspecified	◇
No. of children of gender indicated	① ② ③ ④ ⑤
Affected individuals	■ ●
Death	⊘
Carrier	⊙
Abortion or still birth	● (small)
Propositus	■ with arrow
Method of identifying persons in a pedigree	☐—● with offspring
Here the propositus is child 2 in generation II	☐ ■ ○ with arrow
Consanguineous marriage	☐═○

Example of writing pedigree

I
II
III

POINTS TO NOTE

- Wash your hands and don PPE if appropriate.
- Introduce yourself including your name and role.
- Greet the child, their parents/carers and any other siblings who are present.
- Confirm the child's name and date of birth.
- Make sure to maintain a comfortable distance from the child at the beginning of the consultation, whilst trying to build rapport with the family as a whole. Young children generally feel more comfortable and secure in their parent's arms or lap and may require some time to feel at ease.
- Observe how the child is playing and interacting with any siblings and their parents/carers.
- Make sure to address questions to the child when appropriate. Be mindful to allow the child time to answer and do not interrupt.
- Negotiating both talking to parents/carers without the child present and talking to the child alone requires tact and consideration.
- Generally, this is done to avoid embarrassing older children or adolescents and to allow for the imparting of sensitive information.

PRACTICE QUESTIONS

1. Master Ravi 3-year-old child admitted with fever for evaluation. Collect the history and write the nursing process.
2. Baby Chitra is admitted with thalassemia in pediatric ward. Frame 10 nursing diagnosis which is appropriate for the child.

MULTIPLE CHOICE QUESTIONS

1. Master Teja, 5-year-old is admitted with suspected rheumatic fever in pediatric unit. When obtaining the child's history, the nurse considers which information to be the most important?
   a. Fever that started 3 days ago
   b. Lack of interest in food
   c. A recent episode of pharyngitis
   d. Vomiting for 2 days
2. A baby will be able to hold it's head by:
   a. 11 months
   b. 1 month
   c. 9 months
   d. 3 months
3. When will be the first two lower central incisors erupts?
   a. At 2 to 3 months of age
   b. Between 1 and 2 years of age
   c. At 10 to 12 months of age
   d. At 6 to 8 months of age

ANSWER KEY

1. c   2. d   3. d

CHAPTER 2

Family Assessment

PRACTICE COMPETENCIES

On completion of the chapter, the students will be able to:
- Assess family functioning.
- Assess coping mechanisms of the family.
- Assess resources.
- Assess family structure.
- Understand a picture of multigenerational patterns of behavior or illnesses.
- Identify the normal crisis or common illnesses to be encountered in each stage of development.
- Provide anticipatory care and guidance.

ABSTRACT

Family assessment is a process of gathering and organizing information in order to determine necessary interventions. The family assessment does this in ways that can help a family prevent and solve problems and also provide information on its strengths, values, and goals. Family assessment is essential for providing adequate family care and support. The nurse begins assessment by determining the child's attitude toward family and the extent to which the family can be incorporated into nursing care. Family assessment is an essential component of the nursing process. Here the nurse collects data by using the methods of observation, interviewing, reviewing records, and reports.

Keywords: Observation, interviewing, patient history.

THE FAMILY HISTORY

Definition

A family history consists of the collection of information about the patient and other family members devoted to an understanding of:
- Heritable illness
- Current family health status
- Psychosocial disorders
- Interactional and relationship data

Areas of Family History

Sl. No	Areas of family history
1.	Composition of family (at least 3 generations for siblings, children, parents)
2.	Names, sex, and age or date of birth
3.	Dates of marriages, divorces, and deaths
4.	Racial and ethnic origins
5.	Members of extended family
6.	Significant others (homosexual or heterosexual partners)
7.	Familial: Heritable diseases
8.	Genetic disorders and congenital malformations
9.	Biochemical or metabolic disorders
10.	Renal and cardiovascular disorders
11.	Family psychiatric history
12.	Neurologic disorders
13.	Interactions, relationships, and psychosocial problems
14.	Roles of family members
15.	Types and strength of relationships
16.	Major stressors
17.	Members living together in the household

Symbols and Notation for Recording a Genogram

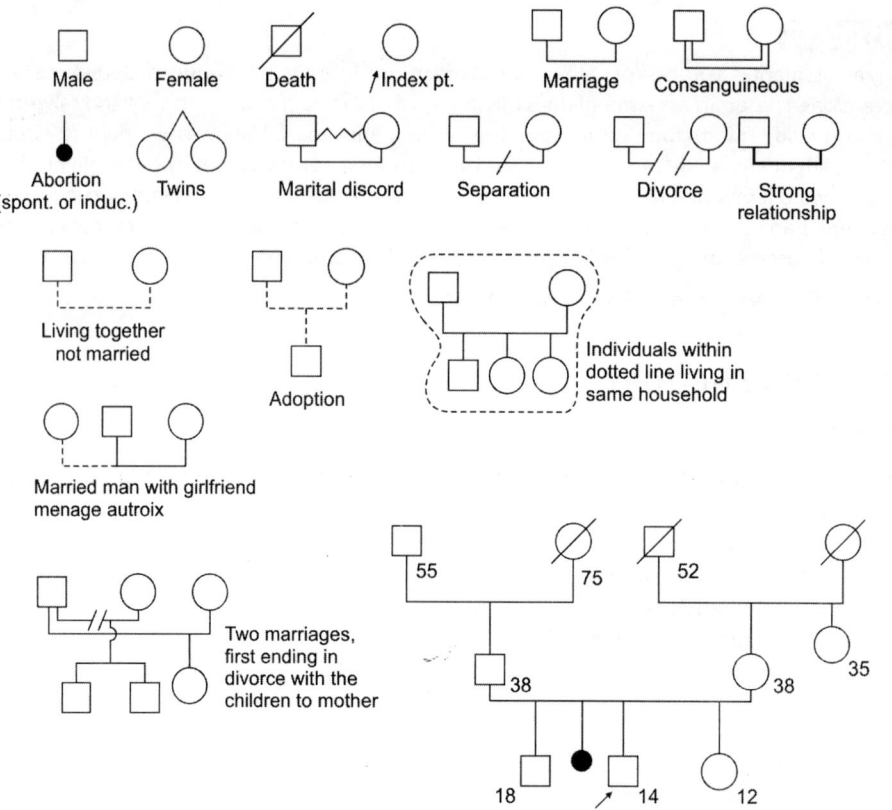

OBSERVATION

- Make a note of family's response—you need to be a good observer of the verbal and nonverbal cues of the family to initiate further action.
- Observing the house and the surroundings will help you to get to know the strong and weak factors that promote or demote the health of the individuals.
- Initiate conversation with the members of the family to know about each individual of the family. Get to know their concern about the prevailing health problems or any other issues about the family and its members.
- During the conversation, nurse also observes for any person with acute or chronic illness, women who is pregnant, children with watering nose or with skin rashes or eruptions or injuries and anyone crying in pain at home.
- Encourage a discussion with the members and get to know their previous and future plans to tackle the prevailing situation (such as water stagnation and mosquito breeding in front of the house).
- Nurse also observes the attitude and practices of family members.

INTERVIEWING TECHNIQUE

Family interview will reveal more information about the individual and family health. Although an understanding of the healthcare values of various cultures are helpful, nurses should remember that persons within a culture are different from each other.

Principles of Interviewing

- Develop trust with the child/family.
- Choose appropriate environment. Provide environment free of distractions.
- Provide privacy.
- Be confidential.
- Make the patient as comfortable as possible.
- Maintain personal distance level of 3 feet.
- Maintain good eye contact and interact at eye level.
- Nurse should be a good listener.
- No preconceived ideas about the child or family.
- Time and duration should be planned.
- Recording the interview
- Evaluation of the interview.
- Setting essential follow up goals.

PHASES OF INTERVIEW

There are three phases of interview. They are:
1. Introduction or initial phase
2. Focus or working phase
3. Termination or recapitulation and transition phase

Introduction or Initial Phase

- Introduce yourself
- Respect the child and family
- Make the child comfortable

Chapter 2: Family Assessment

- ❖ Watch for signs of child discomfort—do not overtire the child or family.
- ❖ Use polite, humble, and professional tone through the interview.
- ❖ Thoroughly explain the interview procedure.
- ❖ Always initiate the interview with general concerns, then move on to specific ones.

Focus or Working Phase

- ❖ Take notes only needed. Do not write throughout.
- ❖ Use effective communication techniques.
- ❖ Control the process of interview, but do not monopolize.
- ❖ Be flexible.
- ❖ Treat the individual and family with respect.
- ❖ Do not contradict the views or beliefs of the child or family.
- ❖ Never try to impose your own moral standards upon the individual.
- ❖ Be compassionate and empathetic.
- ❖ Create conducive atmosphere.

Termination or Recapitulation and Transition Phase

- ❖ Recap the interview results.
- ❖ Set further goals and discuss about the follow-up plans or care.
- ❖ At the end find out from the individual if anything else he/she wishes to discuss.

■ FAMILY HISTORY

The health details of all the family members must be obtained. This includes their age, sex, present health status, treatment taken, and their proximity to the child (in case of communicable diseases). The consanguinity pattern (with degree of relationship) of the parents and the details of the other siblings must be noted. History of previous abortions/still births and their causes also, may give a clue to the diagnosis (habitual abortions occur with maternal syphilis). The birth of abnormal children and the cause of death of children in the family must be asked for. The age of the mother at the time of delivery is important as very young mothers, i.e., <18 years have an increased chance of preterm and IUGR babies while older mothers, i.e., >32 years have an increased chance of babies with Down syndrome and Klinefelter syndrome. In case of diseases exhibiting hereditary traits, an enquiry must be made regarding a much wider circle of relatives than the child's immediate family. A genetic chart (family tree) must be prepared using accepted symbols.

Describe any Family Health Problems: Hereditary/Communicable Diseases.

....
....
....
....
....
....

Chapter 2: Family Assessment

POINTS TO NOTE

- Most subjective data are collected through interviewing the family caregiver and the child.
- The interview helps establish relationships between the child, family and the nurse.
- Listen and communicate. Listening and using appropriate communication techniques help promote a good interview.
- Introduce and explain your purpose. The nurse should be introduced to the child and caregiver and the purpose of the interview stated.
- Establish rapport. Calm, reassuring manner is important to establish trust and comfort; the caregiver and the nurse should be comfortably seated, and the child should be included in the interview process.
- Family caregiver provides most of the information needed in caring for the child, especially the infant or toddler.
- Ask questions and note them. Rather than simply asking the caregiver to fill out a form, the nurse may ask the questions and write down the answers; this process gives the opportunity to observe the reactions of the child and the caregiver as they interact with each other and answer the questions.
- Avoid being judgmental. The nurse must be nonjudgmental, being careful not to indicate disapproval by verbal or nonverbal responses.
- Be age-appropriate. Use age-appropriate toys and questions when talking with the child.
- Establish rapport. Showing interest in the child and in what he or she says helps both the child and caregiver to feel comfortable; by being honest when answering the child's questions, the nurse establishes trust with the child.
- The child's comments should be listened to attentively, and the child should be made to feel important in the interview.

■ PRACTICE QUESTION

1. You are posted in primary health center. Baby Roshini 4-year-old has come to PHC with cough and fever. How will you do the family assessment?

■ MULTIPLE CHOICE QUESTIONS

1. **Effective communication between the healthcare team and family members has been shown to:**
   a. Increase hospital costs from increased staff time spent talking to family members

Chapter 2: Family Assessment

    b. Decrease hospital costs from decreased staff time spent resolving conflict
    c. Increase hospital stays because of better communication with family members about their concern regarding early discharge
    d. Increase the number of phone calls from family members because of comfort with the healthcare team

2. When considering feeding management for child bearing families, it is important to:
    a. Inform all mothers that they should breastfeed
    b. Assist all parents in forming a nurturing relationship surrounding feeding of an infant
    c. Encourage fathers to leave feeding up to mothers, because mothers are naturally better at breastfeeding and bottle feeding of an infant
    d. Encourage mothers to bottle feed their infants to guarantee proper nutrients are provided to the infant

3. Nurses use genetic knowledge:
    a. In all healthcare settings
    b. Only after becoming credentialed as genetics nurses
    c. Primarily with child bearing families
    d. After others have determined whether a genetic condition is present in the family

ANSWER KEY

1. b   2. b   3. a

CHAPTER 3

Nutrition Assessment

PRACTICE COMPETENCIES
On completion of the chapter, the students will be able to:
- Know different methods of assessing nutritional status.
- Understand the basic anthropometric techniques, applications, and reference standards.

ABSTRACT
Nutritional assessment is an integral part of optimal pediatric care. Undernutrition, which may be primarily due to inadequate food intake or secondary to infection, injury or disease, is the most important cause of growth retardation in children. Comprehensive nutritional assessment involves evaluation by clinical, anthropometric, biochemical, and dietary methods. Nutritional parameters include those reflecting changes in body size, composition, and/or function. All patients should be nutritionally screened. If malnutrition is suspected, comprehensive nutritional assessment should be performed.

Keywords: Patient history, anthropometric, biochemical indices.

INTRODUCTION

Nutrition is the essential component of caring ill children. Nutritional interventions can improve patient recovery and survival.

The risk of malnutrition for ill children is increased by their higher metabolic needs and by other associated by their higher metabolic needs and by other associated conditions, such as congenital heart disease, bronchopulmonary dysplasia, gastrointestinal reflux, and other chronic conditions commonly lead to feeding difficulties and can predispose ill children to under nutrition and growth failure.

NUTRITION ASSESSMENT

The nutritional assessment of an ill child requires various methods and tests. No single clinical, biochemical or growth measurement gives a complete picture of a child's nutrition status. The process of nutritional assessment is dynamic and must allow selection of varying assessment methods throughout the child's stay.

Patient History

A reliable and complete history is the first step in accomplishing a nutritional assessment (**Box 3.1**).

Box 3.1: Patient and family history.

- Birth date and prenatal history:
  » Gestational age
  » Birth weight, length, head circumference
  » Maternal nutrition
- Chronic illness
- Congenital or chromosomal abnormalities
- Relevant trauma, illness, surgery
- Level of gastrointestinal function:
  » Oral feedings
  » Tube feedings
  » Parental nutrition
- Feeding history:
  » Ability to suck
  » Frequency of amount intake
  » Vomiting or spitting up
  » General appetite
  » Food preparation
  » Who feeds child
- Bowel pattern (diarrhea, constipation)
- Weight loss or gain
- Medications
- Family or lifestyle factors:
  » Socioeconomic status
  » Hygiene practice
  » Stress within family

Dietary History

The child's dietary history and analysis of the child's current diet to determine nutritional composition and quantity are important. Knowledge of the child's preadmission intake may be particularly helpful.

To collect information regarding the child's preadmission diet, parents can be asked to recall the child's intake in the past 24–48 hours.

■ PHYSICAL ASSESSMENT

A careful physical examination is performed with a specific interest in uncovering subtle signs of deficiencies in macronutrients (protein, energy) and micronutrients (vitamins, minerals, and trace elements) **(Table 3.1)**. The goal of the physical examination is to corroborate and add to findings of the history.

■ ANTHROPOMETRIC MEASUREMENTS

Assessment of growth is a vital component in the care of critically-ill children. Anthropometric measurements including weight, length, height, and head circumference are noninvasive and easily taken.

Weekly weight trends are more relevant than daily fluctuations in assessing a critically-ill child's growth. An unexplained weight loss of >10% of the child's admission weight places the child nutritionally at risk. Length and height are affected when under nutrition occurs chronically.

Triceps skinfold (TSF) and mild-arm circumference (MAC) assist in the assessment of muscle mass and subcutaneous fat content respectively.

Chapter 3: Nutrition Assessment

Table 3.1: Clinical findings associated with nutritional deficiencies.

Sl. No.	Component	Clinical findings	Nutritional deficiencies
1.	General	• Underweight, short stature • Edematous, decreased activity level	• Calorie • Protein
2.	Face	Malar pigmentation (dark skin over cheeks and under eyes), bitemporal wasting, pale	Niacin, B-vitamins, riboflavin and vitamin B6, iron
3.	Lips	• Angular stomatitis: Lesions (cracks) appearing on both side of the mouth • Angular scars: Healed lesions of angular stomatitis • Cheilosis: Lips develop cracks and become red	Niacin and riboflavin, vitamin B6, and iron
4.	Hair	Lack of luster: Dull dry hair, sparseness, discoloration, easily pluck ability	Protein, zinc, biotin, essential fatty acids, vitamin A, ascorbic acid
5.	Gums	Spongy, bleeding, abnormal redness	Vitamin C
6.	Tongue	• Glossitis (red, raw, fissured) • Pale, atrophic, smooth/slick (filiform papillae atrophy) • Magenta color	Folate, niacin, riboflavin, iron, vitamin B6, and B12
7.	Teeth	• Mottled enamel: Mottled teeth with chalky white and brown color, with/without erosion of enamel • Caries	• Excess fluoride • Fluoride
8.	Eyes	• Conjunctival xerosis: Dryness of the transparent membrane that covers the cornea and lines inside of the eyelid, the conjunctiva becomes discolored (muddy colored and loses its brightness) • Xerophthalmia (including keratomalacia): Cornea becomes soft and raw and easily infected. • Bitot's spot: Dry, foamy, triangular spots appearing on the temporal side of the eye • Night blindness: Inability to see in dim light	Vitamin A, zinc, iron
9.	Skin	• *Xerosis*: Generalized dryness with desquamatization • *Dermatosis*: Skin lesions which are symmetrical and are evident only on the part of the body exposed to the sun (such as forearm, legs, face, exposed part of the neck). The skin becomes dry and scaly. Petechiae, purpura, and ecchymosis	• Zinc, biotin, essential fatty acids, tryptophan, niacin • Ascorbic acid, vitamin K
10.	Nails	Brittle and spoon shaped	Iron deficiency
11.	Endocrine system	• *Thyroid enlargement*: Gland is visible and enlarged. Enlargement might be diffused or nodular • Glucose intolerance	• Iodine • Chromium
12.	Skeletal system	Iron, vitamin D	Beading of ribs, pigeon chest: Protruding breast bone, knock knees or bow legs
13.	Gastro-intestinal system	Hepatomegaly	Protein
14.	Nervous system	Irritability, forgetfulness, headache, sleepiness, mental depression, lack of orientation	Vitamin B12, vitamin E, chromium, protein, thiamine, pyridoxine
15.	Glands	Parotid enlargement	Protein
16.	Subcutaneous tissue	Decreased fat fold, edema	Calorie, protein, thiamine
17.	Muscles	Decreased muscle mass (wasting)	Protein, calorie
18.	Others	Altered taste, delayed wound healing	Zinc, vitamin C, and protein

BIOCHEMICAL INDICES

Plasma Proteins

Serum albumin, the major protein synthesized by the liver, was one of the first biochemical markers identified for malnutrition. A low level of serum albumin has been associated with a decrease in dietary protein intake and an increase in morbidity and mortality.

Urine Screening for Somatic Proteins

Creatinine, the metabolic product of creatine, is stored in muscle and excreted by the kidney at a relatively constant rate. Creatinine excretion is measured in 24-hour urine collection.

The 24-hour creatinine excretion of the patient is divided by a 24-hour creatinine excretion of the same-height child and multiplied by 100 to obtain an index:

$$\frac{\text{24-hour urine creatinine excretion (mg)}}{\text{24-hour urine creatinine excretion of same height child (mg)}} \times 100$$

In the well-nourished child, the creatinine height index (CHI) is 90–100%. Severe protein-calorie malnutrition is indicated by CHI under 40%, moderate depletion is indicated by a CHI of 40–60%, and mild depletion is indicated by CHI of 60–80%. Creatinine excretion can be affected by hydration state and catabolic states. Patients taking diuretics and those with renal disease are likely to have low excretions of creatinine.

POINTS TO NOTE

➤ The frequency of nutrition assessment depends on a client's age and pregnancy and disease status and on national policies.
➤ The recommendations below should be adjusted based on national guidelines.
➤ **Pregnant/postpartum women:** On every antenatal visit
➤ **Infants 0–6 months of age:** At birth and on every scheduled postnatal visit.
➤ **Infants 6–59 months of age:** During monthly growth monitoring sessions for children under 2 and every 3 months for older children.
➤ **Children 5 years of age and over:** On every clinic visit.
➤ **Adolescents and adults:** On every clinic visit.
➤ **People with HIV:** On every clinic visit and when initiating or changing antiretroviral therapy (ART).

MULTIPLE CHOICE QUESTIONS

1. Angular stomatitis is due to deficiency of:
   a. Protein b. Niacin
   c. Zinc d. Vitamin C
2. Mottled enamel is due to deficiency of:
   a. Calories b. Vitamin A
   c. Vitamin C d. Excess fluoride
3. Thyroid enlargement is due to deficiency of:
   a. Zinc b. Vitamin C
   c. Iodine d. Protein

4. Delayed wound healing is due to deficiency of:
   a. Vitamin C
   b. Vitamin B12
   c. Calcium
   d. Vitamin D
5. Pigeon chest is the deficiency due to:
   a. Vitamin B12
   b. Vitamin D
   c. Vitamin C
   d. Protein
6. Which of the following is a rich source of vitamin A?
   a. Orange
   b. Apple
   c. Ground nuts
   d. Apricots
7. Which disease is caused by the deficiency of protein?
   a. Pellagra
   b. Marasmus
   c. Beri-Beri
   d. Rickets
8. Which nutrient deficiency is main reason for microcytic anemia?
   a. Folic acid
   b. Amino acids
   c. Iron
   d. Vitamin C

ANSWER KEY

1. b
2. d
3. c
4. a
5. b
6. d
7. b
8. c

CHAPTER 4

Newborn Assessment

PRACTICE COMPETENCIES

On completion of the chapter, the students will be able to:
- Identify the newborn's abnormalities and problems in adapting to life outside the uterus.
- Determine the health of the newborn's central nervous system through the assessment of the presence and strength of the reflexes.
- Evaluate the gestational maturity of the newborn.
- Determine intactness of the central nervous system and provide information about the infants ability to respond to care taking activities.
- Perform early maternal—infant attachment.

ABSTRACT

Babies are inspected soon after birth to identify and obvious visible unexpected features or abnormalities and to reassure parents. The midwife in attendance at the birth usually conducts this initial inspection. It is established as good practice to carry out a more detailed examination of the baby within 24 hours of birth as part of the core health program for under five's. During this routine examination problems can be identified and if appropriate referred for investigation, specialist assessment and treatment as well as being fully discussed with the parents.

Keywords: Vernix caseosa, milia, erythema toxicum, Mongolian spot, caput succedaneum, cephalohematoma, rooting reflex, doll's eye, reflexes of newborn, jaundice, hypoglycemia, Moro reflex, Babinski reflex, plantar grasp, palmar grasp, extrusion, gagging reflex, sucking reflex.

PURPOSES AND PRECAUTIONS

The main purposes are:
- To identify normal characteristics in the neonate.
- To identify existing abnormalities, if any.
- To carry out immediate action if there is any deviation.
- To establish a baseline for future physiological changes.

Precautions to be taken during the procedure of carrying out physical examination:
- Keep your hands clean, dry, and warm.
- Keep your nails short and free of nail polish.
- Do not expose the baby unnecessarily.

- ❖ Do not expose the baby to drafts and chills.
- ❖ Examine the baby swiftly not more than 8 to 10 minutes.
- ❖ If neonate is irritable/crying during examination allow him to suck on a nipple.
- ❖ Inform the mother about outcome of examination.

■ IMMEDIATE EXAMINATION AT BIRTH

Before carrying out examination collect the following articles and practice on a manikin. The articles are tape measure, weighing machine, thermometer, manikin, etc.

Apgar Score

i. As soon as baby is born, a quick visual inspection is done for which an Apgar score is used. It is the best available indicator to tell the physiological status of the neonate and its ability to adjust to extrauterine life immediately.

ii. You need to check the respiratory rate, heart rate appearance, and activity of the neonate. We shall review here the Apgar scoring system in order to get a quick visual inspection of the neonate to help him to establish respiration.

iii. Record the Apgar score of the neonate at 1 minute and 5 minute after birth.

Table 4.1: Apgar score.

Sign	2	1	0
Appearance (color)	Completely pink	Body pink, extremities blue	Completely blue pale
Grimace (response to nasal catheter)	Coughing/sneezing	Facial grimace	No response
Activity (muscle tone)	Activity movements	Some flexion of extremities	Limp, no response
Respiratory effort (cry)	Good strong cry	Weak irregular cry	No cry
Heart rate	100 beats/minute	Less than 100 beats/minute	Absent

The low score at 1 minute indicates respiratory distress and the neonates need resuscitative measure. If score is less even after 5 minutes it indicates neurological damage due to hypoxia and brain damage.

Score: 7–10 indicates the neonate is normal
    4–6   Moderate asphyxia
    0–3   Severe distress/asphyxia

If the score is moderately low, i.e., 4–6 or if severe distress, i.e., 0–3, the neonate requires immediate resuscitation. If the Apgar score is good then go to next step assessment estimating the gestational age. If score is lower than 7 at 1 minute then repeat it again at 5 minutes and record.

After quick assessment of baby by evaluating him on the basis of Apgar scoring at 1 minute and 5 minutes if you are convinced that the neonate is stable. Then you can assess the gestational age and neurological assessment and functions. Make sure that child is quiet during examination.

Estimation of Gestational Age of Neonate

It is essential to estimate the gestational age of neonate as it "tells" the maturity of the systems. Assessment of gestational age is important because perinatal morbidity and mortality are related to gestational age and birth weight. A newborn at each gestational age has its special problems. A premature infant may have certain serious problems such as hyaline membrane disease, asphyxia, and necrotizing enterocolitis.

Chapter 4: Newborn Assessment

It is essential as expected date of delivery and/or date of last menstrual period are often inaccurate and neonatal weight, length, and head-circumference, indicate the intrauterine growth and development.

Dubowitz and Ballard scoring are the most widely used scoring system to assess gestational age.

Dubowitz scoring scale consists of eleven physical characteristics used in the first 24 hours, and these are rated on a 4 point scale, i.e., 0–4.

This clinical estimation of gestational age is accurate. There may be difference of plus or minus 2 weeks.

The external characteristics assessed are breast size and nipple formation, skin texture and opacity, ear cartilage formation and firmness, plantar skin creases texture and hair distribution and genitalia. If this guideline is used as given in **Table 4.2** a rough estimate of maturity can be made.

Table 4.2: Maturity estimate using Dubowitz system.

Physical Characteristics	Gestational age		
	Premature	Transitional	Term
Breast tissue	Below 5 mm	6–10 mm	More than 10 mm may have breast milk
Nipple level formation	No areola	Areola present but not raised	Raised above skin
Skin texture and opacity	Abdominal veins clearly visible, including tributary venules	Veins and some tributaries seen	Some large veins distinctly seen
Ear form and cartilage	Soft little or no cartilage	Antitragus cartilage perhaps cartilage in antihelix	Firm cartilage in tragus and helix
Hair texture and distribution	Wooly or fuzzy very fine hair	Silky or coarser hair	Individual strands seen
Genitalis			
Male	Scrotum empty, no rugae	Descending testis few rugations	Testes in canal scrotum rugated
Female	Prominent labia and clitoris	Labia major a not covering labia minor	Clitoris and labia minora skin covered vaginal discharge or occasional bleeding seen at introitus
Plantar creases	Few if any	Creases up to the anterior 1/3 of sole	Entire sole creased

Neurological Assessment

The neurological assessment is made up of eight neurological criteria which have high significance with gestational age.

In order to perform the neurological assessment you need to develop good experience. Go through the following characteristics you will gain an idea of how it is to be performed then practice it at your work place.

i. **Posture:** Place the infant in supine and quiet. Observe the arm, hip and knee extension, and flexion.
ii. **Square window:** The hand is flexed upon the wrist. Gentle pressure is exerted to obtain as much flexion as possible. The wrist should not be rotated. The square window is the angle formed between the hypothenar eminence and the anterior forearm.

iii. **Ankle dorsiflexion:** The food is flexed in the ankle with gentle but sufficient pressure to obtain maximum flexion. The angle between the top of the foot and the front of the leg is measured.
iv. **Popliteal angle:** The infant is placed on his back, with the pelvis flat on a firm surface. The leg is first flexed on the thigh. Then flex the thigh fully with one hand. With the other hand, extend the leg until the maximum angle is obtained.
v. **Heel to ear:** With infant on his back, move the foot as near to the ipsilateral ear as possible without exerting force, the pelvis must be kept flat in a firm surface.
vi. **Scarf sign:** With infant on his back, draw one of his arm across the neck, as far as possible to the opposite shoulder. The elbow can be lifted across the baby's body.
vii. **Head lag:** The infant still lying on his back. Grasp each forearm just above the wrist and gently pull the infant to a sitting position. Observe the relation between the head and the trunk as the infant is raised forward beyond 90° from the bed surface.
viii. **Ventral suspension:** Lay the infant on his abdomen, with the chest resting on your hand. Then lift the infant perpendicularly from the examining surface. Score is based on the amount of caudal and cephalic muscle tone activity select a newborn and exhibited.

Using the **Table 4.3** given below score the neurological status of the neonate.

Using the tables helps to know if the neonates is at term (38–41 weeks of gestation), transitional (35–38 weeks), premature (30–35 weeks) and below 30 weeks or very premature.

Table 4.3: Scoring of neurological status.

Maneuver	Very premature	Premature	Transitional	Term
Posture	Arm and legs extended	Slight arm moderate leg flexion	Legs abducted arms flexed	Completely flexed
Square window	90°	45–60°	30°	0°
Ankle dorsiflexion	90°	45–75°	20°	0°
Popliteal	180°	160–130°	110–90°	Less than 90°
Heel to ear	Easily, and completely touching ear	Foot almost to face	Half way from 90° to face	90°
Scarf sign	Elbow to opposite axilla	Elbow beyond midline thorax	Elbow to midline	Elbow unable to reach midline
Head lag	No head support	Little head support	Head in same plane as body	Head held forward
Ventral suspension	Complete hypotonia	Slight caudal tone	Moderate caudal, slight cephalic tone	Considerable caudal and cephalic tone

Ballard Scoring system: New Ballard scale for newborn maturity rating assesses six external physical and six neuromuscular characteristics.

It can be used with newborn as young as 20 weeks gestation. Each sign has a number score and the cumulative score correlates with maturity rating from 26-44 weeks of gestation.

Physical Maturity

Skin	Gelatinous red transparent	Smooth pink, viable veins	Superficial peeling and/or rash few veins	Cracking pale area rare veins	Parchment deep cracking no vessels	Leathery cracked wrinkled
Lanugo	None	Abundant	Thinning	Bald areas	Mostly bald	
Plantar creases	No crease	Faint red marks	Anterior transverse crease only	Crease anterior 2/3	Creases cover entire sole	

Chapter 4: Newborn Assessment

Breast	Barely percept	Flat areola no bud	Stippled areola 1–2 mm bud	Raised areola 3–4 mm bud	Full areola 5--0 mm bud	
Ear	Pinna flat stays folded	Slow curved pinna; soft with slow recoil	Well-curved pinna; soft but ready recoil	Formed and firm with instant recoil	Thick cartilage ear still	
Genitals ♂	Scrotum empty no rugae		Testes descending few rugae	Testes down good rugae	Testes pendulous deep rugae	
Genitals ♀	Prominent clitoris and labia minora		Majora and minora equally prominent	Majora large minora small	Clitoris and minora completely covered	

Apgar: ____1 min____ 5 min
Age at examination _____ hrs
Race _____ Sex _____
BD _____
LMP _____
EDC _____
Gestational age by dates _____ wks
Gestational age by examination _____ wks
Birth weight _____ g _____ %
Length _____ cm _____ %
Head circumference _____ cm _____ %
Cn. Diet. None _____ Mild _____
          Moderate _____ Severe _____

Neuromuscular maturity

Neuromuscular maturity sign	Score							Record score here
	–1	0	1	2	3	4	5	
Posture								
Square window (wrist)	>90°	90°	60°	40°	30°	0°		
Arm recoil		180°	140–180°	110–140°	90–110°	<90°		
Popliteal angle	180°	160°	140°	120°	100°	90°	<90°	
Scarf sign								
Heel to ear								

POINTS TO NOTE

- Observation should be made when newborn is quiet and awake.
- Ensure adequate light in examination room.
- The temperature of the examination room is maintained at 28 +/- 2°C.
- Avoid draft and chills in the examination room.
- Wash your hands till elbow for 3 minutes before and after handling the newborn.

WRITE SHORT NOTES ON

1. APGAR score.
2. New Ballard scale for assessing maturity of newborn.

MULTIPLE CHOICE QUESTIONS

1. The recommended room temperature for maintaining warmth for neonates is:
   a. 28°C
   b. 34°C
   c. 25–28 °C
   d. 25°C
2. A nurse in the newborn nursery is monitoring a preterm newborn infant for respiratory distress syndrome. Which assessment signs if noted in the newborn infant would alert the nurse to the possibility of this syndrome?
   a. Hypotension and bradycardia
   b. Tachypnea and retractions
   c. Acrocyanosis and grunting
   d. The presence of a barrel chest with grunting
3. When determining a newborn's gestational age using the Ballard Score, which of these findings would indicate low neuromuscular maturity?
   a. 30° flexion of the wrist
   b. Frog-like posture
   c. Arm pulled across midline of chest
   d. A brisk 90° arm recoil

ANSWER KEY

1. c   2. c   3. c

CHAPTER 5

Anthropometry Measurements

PRACTICE COMPETENCIES
On completion of the chapter, the students will be able to:
- Provide objective health data which enable one to assess physical growth and development.
- Identify potential health problems.
- Evaluate an individual's nutritional status.
- Identify individuals in need of treatment and follow-up care.
- Plan an accurate assessment of the growth pattern and/or nutritional status of those being measured.

ABSTRACT
Growth assessment is the single most useful tool for defining health and nutritional status at both the individual and population level. This is because disturbances in health and nutrition, regardless of their etiology, almost always affect growth. Growth monitoring strives to improve nutrition, reduce the risk of inadequate nutrition educate care givers, and produce early detection and referral for conditions, manifested by growth disorders. At the population health level, cross sectional surveys of anthropometric data help define health and nutritional status for purpose of program planning, implementation and evaluation. Growth monitoring is also used in all settings to assess the response to intervention. This chapter contains the procedures related to anthropometric measurements such as weight, height, head, circumference, chest circumference, mind-arm circumference, skin fold thickness, abdominal circumference, fontanelle and dentition.

Keywords: Anthropometry, weight, infant weighing scale, length and height, stadiometer, head circumference, mid-arm circumference, Shakins tape, skin folding lange calipers, fontanelle, canine, premolars, teeth eruption, incisors, temporary teeth.

INTRODUCTION

The term anthropometric refers to comparative measurements of the human. The anthropometric measurements commonly used as indices of growth and development for infants include length, weights and head circumference. Typically growth is evaluated by comparing individual measurements to reference standards, represented by percentile curves on a growth charts.

DEFINITIONS

1. **Anthropometry:** Anthropometry is a system of measurements of the size and make-up of the body and specific body parts.
2. **Anthropometric:** The term anthropometric refers to comparative measurements of the human body.

ANTHROPOMETRIC MEASUREMENTS

Measurements of physical growth in children is a key elements in evaluation of the health status of children.

Physical Growth Parameters

1. Weight
2. Height
3. Head circumference
4. Chest circumference.
5. Mid-arm circumference
6. Skin folding
7. Abdominal circumference
8. Frontanelle
9. Dentition.

General Instruction to be followed during techniques of measurement are:
1. Welcome parents and the child to a neat and clean physical environment.
2. Sit in front of the child at eye level and explain the reasons for carrying out the procedure to parents and child.
3. Approach the child in a positive manner.
4. Allow the child to handle equipment.
5. Allow the older child to participate in certain activities of physical measurements.
6. Assure the child that none of the equipment hurts.
7. Obtain cooperation of small children by offering toys to them.
8. Young child can be allowed to sit in parents lap.
9. Educate the school age child by informing the findings of physical measurements.

Note: Carrying out the measurements, skill fully, accurately and quickly.

You can carry out these activities in various setting such as hospitals and field.

Areas are included in hospitals and field

- Under five clinic of hospital
- Hospitals: Wards
- Under five clinic of primary health care
- Child guidance clinic
- School health clinic
- Field: home, community.

1. Weight

Average birth weight is 2.5–3.5 kg. Infants weighed shortly after birth and each day if they remain in the birth center.

Purposes
- It helps to assess nutritional status and to calculate doses
- To determine whether weight loss of child after birth is normal
- It help to provide a basis for evaluating further growth and daily thereafter.

Equipment
- Infantometer
- Weighing scale
- Beam balance/electronic weighing machine
- Clean cloth or paper to prevents cross infection and to lessen of infants body heat to the scale through conduction.

Procedure
- Infants is measured on infantometer.
- Selects an appropriate sized beam balance with measures weights to the nearest 10 g and for infants and 100 g for children.
- Balance the scale by setting it at zero before checking the weight.
- Measure the weight in a comfortably warm room to prevents hypothermia.
- Weight the infants and toddlers without dress.
- Older children are usually wear under pants.
- Cover place a clean sheets or paper on beam with each infant's measurements.
- When weighing infant place hand slightly above body to prevent accidental falling.
- Take reading at eye level.
- If the child is wearing some types of special devices such as splint or cast record on chart with weight.
- If weight scale indicates weight in pounds you can convert it into kilogram by dividing it by 2.2 as 1 kg – 2.2 pounds.
- Record the weight on appropriate chart.

Weight
- Average birth weight is 2.5–3.5 kg
- 1st weeks 10% weight loss, regains with in 10 days of life
- 0–3 months—30 g/day weight gain
- 3–6 months—20 g/day
- 6 months—weight doubles birth weight
- 1 year—weight triples

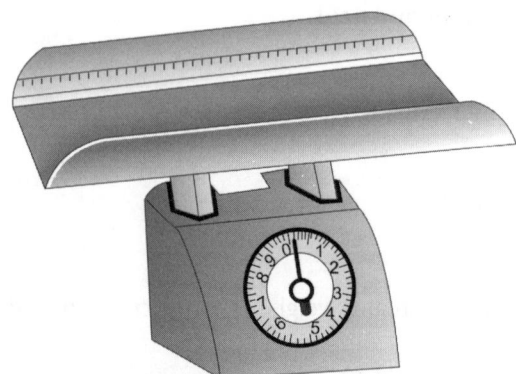

Fig. 5.1: Infant weighing scale.

- ❖ 2 years—4 times
- ❖ 3 years—5 times
- ❖ 10 years—10 times.

Formula for calculating weight
3–12 months weight = age in month + 9/2
1–6 years weight = Age in years × 2 + 8
7–12 years weight = Age in years × 7 – 5/2.

2. Length and Height

Length of the newborn is 45–50 cm.

Purposes
- ❖ It helps to assess nutritional status
- ❖ It helps to assess growth of the child.

Equipment
- ❖ Tape measure
- ❖ Stadio measure.

Procedure: Up to 2 years of age length is measured by lying down, head and touching head of the scale. Grasp knee and together gently and pushdown knees and legs are extended and heel of the against the board.
- ❖ Measure from the crown of the head to heel of the feet with tape.
- ❖ In order children height is measured by stadio meter or tape measure.
- ❖ Measure height by having the child stand with head in midline.
- ❖ Be sure that child back to the wall, heels, buttock and back of shoulder touching wall, arms hand freely.
- ❖ Flat object placed on top of head and height measured using tape measure.
- ❖ Record length/height on the charts.

Length: The average length of term infant at birth is 50 cm.
- ❖ 3 months—60 cm
- ❖ 9 months—70 cm
- ❖ 1 year—75 cm

Formula: Height formula for 2–12 years
Height (cm) = Age in years × 6 + 77.

3. Head Circumference

Head circumference is related to the rate of the growth of the brain. In the newborn, it is 2.5 cm larger than the chest circumference.

Purpose
- ❖ It helps to evaluate the diagnostic procedure
- ❖ It is an important screening procedure for detecting abnormalities of head growth.

Procedure: Head circumference is measured by placing the measuring tape above the eyebrows and

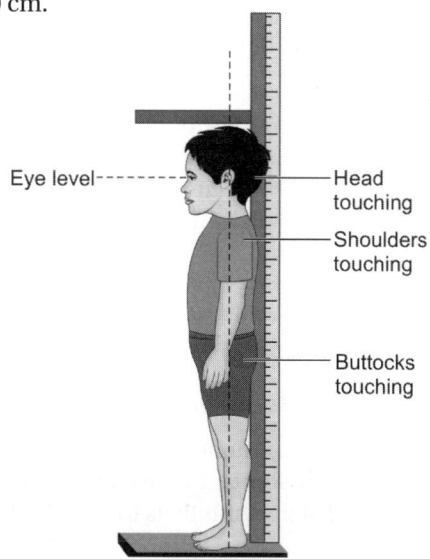

Fig. 5.2: Height measurement.

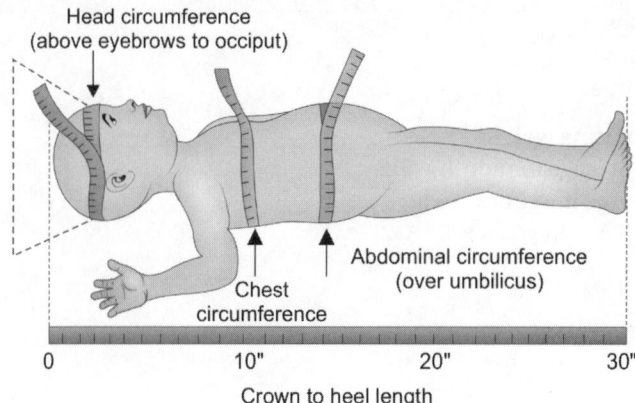

Fig. 5.3: Length, HC, CC, AC measurement.

pinna of the ears and around the occipital prominence at the back of the skull and recording is done in cm.

Head circumference
- At birth 33—35 cm
- At 3 months—40 cm
- At 6 months—43 cm
- At 2 years—48 cm
- At 7 years—50 cm
- At 12 years—52 cm.

4. Chest Circumference

The chest is barrel shaped at birth, and anteroposterior and transverse diameters are equal. Gradually transverse diameter increases. At the end of the one year of the age, head circumferences and chest circumferences are equal. The chest circumferences increases.

Equipment: Tape measures.

Procedure
- Place the tape around the chest at the level of nipples
- Record in mid respiration (inspiration and expiration)
- At birth chest circumference is 30.5–33.0 cm
- At birth head circumference is greater than chest, i.e. 2 to 3 cm
- 1 year head and chest circumference equal
- 2 years chest circumference is grater than head circumference about 2 to 3 cms

Note: Don't compress the measuring tape on the chest wall it would compress the soft tissue underneath.

5. Abdominal Circumference

Abdominal circumference is measured and recorded as a base line value for fetus assessment. It is usually similar to the chest circumference and abdominal circumference is measured at the level of the umbilicus the top edge of tape is at the lower level of the umbilical card stump.

Procedure
- ❖ To measure abdominal circumference place the paper tape under the newborn abdomen at umbilical level.
- ❖ Note abdominal circumference and record, it in the infants chart. Abdominal circumferences vary but are typically similar to the chest circumference.
- ❖ Recording provides baseline value facilitates detection of abnormalities.
  For example, distension.

6. Mid-arm Circumference

The mid-arm circumference determines muscle wasting. It is a useful indicator of nutritional status of children.

Purpose
- ❖ It helps to assess the nutritional status of the child
- ❖ It helps to assess the indirect measure of muscle mass in children of 1–6 years.

Equipment
- ❖ Shakir's tape
- ❖ Tape measures.

Procedure
Shaikir's tape used for mid-arm circumference. This is plastic tape with colored zones.
  Green—more than 13.5 cm
  Yellow—between 12.5 cm and 13.5 cm
  Red—less than 12.5 cm.
- ❖ Hang left arm freely
- ❖ Measurements taken at midpoint of upper arm between tip of acromion process and olecranon process.
- ❖ Tape is used around the arm

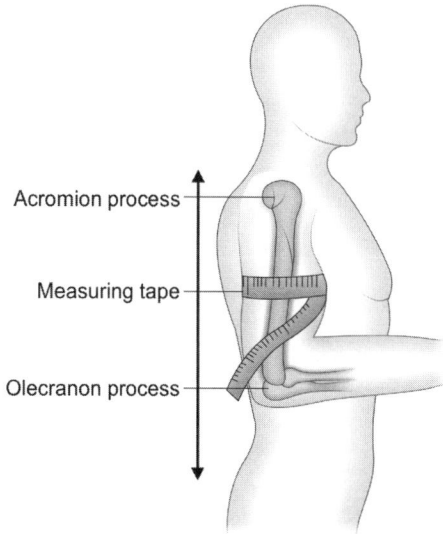

Fig. 5.4: Mid-arm circumference measurement.

- ❖ At birth—11-12 cm
- ❖ 1 year—12-16 cm
- ❖ 1 to 5 years—16-17 cm
- ❖ 12 years—17-18 cm
- ❖ 15 years—20-21 cm.

7. Skin Foldings

Skin fold measurements are used to determine the fat contents of subcutaneous tissue.

Measures of relative weight and stature can not distinguish between adipose tissue or muscle.

Equipment: Lange calipers.

Procedure
- ❖ One convenient measures of body fat is skin fold thickness which increasingly recommended.
- ❖ Skin fold thickness is measured with special calipers. Such as the lange calipers.
- ❖ The most common sites for measuring are the triceps, sub-scapula, supraluminal, abdomen and upper thigh calf.
- ❖ It is recorded skin fold area on the left side.
- ❖ Hold a fold of skin between thumb and index finger and measures.

8. Examination of Fontanelles

Wide gap in suture line is called fontanelles.

Two fontanelles has clinical significant.
1. Anterior fontanelle: It is diamond shaped and measures 3 × 3 cm. It closes at 18 months (1½ years).
2. Posterior fontanelle: It is triangular in shape and measures about 1.2 × 1.2 cm. It closes at 6 weeks of age (1½ months).

9. Dentition

Temporary (deciduous) teeth:
The temporary teeth are 20 in number. They are:

Canines-2
Incisors-4 } in each jaw
Molars-4

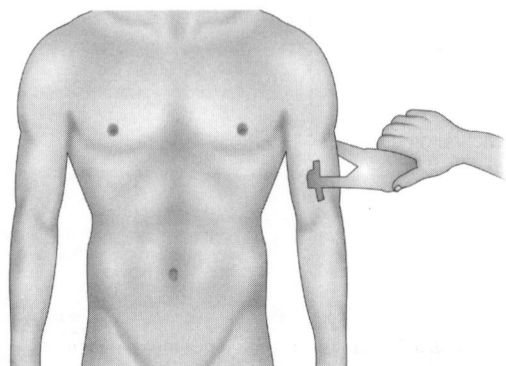

Fig. 5.5: Skin fold thickness measurement.

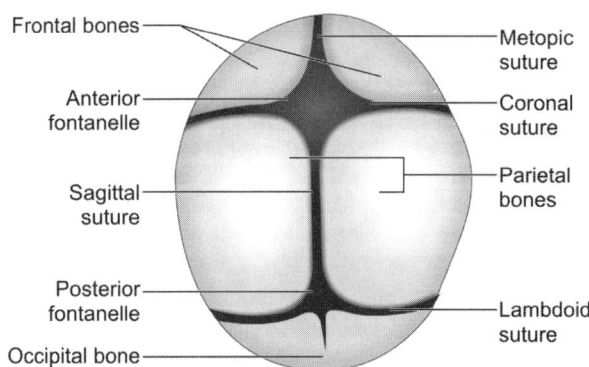

Fig. 5.6: Fontanelles.

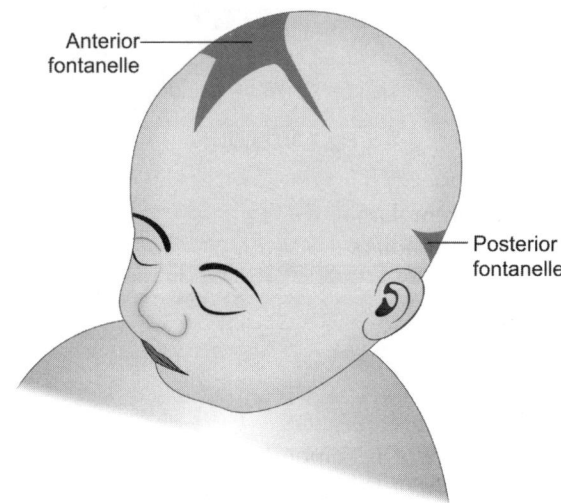

Fig. 5.7: Fontanelles of newborn.

Time of eruption of temporary (deciduous) teething:
Birth–Nil
6–8 months   :   Lower central incisors
7–9 months   :   Upper central incisors
10–12 months   :   Lower lateral incisors
7–9 months   :   Upper lateral incisors
18 months   :   Canines
12–14 months   :   1st molar
20–30 months   :   2nd molar

Permanent (secondary) teeth:
The permanent teeth are thirty two in number. They are:
6–8 years   :   Central incisors
7–9 years   :   Lateral incisors
11–12 years   :   Canines

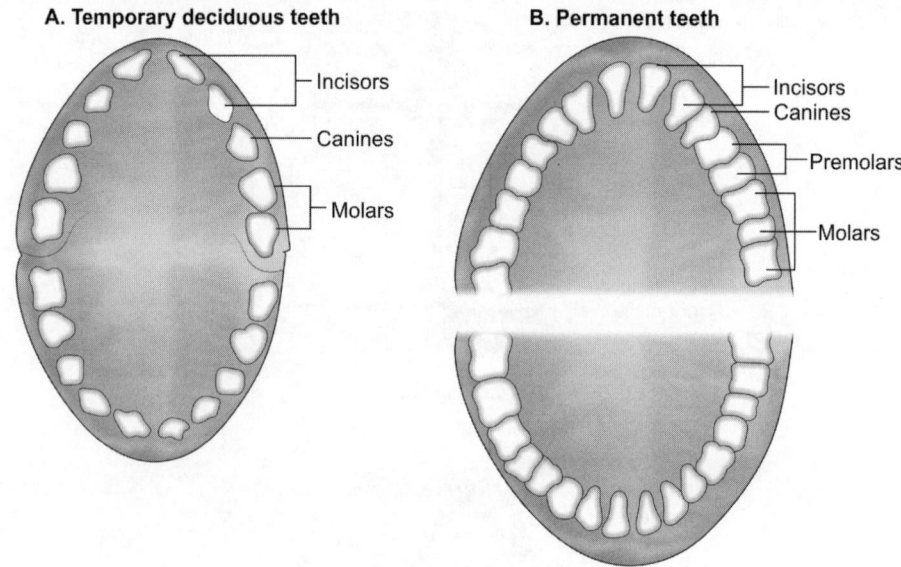

Fig. 5.8: Dentition.

9–11 years   : Anterior premolars
10–12 years : Posterior premolars
6–7 years   : 1st molar
12–14 years : 2nd molar
17–25 years : 3rd molar

FILL IN THE BLANKS

1. Formula for calculating weight of 3–12 months old baby _____
2. Formula for calculating weight of 1–6 years old child _____
3. Formula for calculating weight of 7–12 years old child _____
4. Formula for calculating height of 2–12 years old child _____
5. Anterior fontanelle closes by _____
6. Posterior fontanelle closes by _____

POINTS TO NOTE

- Firstly, explain the process to the parent and child.
- The weighing scales must be accurate.
- The baby scales platform must be safe and secure to prevent the child from falling.
- The mother or nurse must stay with the child when he is being weighed to prevent falling.
- To prevent cross infection, the nurse should stand behind or to the side of the person being weighed to prevent contact with the person's face and mouth.
- If a mother is very heavy (e.g., more than 100 kg) and the baby's weight is relatively low (e.g., less than 2.5 kg), the baby's weight may not register on the scale. In such cases, have a lighter person hold the baby on the scale.

MULTIPLE CHOICE QUESTIONS

1. A six year old infant cannot:
    a. Grasp dangling objects
    b. Fix gaze
    c. Lift and hold head
    d. Turn head towards sound
2. Number of deciduous teeth is:
    a. 20
    b. 24
    c. 32
    d. 28
3. Shakir tape is used for:
    a. Measurement of height
    b. Measurement of length of infant
    c. Measurement of mid arm circumference
    d. Measurement of skin pad thickness

ANSWER KEY

1. a   2. a   3. c

CHAPTER 6

Developmental Assessment

PRACTICE COMPETENCIES

On completion of the chapter, the students will be able to:
- Assist in early diagnosis of conditions with a genetic basis, such as Duchenne muscular dystrophy and fragile X syndrome, facilitates genetic counseling for families.
- Provide care givers with reliable information before a developmental problem becomes obvious.
- Understand the child's difficulty and make appropriate management plans for their family.
- Counsel care givers if assessment shows that the child is within the normal range by reassuring and relieving anxiety.
- Compare early assessments with the later ones.
- Provide an opportunity to encourage good parenting and developmental stimulation.

ABSTRACT

A careful history is necessary to identify parental concerns. These should always be listened to and taken into consideration, as parental observation has been shown to be as effective as assessment by health professionals in detecting problems in many areas of child health and development. The assessment starts the moment the health professional meets the child and parents. A good overview of developmental skills can be obtained by watching the child play. A few simple toys, such as some bricks, a car, a doll, ball, pencil, and paper are all that are required, as they can be adapted for any age. It is important to talk and listen to the child and the parents, as well as observing eye contact and other social interactions during play. This chapter contains the assessment of development in the areas of gross motor, fine motor, language and personal or social developments and also reflexes of the newborn, important mile stones at a glance. The Denver Developmental Screening Test described.

Keywords: Gross motor, fine motor, language, personal or social, rooting reflex, sucking reflex, Moro reflex, grasp reflex, grossed extension reflex, Glabellar reflex, tonic neck reflex, stepping reflex, plantar reflex, mile stones, Denver Developmental Screening Test (DDST).

DEVELOPMENT

Development is the functional maturation of organs and particularly of the central nervous system. In contrast to measuring physical growth, the measurement of behavioral development is subjective, widely variable and tend to be in exact controversial.

Environment, sociocultural pattern, nature versus nurture and genetic factor also influence the pattern of individual development.

ASSESSMENT OF DEVELOPMENT

Developmental assessment is a part of clinical examination. It is based on observation related to achievements which are normal expected at given chronological age.
1. Gross motor
2. Fine motor
3. Language
4. Personal or social.

1. *Gross motor*: This includes control of head, trunk and extremities.
2. *Fine motor:* It pertains to control of the fine movement of fingers.
   Motor control indicates neurologic inferiority, acceleration or delay, however, need not necessarily be related to intellectual abilities.
3. *Language:* Language development is related to the perception of sounds and production of words and language is in the form of speech.
4. *Personal and social*: This is widely variable, depends upon social and environmental factors.

However, some personal factors like control of bowel and bladder are related to neurologic integrity and have established value.

DEVELOPMENT OF NEWBORN

Assessment of newborn for appropriate development will primarily depend upon a variety of reflexes.

REFLEXES OF NEWBORN

Rooting Reflex (Fig. 6.1)

When a corner of mouth or lip touches with finger mouth turns towards the stimulated side.

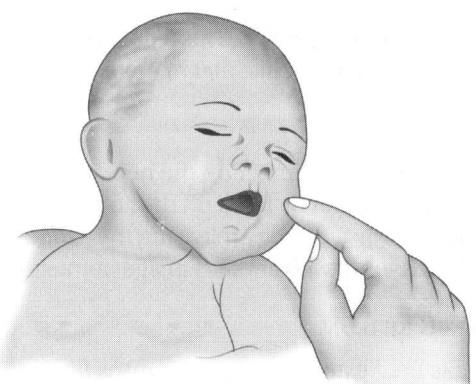

Fig. 6.1: Rooting reflex.

Sucking and Swallowing Reflex (Fig. 6.2)

It is a movement of lips and tongue in the direction of stimulus.

Moro Reflex (Fig. 6.3)

When the examiner bangs the table, there is a sudden abduction at shoulders and extension at elbows of the arms as also complete opening of hands followed by adduction and flexion.

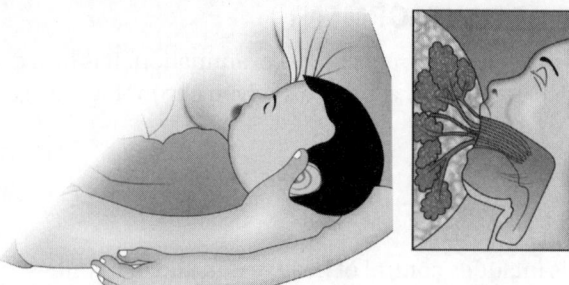

Fig. 6.2: Sucking reflex.

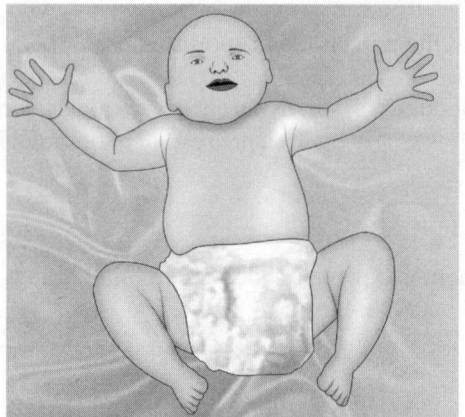

Fig. 6.3: Moro reflex.

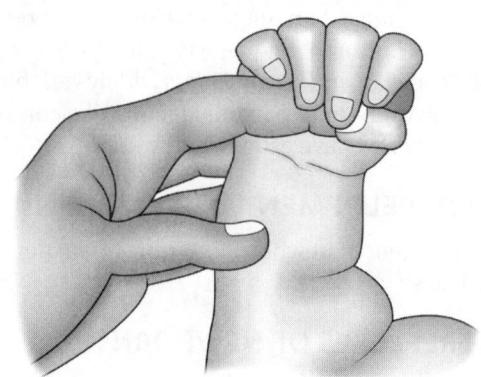

Fig. 6.4: Grasp reflex.

The baby seems to be attempting to embarrass. This reflex normally disappear after four months. If it is persistence, suggest a damaged brain like that in mental retardation or cerebral palsy.

Grasp Reflex (Fig. 6.4)

It consists in placing the examiner index finger on the neonates palm. The infant immediately grasps it. The grasp is so firm that he can be lifted off the cot by means of this only, on strocking dorsum of the hand, he opens the fist, thereby releasing the examiners fingers.

Persistence of grasp reflex beyond twelve weeks of age points to brain damage.

Crossed Extension Reflex (Fig. 6.5)

Stroking the foot as the leg is held extended at knee causes flexion, abduction, extension and adduction together with fanning of the toes of the other leg. The response stimulates wording painful stimuli.

Glabellar Reflex or Tape (Fig. 6.6)

It comprises tapping of the glabellar or nasion (the meeting point of forehead and nose). The neonate reacts by closure of eyes or blinking.

Tonic Neck Reflex (Fig. 6.7)

On suddenly turning a supine neonates head to one side, the arm and the leg of the same side extend and those of the other side get flexed.

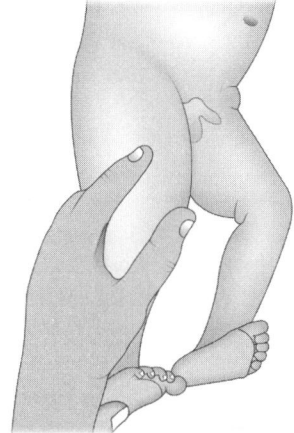

Fig. 6.5: Crossed extension reflex.

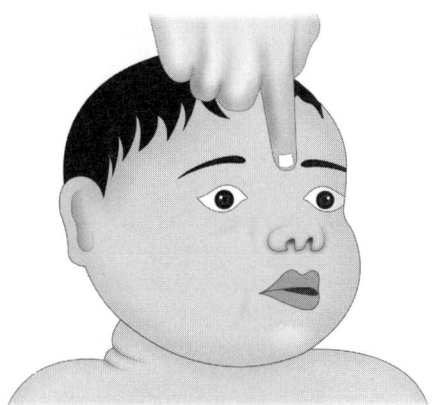

Fig. 6.6: Glabellar reflex.

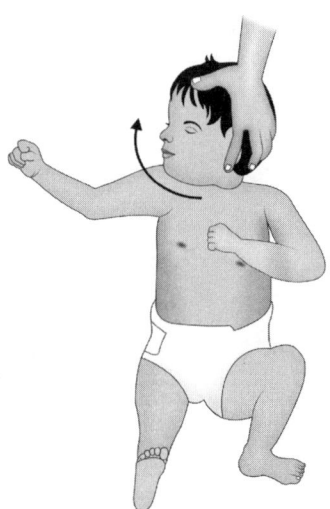

Fig. 6.7: Tonic neck reflex.

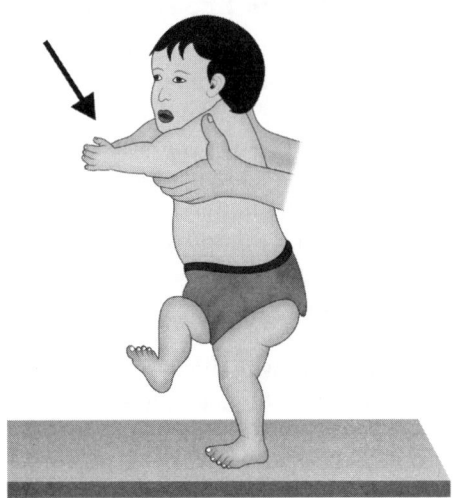

Fig. 6.8: Stepping reflex.

Persistence of the reflex beyond the age of six to nine months or maintenance tonic neck posture constantly even at an early age point to existence of cerebral palsy.

Stepping Reflex (Fig. 6.8)

The neonate shows movements of walking when held upright and inclined forward with soles touching a flat surface.

Plantar (Babinski) Reflex (Fig. 6.9)

It is elicited by stimulating the lateral aspects of sole of the foot, beginning at the heel and extending to the base of the toes with a firm objects such as examiners thumb or a hand key. A positive response is characterized by extension of the great toe and fanning of the other toes.

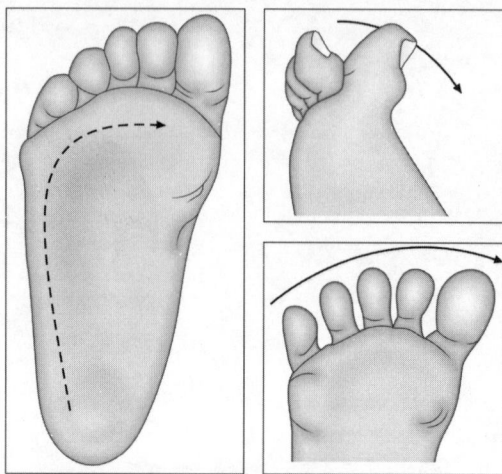

Fig. 6.9: Babinski reflex.

IMPORTANT MILESTONES AT GLANCE

- Social smile—4 to 6 weeks
- Head holding—3 months
- Sit with support—6 months
- Sit without support—7 months
- Reaches out for a bright object and get it—5 to 6 months
- Crawls—8 to 10 months
- Creeps—10 to 11 months
- Stands holding furniture—9 months
- Walks holding furniture—12 months
- Stands without support—10 to 11 months
- Says one word with meaning—12 months
- Says 3 words with meaning—13 months
- Joins 2 or 3 words into sentence—15 to 18 months
- Feeds self with spoon—13 months
- Climbs stairs—15 to 18 months
- Takes shoes and socks off—15 to 18 months
- Put shoes and socks on—24 months
- Takes some cloths off—24 months
- Dresses self fully—3 to 4 years
- Dry by day—2 years
- Dry by night—3 years
- Knows full name and sex—3 years
- Rides tricycle—3 years

LANGUAGE DEVELOPMENT

The development of language is a complex phenomena that involves coordination of the cognitive, psychological and physiological capacity of the child. Several basic physiologic requirements are needed in order to develop speech. They must have normal respiratory function, neurological function of the speech center and cerebral cortex. Skeletal development of the mouth and nasal cavities must be intact for articulation of words.

Lastly, the child must have sufficient hearing capacity for normal development of language to occur. In terms of cognitive capacities, a child must have the ability to symbolize before the use of language occurs. Basically child must understand what the meaning of the words before using them. The infant does not initially possess this ability. As the child mental capacities develop, words become associated with significant figures and objects in the environment.

Speech Development of the Child

1–12 months	:	Cooing, babying, initiation of sounds, such as: Goo, aha, ba, maa.
1–2 years	:	One word sentence, such as: Out, ball, kite.
2–3 years	:	Multiword sentences, locate, name, demand, indicates, possession, question, such as: Their book, more milk, my shoe.
3–4 years	:	Grammatically correct verbal utterances, such as: I want my shoe, this is my bag.

■ DEVELOPMENTAL SCREENING TEST

DENVER II TEST: Denver II test has been shown in **Figure 6.10**.

Directions for Administration

1. Try to get child to smile by smiling, talking or waving. Do not touch him/her.
2. Child must stare at head several seconds.
3. Parent may help guide toothbrush and put toothpaste on brush.
4. Child does not have to be able to tie shoes or button/zip in the back.
5. Move yarn slowly in an arc from one side to the other, about 8'above child's face.
6. Pass if child grasps rattle when it is touched to the backs or tips of fingers.
7. Pass if child tries to see where yarn went. Yarn should be dropped quickly from sight from testers hand without arm movement.
8. Child must transfer cube from hand to hand without help of body, mouth or table.
9. Pass if child picks up raisin with any part of thumb and finger.
10. Line can vary only 30° or less from testers line.
11. Make a fist with thumb pointing upward and wiggle only the thumb. Pass if child imitates and does not move any fingers other than the thumb.

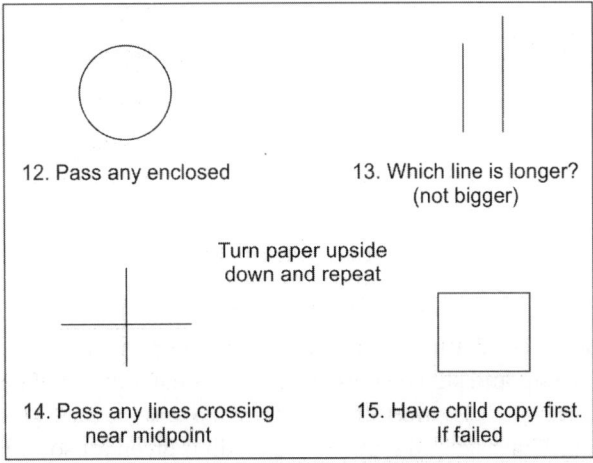

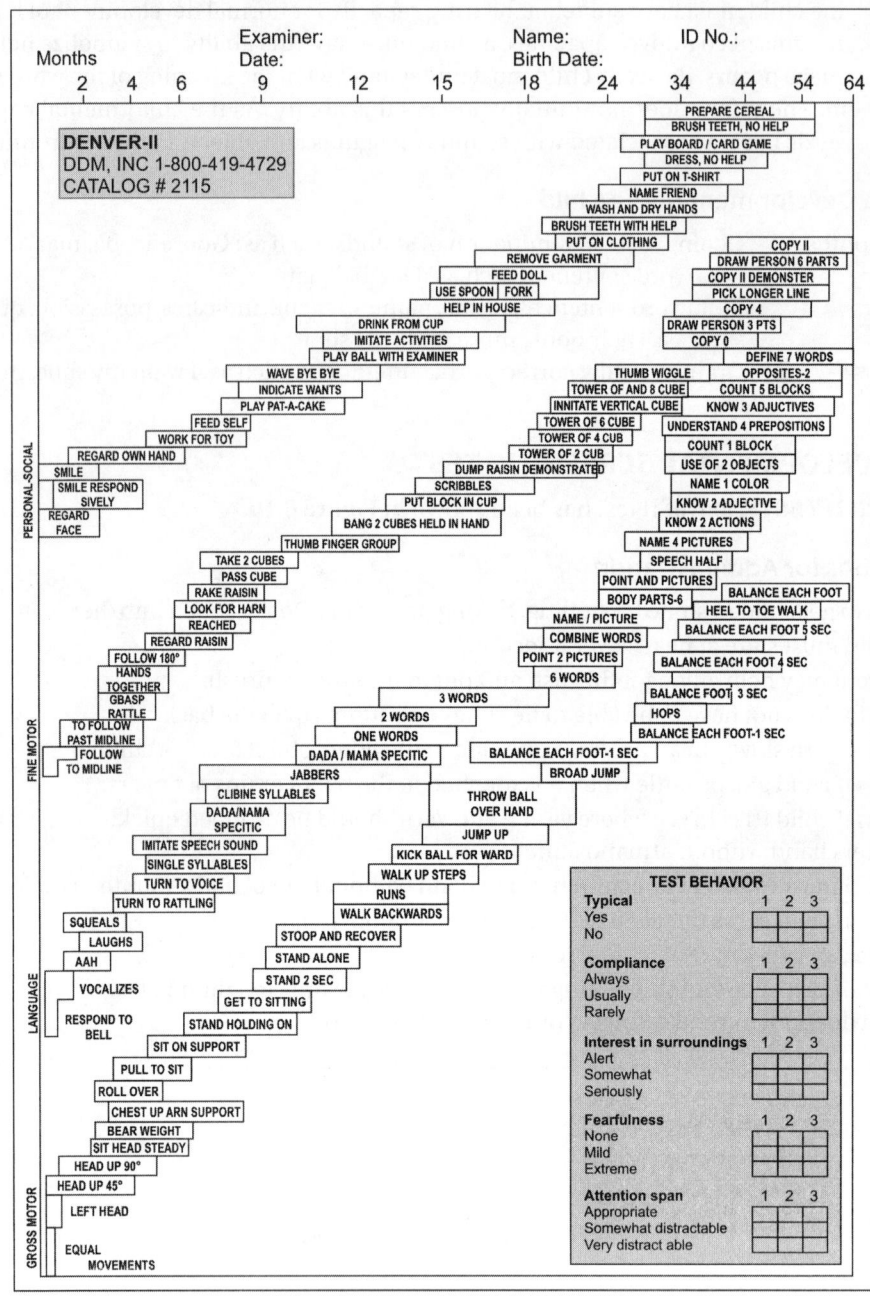

Fig. 6.10: Denver II test.

When giving items 12, 13, 14 and 15, do not name the forms. Do not demonstrate 12 and 14.
16. When scoring each pair (2 arms, 2 legs, etc.) count as open part.
17. Place one cube in cup and shake gently near child's ear, but out of sight. Repeat for other ear.
18. Point to picture and have a child name it (no credit is given for sounds only)

If less than 4 pictures are named correctly, have child point to picture as each is named by tester.

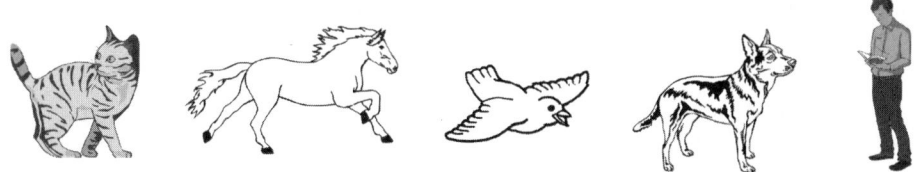

19. Using doll, tell child: Show me the nose, eyes, ears, mouth, hands, feet, tummy, hair. Pass 6 of 8.
20. Using pictures, ask child: which one flies?........says meow? ...... Talks?....... barks?......gallops? Pass 2 of 5, 4 of 5.
21. Ask child: what do you do when you are cold?.....tired?.....hungry? pass 2 of 3, 3 of 3.
22. Ask child: what do you do with a cup? What is a chair used for? What is a pencil used for? Action words must be included in answers.
23. Pass if child correctly place and says how many blocks are on paper (1,5).
24. Tell child: put block **on** table; **under** table; **in front of** me; **behind** me. Pass 4 of 4. (Do not help child by pointing, moving head or eyes.)
25. Ask child: what is ball? ....Lake? ......desk? ......house? .... banana? ....curtain? .... fence? ....ceiling? ..... pass if defined in terms of use shape, what it is made of, or general category (such as banana is fruit, not just yellow). Pass 5 of 8, 7 of 8.
26. Ask child: if horse is big, a mouse is ----? If fire is hot, ice is ----? If the sun shines during the day, the moon shines during the ------? Pass 2 of 3.
27. Child may use wall or rail only, not person. May not crawl.
28. Child must throw ball overhand 3 feet to within arms reach of tester.
29. Child must perform standing board jump over width of test sheet (8½ inches).
30. Tell child to walk forward ⇨ heal with one inch of toe. Tester may demonstrate.
31. In the second year, half of normal children are noncompliant.

Observations

Write any observations while performing the test.

DENVER DEVELOPMENT EXAMINATION

Overviews

- Administered to children at birth—6 years
- Assesses the child's performance on age appropriate tasks
- Screen for possible problems
- Not a predictor of later development

The Test

Test consists of 125 tasks or items covering four areas:
1. Personal—social
2. Fine motor —adaptive
3. Language

4. Gross motor
   - Children are tested on the tasks or items pertinent to their age
   - It must be conducted in a standardized manner
   - Kit comes with the necessary supplies and scoring sheets.

Prior to the Test

- Know four types of tests on the right side of DDST
- Directions of the test is given at the back
- Determine testable tasks and items based on the child's age
- Ensure your supplies are in order
- Set up an appropriate testing location.

The Test

- Give her/him blocks to arrange
- Give doll and bottle for feeding
- Ask baby about body parts of doll (e.g., nose, mouth, legs, arm, etc.)
- Ask him to name the figures
- Give a ball and ask him to throw.

Scoring

- Assign each tested task/item a pass, fail, no opportunity or refusal score
- Mark on DDST chart against each task as P (pass), F (fail), No (no opportunity), R (refusal)
- Interpret the test based on findings:
  Normal: No delays and max of one caution.
  Suspect: Two or more caution and/or one or more delays
- Schedule follow-up
- Repeat test and/or follow-up with appropriate healthcare provider.

POINTS TO NOTE

These indicators suggest that development is seriously disordered and that the child should be promptly referred to a developmental or community pediatrician:
- Loss of developmental skills at any age.
- Parental or professional concerns about vision, fixing, or following an object or a confirmed visual impairment at any age (simultaneous referral to pediatric ophthalmology).
- Hearing loss at any age (simultaneous referral for expert audio logical or ear, nose, and throat assessment).
- Persistently low muscle tone or floppiness.
- No speech by 18 months, especially if the child does not try to communicate by other means such as gestures (simultaneous referral for urgent hearing test).
- Asymmetry of movements or other features suggestive of cerebral palsy.
- Increased muscle tone persistent toe walking complex disabilities.
- Head circumference above the 99.6th centile or below 0.4th centile.

■ PRACTICE QUESTIONS

1. Identify the following:
   a. Rooting reflex
   b. Glabellar reflex

c. Moro reflex
   d. Tonic neck reflex
   e. Crossed extension reflex
2. Write short notes on:
   a. Mile stones of an infant

MULTIPLE CHOICE QUESTIONS

1. Which of the developmental milestone puts the 4-months-old infant at greatest risk for injury?
   a. Switching objects from one hand to another
   b. Crawling
   c. Standing
   d. Rolling over
2. The nurse notes a swelling on the neonate's scalp that crosses the suture line. What is this assessment finding?
   a. Cephalhematoma
   b. Caput succedaneum
   c. Hemorrhage edema
   d. Perinatal caput
3. What is the use of the administration of the Denver Developmental Screening Test or (DDST) to a five months old infant?
   a. To assess the intelligent quotient
   b. To assess the emotional development
   c. To assess the social and physical activities
   d. To assess the predisposition to genetic and allergic

ANSWER KEY

1. d   2. b   3. c

CHAPTER 7

Assisting with Common Diagnostic Procedures

PRACTICE COMPETENCIES
On completion of the chapter, the students will be able to:
- Identify indications and contraindications for carrying out any diagnostic procedure.
- Carry out physical examination of a child.
- Place the child in appropriate position during procedures.
- Assist the physician in various specialized procedures.
- Identify any adverse reaction in child during procedure.
- Monitor vital signs.
- Provide nursing care as per needs of the child.

ABSTRACT
A laboratory (lab) test is a procedure in which a healthcare provider takes a sample stool, throat swab, urine, blood or any other body fluid, or body tissue. The tests can provide important information about child's health. They may be used to help diagnose diseases and conditions, monitor treatments for a disease, or check the health of organs and body systems. But lab tests can be scary, especially for children. Fortunately, children don't need to be tested as often as adults. But if the child does need testing, steps can be taken to help him or her feel less scared and anxious. Preparing in advance may also help keep the child calm and less likely to resist the procedure.

Keywords: Blood, urine, stool, throat swab, venepuncture, specimens, culture and sensitivity.

INTRODUCTION

The most important step in the recovery of pathogenic organisms responsible for infectious disease is the proper specimen collection, processing and handling by you, the healthcare professional. It is one way of knowing about the patient's health status by identifying pathogens and analyzing **urine, blood, sputum, and feces**. One of the many responsibilities assigned to us, as nurses, is to collect and label specimen for analysis and to ensure their delivery to the lab. And knowing the proper way of gathering specimen is necessary for self-protection and to prevent the spread of disease.

DEFINITION

Diagnostic tests help in detection and confirmation of the presence or absence of any disease, injury or any other health condition that requires medical attention.

There are thousands of diagnostic tests for various diseases that are being carried out in different diagnostic centers and hospitals every day.

Objectives

- Specify most common specimen collection procedures
- Know the importance of various specimen collection for patient care and satisfaction
- Emphasize the importance of protecting yourself against exposure to bloodborne pathogens.

Concepts of Specimen Collection

- Collect the specimen from the actual site of infection without contaminating adjacent tissues and secretions.
- Collect the specimen at the best time possible (e.g., early morning sputum for AFB culture)
- Collect ample amount of sample by using appropriate collection devices such as sterile, leak-proof specimen containers.
- Use appropriate transport media such as anaerobic transport vials, culturette for bacterial culture, and the like.
- Check expiration date before inoculating collection device.
- Collect specimens before administration of antimicrobial agents whenever possible.
- Label the specimen properly and fill out test request form completely.
- Lessen transport time and maintain an appropriate environment between collection of specimens and delivery to the laboratory.

Importance of Specimen Collection

The following could affect the hospital's reimbursement under recent healthcare reform laws and regulations:
- Poor specimen quality can affect key quality reporting requirements and metrics
- Reduced power to act upon infection
- Decreases patient satisfaction from improper collection technique
- Expanded cost-per-medicare beneficiary due to repeated specimen collections and unnecessary treatment.

Specimen collection is also key to **patient's satisfaction** and poor collection practice can lead to:
- Defective results and improper treatment
- Duplicated specimen collections and re-testing
- Vessel trauma and pain

Poor specimen collection may also affect **nurses** professionally and personally by:
- Decreased ability to provide up-to-date, proper patient care
- Exposure to bloodborne pathogens
- Unnecessary repeated specimen collection and patient dissatisfaction.

Nurses' Roles in Specimen Collection

- Patient interaction
- Suitable selection of supplies
- Appropriate and proper collection
- Precise sample identification
- Up-to-date transfer to the lab

■ THROAT SWAB SPECIMEN COLLECTION

A throat swab culture is a laboratory diagnostic test that evaluates for the presence of a bacterial or fungal infection in the throat. It is done to isolate and identify any pathogens, which may be medium. A sample of mucus and secretions from the back of the throat is collected on a cottontipped applicator and applied to a slide or a special cup that allows infections to grow. These infections can include strep throat, *pneumonia, tonsillitis*, whooping *cough*, and *meningitis*.

Purpose

Throat swab culture is done to detect the presence of organisms in the throat that could cause infection. For instance, the presence of group A *Streptococcus* bacteria in your throat is a key sign that you may have strep throat.

Supplies and Equipment

The supplies and equipment required to obtain a sample for throat culture are:
- Sterile cotton-tipped applicator specimen collection tip (culturette)
- Tongue depressor
- Laboratory request form
- Flashlight

Procedure

- Always observe proper hand hygiene prior to the test.
- Have the patient sit comfortably either on bed or chair while explaining the procedure.
- Allow the patient to tilt his head back and ask him. *Antiseptic mouthwash should be avoided before this test.*
- Make use of the flashlight to light up the back of the throat and check for presence of inflammation using the tongue depressor.
- *Swab the tonsillar areas from side to side and make sure to include any inflamed or purulent sites.* The test may cause momentary gagging because the back of the throat is a sensitive area, but it should not be painful.
- Refrain from touching the tongue, cheeks, or teeth with the applicator, due to possible contamination with oral bacteria.
- Place the cotton-tipped applicator into the culture tube immediately.
- Label the culture tube with the patient's name, SSN, and ward number if applicable.
- Fill out the request form completely with the following information:
  - Patient's name
  - Patient's rank or status
  - Family member prefix and sponsor's social security number
  - Ward number if inpatient, or mobile number if outpatient
  - Source of the specimen (e.g., throat)
  - Any antibiotics the patient is taking
  - Date and time the specimen was obtained
  - Name of the physician who ordered the culture
- The sample is then taken to the laboratory for culture.

SPUTUM SPECIMEN COLLECTION

A sputum specimen is a sample of material expelled from the respiratory passages taken for laboratory analysis to determine the presence of pathogens. A specimen of mucus from the lungs expectorated through the mouth or obtained via tracheal suctioning with an in-line trap or bronchoscope. Specimens are often taken for three consecutive days because it is difficult for the patient to cough up enough sputum at one time, and an organism may be missed if only one culture is done.

Purpose

A sputum specimen is obtained for culture to identify the microorganism responsible for lung infections; identify cancer cells shed by lung tumors; or aid in the diagnosis and management of occupational lung diseases.

Supplies and Equipment

Supplies and equipment required to collect a sputum specimen are:
- Sterile container with tight-fitting lid
- Emesis basin
- Box of tissues
- Gloves
- Goggles
- Aerosol of 10% sodium chloride or sterile water (optional)
- Nebulizer (optional)
- Laboratory request form

Preparation

To prepare your patient, have him drink enough fluids on the night before the test, provided that he is not on fluid restriction. The additional intake will further increase sputum production overnight and assure that you'll get a good sample.

For best results, obtain the sample first thing in the morning. If you can't obtain the sample before the patient has breakfast, though, wait at least an hour after he has eaten before trying. Before you begin, describe the procedure to him.

10 to 15 mL of sputum is typically needed for laboratory analysis. A specimen will be rejected by the laboratory if it contains excessive numbers of epithelial cells from the mouth or throat or if it fails to show adequate numbers of neutrophils on gram staining. If the patient cannot cough up a specimen, the respiratory therapist can use sputum induction techniques such as heated aerosol (nebulization), followed in some instances by postural drainage and percussion.

Procedure

- Observe proper hand hygiene and gather equipment.
- Provide privacy for the patient and explain the entire procedure.
- Position your patient in a chair or on the side of bed. If he is not capable of sitting alone, place him in a high-Fowler's position. Remove dentures, if he has them.
- Place the tissues nearby and have the patient rinse his mouth with clean water to remove any food particles. Don't allow him to brush his teeth or use mouth wash. Doing so could kill bacteria in the sputum, rendering it useless.
- Don gloves and goggles. Uncap the container but avoid touching the inside to ensure that it is sterile.

- Using the sterile collection container provided, instruct the patient to take three deep breaths, then force a deep cough and expectorate into a sterile screw-top container. To prevent contamination by particles in the air, keep the container closed until the patient is ready to spit into it.
- If you don't get an adequate sample on the first try, have him continue to cough until you're able to collect a minimum of 15 mL. If the patient has trouble bringing up secretions, however, have him breathe into the nebulizer and try again.
- Once you've collected the specimen, securely cap the container. Remove and discard your gloves and wash your hands thoroughly. Allow the patient to rinse out his mouth and provide a tissue.
- Record the amount, consistency, and color of the sputum collected, as well as the time and date in the nursing notes.
- Send the sample to the lab immediately, without refrigeration.

STOOL SPECIMEN COLLECTION

A stool culture is the process of growing or culturing organisms existing in feces to see if any of them cause disease. The most common is the ova and parasites test, a microscopic examination of feces for detecting parasites such as amoebas or worms. Stools specimen are often tested for blood. Guaiac fecal occult blood test may be done in the laboratory but are sometimes done at the nursing station to test a stool for occult blood.

Purpose

Stool cultures play an important role in understanding and treating intestinal illness. It can confirm the presence of harmful bacteria. It may also show what treatments may work to kill an invasive organism. If no dangerous bacteria are present in the stool culture but symptoms still exist, other explanations like irritable bowel syndrome, a parasitic infection, or other diagnosis can be explored.

Supplies and Equipment

Supplies and equipment required to collect a stool specimen are:
- Gloves
- Clean bedpan and cover (an extra bedpan or urinal if the patient must void)
- Specimen container and lid
- Wooden tongue blades
- Paper bag for used tongue blades
- Labels
- Plastic bag for transport of container with specimen to laboratory

Procedure

- Discuss the test and the procedure with the patient. Ask him to tell you when he feels the urge to have a bowel movement.
- Wear gloves when handling any bodily discharge.
- Bedpan should be provided when the patient is ready. If the patient wants to urinate first, provide the urinal for a male patient or provide the extra bedpan for a female patient. Avoid mixing urine or regular toilet paper into the sample.

- With the use of a tongue blade, transfer a portion of the feces to the specimen container. Don't touch the specimen because it is contaminated. It is not necessary to keep the specimen sterile because the gastrointestinal tract is not sterile.
- Immediately cover the container and label it with the patient's name and other needed information.
- Fill out the appropriate laboratory request form completely, noting any special examination ordered.
- Take the specimen to the lab immediately; examination for parasites, ova, and organisms must be made while the stool is warm.
- With regard to an infant patient, place the diaper in a leakproof bag, label it, and take the diaper and request form to the lab as soon as possible. However, it can be difficult to keep urine away from the stool sample.

Guaiac Fecal Occult Blood Test (gFOBT)

The stool guaiac test finds hidden (occult) blood in the stool (bowel movement). It is the most common form of fecal occult blood test (FOBT) in use today.

Purpose

This test uses guaiac as reagent to detect the presence of occult blood (blood that appears from a nonspecific source, with obscure signs and symptoms), which is not visible.

Supplies and Equipment

- Test kit (with detailed instructions)
- Test cards
- Brush or wooden applicator
- Gloves

Preparation

Do not allow the patient to eat red meat, any blood-containing food, cantaloupe, uncooked broccoli, turnip, radish, or horseradish for 3 days prior to the test. The patient may need to stop taking medicines that can interfere with the test. These include vitamin C and nonsteroidal anti-inflammatory medicines such as ibuprofen and aspirin. However, never let the patient stop such medication without consulting the physician. There is no discomfort when the test is done since it only involves normal bowel function.

Procedure

- Discuss the test and the procedure with the patient. And prepare himself when he feels the urge to have a bowel movement.
- Tell the patient that he needs to collect a sample from his bowel by placing a sheet of plastic wrap or paper loosely across the toilet bowl to catch the stool or he can use a dry container to collect the stool.
- Inform the patient to not mix the sample with urine. Tell him to flush the remaining stool down the toilet. Remind the patient not to take samples from the toilet bowl water.
- Allow the patient to use the wooden applicator or a brush to smear a thin film of the stool sample onto one of the slots in the test card or slide.
- Next, the patient needs to collect a specimen from a different area of the same stool and smear a thin film of the sample onto the other slot in the test card or slide.
- Close the slots and put the name of the patient and the date on the test kit.

- Instruct the patient to repeat the test on his next two bowel movements to improve the accuracy of the test.
- Remove gloves and wash hands thoroughly.
- Send the specimen to the laboratory.
- Inform the patient that he may resume his usual diet and medications as ordered.

VENEPUNCTURE

Venepuncture is the preferred method of blood sampling for term neonates, and causes less pain than heel-pricks.

Equipment and Supplies for Pediatric Patients

- Use a winged steel needle, preferably 23 or 23 gauge, with an extension tube (a butterfly): avoid gauges of 25 or more because these may be associated with an increased risk of hemolysis; use a butterfly with either a syringe or an evacuated tube with an adaptor; a butterfly can provide easier access and movement, but movement of the attached syringe may make it difficult to draw blood.
- Use a syringe with a barrel volume of 1–5 mL, depending on collection needs; the vacuum produced by drawing using a larger syringe will often collapse the vein.
- When using an evacuated tube, choose one that collects a small volume (1 mL or 5 mL) and has a low vacuum; this helps to avoid collapse of the vein and may decrease hemolysis.
- Where possible, use safety equipment with needle covers or features that minimize blood exposure. Auto-disable (AD) syringes are designed for injection, and are not appropriate for phlebotomy.

Preparation

Ask whether the parent would like to help by holding the child. If the parent wishes to help, provide full instructions on how and where to hold the child; if the parent prefers not to help, ask for assistance from another phlebotomist.
Immobilize the child as described below.
- Designate one phlebotomist as the technician, and another phlebotomist or a parent to immobilize the child.
- Ask the two adults to stand on opposite sides of an examination table.
- Ask the immobilizer to:
  - Stretch an arm across the table and place the child on its back, with its head on top of the outstretched arm;
  - Pull the child close, as if the person were cradling the child;
  - Grasp the child's elbow in the outstretched hand;
  - Use their other arm to reach across the child and grasp its wrist in a palm-up position (reaching across the child anchors the child's shoulder, and thus prevents twisting or rocking movements; also, a firm grasp on the wrist effectively provides the phlebotomist with a "tourniquet").

If necessary, take the following steps to improve the ease of venepuncture.
- Ask the parent to rhythmically tighten and release the child's wrist, to ensure that there is an adequate flow of blood.

- ❖ Keep the child warm, which may increase the rate of blood flow by as much as sevenfold (65), by removing as few of the child's clothes as possible and, in the case of an infant, by:
  - Swaddling in a blanket; and
  - Having the parent or caregiver hold the infant, leaving only the extremity of the site of venepuncture exposed.
- ❖ Warm the area of puncture with warm cloths to help dilate the blood vessels.
- ❖ Use a transilluminator or pocket pen light to display the dorsal hand veins and the veins of the antecubital fossa.

Drawing Blood

- ❖ Follow the procedures
  - Hand hygiene;
  - Advance preparation;
  - Patient identification and positioning;
  - Skin antisepsis (but DO NOT use chlorhexidine on children under 2 months of age).
- ❖ Once the infant or child is immobilized, puncture the skin 3–5 mm distal to (i.e., away from) the vein; this allows good access without pushing the vein away.
- ❖ If the needle enters alongside the vein rather than into it, withdraw the needle slightly without removing it completely, and angle it into the vessel.
- ❖ Draw blood slowly and steadily.

BLOOD CULTURES

A blood culture is a fairly routine test that identifies a disease-causing organism in the blood, especially in patients who have temperatures that is higher than normal, for an unknown reason. The test is relatively simple for the patient and involves a simple blood draw.

Purpose

A blood culture is being done to determine which specific organism or bacteria is causing the problem and how best to combat it.

Supplies and Equipment

Supplies and equipment required for a blood culture are:
- ❖ Sterile syringe (20 cc) and three needles (usually 20 gauge)
- ❖ Two blood culture bottles (one for anaerobic and one for aerobic specimens)
- ❖ Betadine solution or alcohol swab
- ❖ Sterile cotton balls or gauze pads
- ❖ Gloves
- ❖ Tourniquet
- ❖ Band-aid
- ❖ Chux (to protect the bed)
- ❖ Laboratory request form

Preparation

The test requires little preparation for the patient. The patient will be asked what kind of medications he is taking, including prescriptions and nutritional supplements. The patient may be asked to stop taking certain medications that may alter the blood culture results.

Procedure

- Discuss the procedure and the reason for doing it to the patient.
- Bring together all supplies and equipment needed to patient's bedside.
- Assist the patient to comfortable position. Ask for someone within the team to assist if the patient is uncooperative.
- Observe proper hand hygiene.
- Clean the top of both culture bottles with betadine solution or alcohol swab.
- Place the needle on the syringe.
- Apply the tourniquet to allow the veins to fill with blood and become more visible.
- Put on gloves and clean the drawing site with betadine solution or alcohol swab.
- Draw at least 10 cc of blood from the patient (5 cc is needed for each bottle).
- Unbind the tourniquet.
- Remove the syringe and needle while applying pressure to the venipuncture site with the cotton ball or gauze pad. Have the patient apply pressure to the site.
- Replace the needle on the syringe with another sterile needle.
- Inject 5 cc of blood into the anaerobic bottle, not allowing air to enter the bottle.
- Replace the needle on the syringe with another sterile needle.
- Inject the remaining 5 cc of blood into the aerobic bottle and while the needle is still in the bottle, disconnect it from the syringe so that air enters the aerobic bottle.
- Gently mix the blood with the solution in both bottles.
- Label both bottles with the patient's identifying information and the type of culture that is, aerobic or anaerobic.
- Fill out the laboratory request form completely and send the specimens to the laboratory immediately.
- Secure a band-aid or some gauze over the puncture site.

The role of nurses in collecting, labelling, and ensuring the timely and proper delivery of specimens to the laboratory plays a very important thing in the hospital setting. With this, nurses should be knowledgeable enough about the hospital's policy and procedures for specimen collection. However, nurses should not only possess the right knowledge, but as well as the skill and understanding in performing necessary procedures in accordance with the organization's protocols, policies, and guidelines.

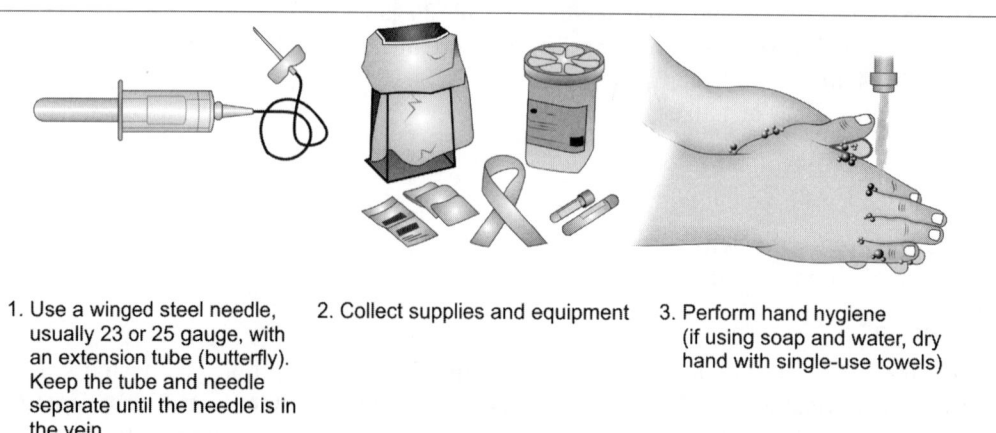

1. Use a winged steel needle, usually 23 or 25 gauge, with an extension tube (butterfly). Keep the tube and needle separate until the needle is in the vein
2. Collect supplies and equipment
3. Perform hand hygiene (if using soap and water, dry hand with single-use towels)

Contd...

Contd...

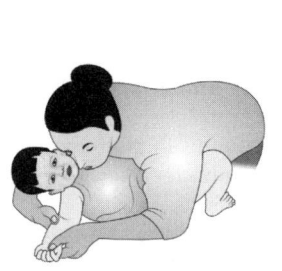

4. Immobilize the baby or child

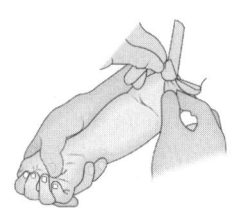

5. Put the tourniquet on the patient about two finger widths above the venepuncture site

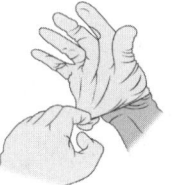

6. Put on well-fitting, non-sterile gloves

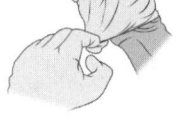

7. Attach the end of the winged infusion set to the end of the vacuum tube and insert the collection tube into the holder until the tube reaches the needle

8. Remove the plastic sleeve from the end of the butterfly

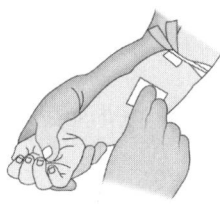

9. Disinfect the collection site and allow to dry

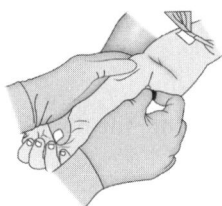

10. Use a thumb to draw the skin tight, about two finger widths below the venepuncture site

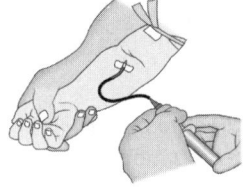

11. Push the vacuum tube completely onto the needle

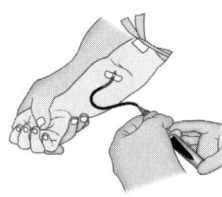

12. Blood should begin to flow into the tube

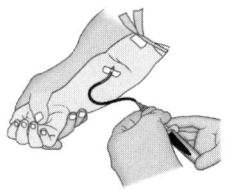

13. Fill the tube until it is full or until the vacuum is exhausted; if filling multiple tubes, carefully remove the full tube and replace with another tube, taking care not to move the needle in the vein

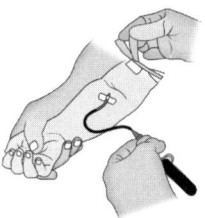

14. After the required amount of blood has been collected, release the tourniquet

Fig. 7.1: Assisting for blood sample collection.

Chapter 7: Assisting with Common Diagnostic Procedures

> **POINTS TO NOTE**
>
> - A blood culture is being done to determine which specific organism or bacteria is causing the problem and how best to combat it.
> - Venepuncture is the preferred method of blood sampling for term neonates, and causes less pain than heel-pricks.
> - Throat swab culture is done to detect the presence of organisms in the throat that could cause infection. For instance, the presence of group A Streptococcus bacteria in your throat is a key sign that you may have strep throat.
> - Swab the tonsillar areas from side to side and make sure to include any inflamed or purulent sites. The test may cause momentary gagging because the back of the throat is a sensitive area, but it should not be painful.

MULTIPLE CHOICE QUESTIONS

1. Throat swab is performed to identify:
   a. Bacterial infections
   b. Fever
   c. Improved circulation
   d. Jaundice

2. Heel pick is performed:
   a. To collect urine
   b. To collect saliva
   c. To collect blood
   d. To collect sweat

3. Normal color of urine is:
   a. Green
   b. Pink
   c. Pale yellow
   d. Red

4. To identify the bacterial invasion in blood, the diagnostic test performed is:
   a. Saline irrigation
   b. Blood culture
   c. CT scan
   d. Chest X-ray

ANSWER KEY

1. a   2. c   3. c   4. b

CHAPTER 8

Monitoring of Babies

PRACTICE COMPETENCIES
On completion of the chapter, the students will be able to:
- Assist in recognizing and responding to clinical deterioration in children
- Monitor clinical observations;
- Perform continuous monitoring of pulse oximetry and cardio-respiratory status
- Carry out appropriate documentation

ABSTRACT
Accurate and safe monitoring of infants and children requires knowledge of their unique physiology, especially cardiovascular function, pulmonary physiology, and metabolic function. These individual features influence the equipment selection, as well as data interpretation. Vascular monitoring in pediatric patients requires specific knowledge of insertion procedures and complications, fluid maintenance, and hemodynamic norms, indexed to body surface area. Likewise, maintenance care for pediatric patients always includes attention to precise fluid balance, thermoregulation, and metabolic needs. Finally, all pediatric patients require constant vigilance to protect the integrity of their monitoring systems and, ultimately, the safety of these patients. Failure to address these concerns may result in complications or invalid data.

Keywords: Temperature, respiratory rate, pain, pulse oximetry, blood sugar.

INTRODUCTION

Neonates are a specialized cohort of patients requiring an individualized approach in nursing care. The four major components of neonatal nursing care are keeping them warm, pink, sweet and calm.

Goals of care include the following:
- Minimizing stress
- Conserving energy and enhancing recovery
- Promotion of growth and well-being
- Protecting sleep pattern

AIM

To provide safe care of a neonate on the ward, when there is no requirement for a Neonatal Intensive Care Unit (NICU) bed.

OBSERVATIONS AND MONITORING

The neonate needs to be admitted onto the monitor profile so that alarm limits are specific to age and weight. For neonatal patient's particular attention should be placed on the following aspects of assessment:

Temperature

- The normal temperature of a neonate ranges from 36.5°C – 37.2°C.
- Temperatures measured per axilla every 4 hours, unless febrile or hypothermic.
- A medical review and full septic work up should be considered for any neonate with a temperature > 38°C
- **A full septic work up includes**: Lumbar puncture, sterile urine culture [suprapubic aspirate (SPA)] or by insertion of urinary catheter), blood cultures, full blood examination, CRP and chest X-ray.
- A temperature of ≤36.5°C is considered hypothermic and a medical review is required.
- An extra layer (clothing/blanket) should be added and the temperature should be repeated hourly. If the temperature remains at 36.5°C or below, the neonate should be considered for transfer to an incubator.

Isolette Use in Pediatric Wards

- Hourly temperatures should be checked until there are two consecutive temperatures equal to or greater than 36.6°C
- SEPSIS assessment and management.

Neutral Thermal Environment

Neonates are particularly vulnerable to heat loss via convection, conduction, evaporation and radiation.
Therefore ensure:
- They are dressed appropriately with a singlet, jumpsuit, socks, wrap, blanket and hat.
- Maintain bed 1 meter distance from window and avoid drafts.
- Minimal handling and clustering of cares
- Consider the need to use an overhead radiant warmer to regulate temperature.
- There are two modes—manual and servo. The manual control should only be used for bed warming and not when patient is in the cot. The servo control should be used to maintain patient's temperature and prevent overheating.
- Consider transfer to an incubator (Isolette) if neonate is hypothermic

Transfers

- If a neonate needs to be transferred between departments, appropriate measures to maintain their temperature need to be ensured.
- As per RCH Policy and Procedures: Isolette use in pediatric wards consider using isolettes/incubator for neonates, immediately postoperatively for a stabilization period as per criteria (4–24 hours)
- Neonates returning from theater to the wards need to have a temperature of ≥36.5, prior to leaving the department.
- Prior to transfer, any potential or active risks for infectious diseases should be advised to the receiving unit to maintain appropriate precautions and use of personal protective equipment for infection control.

Respiratory Rate

The respiratory rate is checked at least once per shift established by counting the patient's breaths over 60 seconds. Further respiratory assessment including the pattern and effort of breathing should also be evaluated at this time. Respiratory distress should be recorded as nil, mild, moderate or severe based on the assessment.

Assessment of Respiratory Distress*

	Mild	Moderate	Severe
Airway	Stridor on exertion/crying	Some stridor at rest	Stridor at rest
Behavior and feeding	• Normal • Talks in sentences	• Some/intermittent irritability • Difficulty taking/crying • Difficulty feeding or eating	• Increased irritability and/or lethargy • Looks exhausted • Unable to talk and cry • Unable to feed and eat
Respiratory rate	Mildly increased	• Respiratory rate in orange zone	• Respiratory rate in purple zone • Increased or markedly reduced respiratory rate as the child tires
Accessory muscle use	Mild intercostal and suprasternal recession	• Moderate intercostal and suprasternal recession • Nasal flaring	Marked intercostal and suprasternal and sternal recession
Oxygen	No oxygen requirement	• Mild hypoxemia corrected by oxygen • Increasing oxygen requirement	Hypoxemia may not be corrected by oxygen
Other		May have brief apneas	• Gasping, grunting • Extreme pallor, cyanosis • Increasingly frequent or prolonged apneas

*__Note:__ Not all features are relevant to all conditions.

Pain

- ❖ Assess pain using mPAT or FLACC scale
- ❖ Assess withdrawal using withdrawal assessment tool (WAT) or NAS scoring, if appropriate
  Clinical guideline (Nursing)—neonatal pain assessment, further information regarding FLACC scale can be found via clinical guideline (nursing) pain assessment and measurement
- ❖ For more information regarding the management of procedural pain for infants please refer to:
  Clinical guideline (Nursing)—sucrose oral for procedural pain management in infants.

Cardio-respiratory Monitoring

Continuous cardio-respiratory monitoring is the technological measurement of heart rate/pulse rate, respiratory rate and SpO_2. Children who are clinically unstable or are at risk of sudden changes in condition should have cardio-respiratory monitoring. Some indications include:
- ❖ Potential or actual apneic or bradycardic episodes
- ❖ Recent unexplained sudden collapse
- ❖ Abnormalities of heart rate and rhythm or high-risk of arrhythmia (e.g., pericardial effusion, altered electrolytes)
- ❖ Temporary pacing

- ❖ Prostaglandin infusion, medications that compromise cardiac function including concentrated electrolyte therapy, administration of pro-arrhythmic drugs with potential to cause QT prolongation or ventricular dysrhythmias, therapies associated with a high-risk of anaphylaxis, administration of toxic medications
- ❖ High-risk of respiratory failure (e.g., infants with severe bronchiolitis)
- ❖ Postoperative assessment as ordered by medical staff (e.g., 24-48 hours postspinal surgery).

Pulse Oximetry Monitoring

Continuous pulse oximetry monitoring measures oxygenation (SpO_2) and pulse rate.

Indications for its use include the child who:
- ❖ is receiving oxygen therapy and clinically unstable
- ❖ is clinically unstable and the need for oxygen therapy is yet to be determined
- ❖ has a nasopharyngeal airway or tracheostomy and requiring acute nursing care
- ❖ is receiving respiratory support (e.g., invasive or noninvasive ventilation)
- ❖ is undergoing a procedure where respiratory depressants are used
- ❖ is a high-risk patient receiving an opioid infusion
- ❖ is in the immediate postoperative period
- ❖ has a decreasing conscious status.

It is important to neither rely on nor ignore monitors. Whenever continuous monitoring of heart rate, SpO_2 or respiratory rate is in use, clinical observations must be documented hourly, at a minimum. The heart rate should be cross checked by palpation of the pulse or auscultation of the heart at least once per shift and whenever there is concern about the child's physiological condition, a change in heart rhythm or when there is doubt about the accuracy of the monitoring technology.

Blood Sugar Level

- ❖ A blood sugar level should be measured on admission for all sick neonates.
- ❖ Further BSL frequency dependent on:
    - Severity of illness
    - Risks of hypoglycaemia
    - Clinical signs of hypoglycaemia
    - Changes made to glucose infusions

Enteral Intake

- ❖ Establish feeding routine and history—breast fed, EBM, formula fed, or on nasogastric tube feeds
- ❖ Assess the most appropriate feeding method (oral/nasogastric)
- ❖ Strict recording of enteral input including duration of breast-feeds and pre-and post-weights and/or, formula volumes and/or EBM volumes should be recorded.
- ❖ If the neonate is too unwell to feed, breastfeeding mothers should be supported to express and store their breast milk.
- ❖ If poor oral intake, the neonate needs to be assessed for insertion of a nasogastric tube or commencement of IV fluids.
- ❖ The following table shows suggested feeding volumes by age, however this table is an approximate guide only and requirements will differ according to gestational age and disease process.

Age	mL/kg/day
Day 1–4	Commence at 30 to 60 mL/kg/day and increase over the next few days as tolerated
Day 5–3 months	150 mL/kg/day; some infants especially preterm may require 180–200 mL/kg/day as clinically indicated
3–6 months	120 mL/kg/day
6–12 months	100 mL/kg/day; some infants may reduce to 90 mL/kg/day as clinically indicated

Output

The following should be assessed and documented:
- Urine output should be measured and nappies weighed
- Urine output should be ≥ 2 mL/kg/hr, variances to this should be considered and signs of clinical dehydration be reported to the treating team.
- Bowel actions—frequency, consistency and color,
- Vomiting—frequency and color.
- If NGT in situ— color, quality, amount of aspirate and regular pH testing

General Considerations
- Check the general child health record
- Immunization record
- Newborn screening test

MANAGEMENT

Intravenous Fluid Management

All intravenous fluids require a current medical order as per usual protocol Intravenous (IV) fluids:

Age	mL/hr	mL/kg/day	Recommended fluid
0–24 hours	Weight x 2.5	60 mL/kg/day	10% Dextrose
25–48 hours	Weight x 2.5	60 mL/kg/day	10% Dextrose
49–72 hours	Weight x 3	72 mL/kg/day	*10% Dextose + NaCl + KCl
> 72 hours	Weight x 4	96 mL/kg/day	*10% Dextose + NaCl + KCl

Note: *Ordered as 10% dextrose 500 mL and 6.5 mL 20% NaCl and 10 mL 7.5% KCl (giving 22 mmol NaCl and 10 mmol KCl per 500 mL)

Considerations if oral or nasogastric feeds are not tolerated or suitable, and IV fluid therapy is initiated. When selecting an appropriate IV fluid the following should be taken into account:
- Neonates require solutions with a minimum of 10% dextrose to meet their increased metabolic demand and decreased energy reserves.
- A maximum fluid rate of 100 mL/kg/day should not be exceeded without consultation/approval from treating medical team and neonatal consultant.
- Restriction of fluids is often required and needs to be considered in the sick neonate.
- Blood gases, BSL and UEC's prior to commencement and 24 hourly (sooner if clinically indicated) for neonates on maintenance IV fluids.

- Baseline weights should be recorded then frequency as clinically indicated. At a minimum twice weekly but for a sick neonate on IV fluids more frequent weights will be necessary.
- Syringe driver and minimum volume tubing should be used for administration of IV fluids and medications (i.e., Intravenous antibiotics).

IV and Central Venous Access Devices (CVAD) Access in Neonates

IV cannula sites should be visible and not covered in crepe bandage must be checked hourly in the neonatal populations as they are at high-risk for pressure injuries and extravasation.

Skin Care

- Assessment of skin integrity should occur on admission and at least once a shift (and at each nappy change as needed).
- Assess neonate for risk factors of skin breakdown, i.e., loose or frequent stools, drug withdrawal, medications that alter stool frequency or composition.
- Nappy area: Maintain skin integrity; apply a thick barrier cream that contains zinc oxide at every nappy change when having frequent or loose bowel actions well as at the first sign of erythema or skin breakdown.
- Report any rashes to medical staff for review.

Sleep Maximization

- Optimal sleep is essential for normal growth and development and aids recovery.
- Term neonates usually sleep 16-18 hours per day for normal growth and development.
- Minimal handling and clustering of cares while the baby is awake.
- Clinical practice guidelines: Minimal handling
- Encourage lighting use to reflect day and night patterns. This helps develop normal transition to night time sleeping patterns
- Supporting quiet times to encourage sleep and settling behaviors.

PARENT ENGAGEMENT

Illness and separation causes increased stress and anxiety on the infant and their family, and this has been proven to affect brain development and subsequent neurodevelopmental progress in childhood. Therefore, it is essential that every effort is made to nurture the parent-infant bond by encouraging families to interact with their babies as much as possible, from as early as possible.

Encourage engagement through:
- Participating in feeding
- Attending to nappy cares
- Facilitating bathing
- Providing routine
- Skin to skin care

Discontinuation of Continuous Monitoring

As the condition of the child stabilizes and the risk of sudden deterioration lessens, the decision to continuously monitor the child should be reviewed by the nursing and medical staff (usually at least once per shift). When no longer necessary the patient can be transitioned to 1-4 hourly observations.

The need for close observation and monitoring should be balanced against unnecessary dependency on the monitors.

> **POINTS TO NOTE**
>
> - Neonates are particularly vulnerable to heat loss via convection, conduction, evaporation and radiation.
> - Term neonates usually sleep 16–18 hours per day for normal growth and development.
> - Nappy area: maintain skin integrity; apply a thick barrier cream that contains zinc oxide at every nappy change when having frequent or loose bowel actions well as at the first sign of erythema or skin breakdown.
> - A maximum fluid rate of 100 mL/kg/day should not be exceeded without consultation/approval from treating medical team and neonatal consultant.
> - Urine output should be ≥2 mL/kg/hr, variances to this should be considered and signs of clinical dehydration be reported to the treating team.
> - Whenever continuous monitoring of heart rate, SpO_2 or respiratory rate is in use, clinical observations must be documented hourly, at a minimum. The heart rate should be cross checked by palpation of the pulse or auscultation of the heart at least once per shift.

MULTIPLE CHOICE QUESTIONS

1. **The temperature of the neonates is maintained by using:**
   a. Ventilator
   b. Infusion pump
   c. Radiant warmer
   d. Phototherapy
2. **Sepsis is formed due to:**
   a. Improper food practice
   b. Aseptic techniques
   c. Breastfeeding
   d. Warmer care
3. **Blood sugar levels are checked to identify:**
   a. Hypertension
   b. Hypoglycemia
   c. Hypomagnesemia
   d. Hyponatremia
4. **Pulse oximetry is used to check:**
   a. Blood sugars
   b. Electrolyte balance
   c. Oxygen saturation
   d. Respiration rate

ANSWER KEY

1. c   2. b   3. b   4. c

CHAPTER 9

Kangaroo Mother Care

PRACTICE COMPETENCIES
On completion of the chapter, the students will be able to:
- Keep the baby warm.
- Promote and sustain breastfeeding.
- Decrease the risk of infection.
- Promote bonding between baby and mother.

ABSTRACT
The term kangaroo mother care (KMC) is derived from practical similarities to marsupial care-giving, i.e., the premature infant is kept warm in the maternal pouch and close to the breasts for unlimited feeding. It is a gentle and effective method that avoids agitation routinely experienced in a busy ward with preterm infants. An important main stay of kangaroo mother care is breastfeeding encouragement. Observational studies have shown reduction in mortality after institution of KMC. Preterm babies exposed to skin to skin contact showed a better mental development and better results in motor tests. It also improves thermal care and with a lesser risk of hypothermia. All stable LBW babies are candidate for KMC. Often this is desirable, until the baby's gestation reaches term or the weight is around 2,500 g. The mother and family members are encouraged to take care of the baby in KMC and should be counseled to come for follow up visits regularly.

Keywords: Kangaroo mother care, skin-to-skin contact, thermal care, low birth weight, breastfeeding.

INTRODUCTION
Caring low birth weight baby is a great challenge for the neonatal care unit and the family. Number of low birth weight babies is still far beyond the expected target in our country. The cost of quality management of these babies is increasing day by day. Kangaroo mother care is a low cost approach for the care of low birth weight baby. This method of care was introduced and popularized by Dr Edger Ray, Dr Martinez and Dr Charpak in late 1970s.

DEFINITION
Kangaroo mother care (KMC) is a special way of caring low birth weight (LBW) infants by skin-to-skin contact. It promotes their health and well being by effective thermal control, breastfeeding and bonding. KMC is initiated in hospital and continued at home.

■ COMPONENTS OF KMC

In KMC, the infant is continuously kept in skin-to-skin contact by the mother and breastfed exclusively to the utmost extent. The two components of KMC are:

1. Skin-to-Skin contact

Direct, continuous and prolonged skin-to-skin contact is provided between the mother and her baby to promote thermal control.

2. Exclusive Breastfeeding

Skin-to-skin contact promotes lactation and feeding interaction with exclusive breastfeeding for adequate nutrition and to improve desired weight gain.

Prerequisites of KMC

Support to the mother

Mother needs support in hospital and home from care-givers and family members. Counseling and supervision should be provided to the mother by the health personnel in hospital, whereas mother requires assistance and cooperation from her family members at home.

Post-discharge follow-up

KMC should be continued at home after discharge from hospital. For safe and successful KMC at home, a regular follow-up should be arranged to solve problem and to evaluate health status of the infant.

Benefits of KMC

1. KMC helps in thermal control and metabolism. Prolonged, continuous and direct skin-to-skin contact between mother and neonate provides effective thermal control and reduces risk of hypothermia.
2. KMC results in increased duration and rate of breastfeeding.
3. KMC satisfies all five senses of the infant. Baby feels warmth of the mother through skin-to-skin contact (touch), sucks the breast to feed (taste), smells the mother's odor (olfaction) and makes eye contact with mother's (vision).
4. During KMC, the baby has more regular breathing and less predisposition to apnea.
5. KMC protects against nosocomial infection and reduces incidence of severe illness including pneumonia during infancy.
6. Daily weight gain is slightly better with KMC, thus duration of hospital stay may be reduced. LBW baby receiving KMC could be discharged from the hospital earlier than conventional care.
7. KMC facilitates better mother-infant bondage due to significantly less stress during kangarooing than the incubator care of the baby.

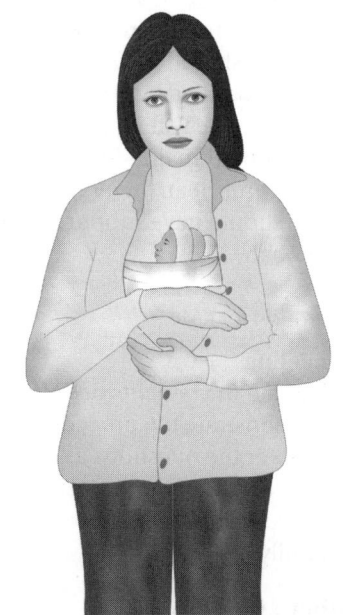

Fig. 9.1: Kangaroo mother care—mother.

8. KMC is one of the best methods of transporting small babies by keeping them in continuous skin-to-skin contact with mother or family members.
9. Mother feels increased confidence, self-esteem, sense of fulfillment and deep satisfaction with KMC. Father feels more relaxed, comfortable and better bonded.
10. KMC does not require additional staff compared to incubator care.

Requirements for KMC Implementation
- Training of nurses, doctors and other staff on KMC, specially who are involved in care of mother and baby.
- Educational material like information book let pamphlets posters video in language local film, etc. on KMC in local language.
- KMC does not require extra staff. Once KMC is implemental, care-givers appreciate it because of health benefits to the babies and the satisfaction expressed by the mothers.

Eligibility Criteria for KMC

For Babies
- All stable LBW babies are eligible for KMC, it is particularly useful for caring LBW infants weighting below 2,000 g.
- In a stable baby, KMC can be initiated soon after birth.
- KMC should be started after the baby is hemodynamically stable.
- Sick LBW infants may take a few days to initiate KMC. So the sick baby needs transfer to a proper facility immediately.
- Infants of birth weight less than 1,200 g with serious prematurity related morbidity may take days to weeks to allow initiation of KMC.
- KMC can be initiated who is otherwise stable but may still be IV fluid therapy, tube feeding and/or oxygen therapy.

For Mothers
- All mothers can provide KMC irrespective of age, parity, education, culture and religion.
- Mother should be free of serious illness and able to take adequate diet and supplements recommended by her doctor.
- She must be willing to provide KMC to her baby.
- She should maintain good hygiene, daily bath/sponge, change of clothes, hand hygiene, short and clean finger nails, etc.
- She should have supportive family and community to be encouraged to continue KMC to her baby.

Preparation for KMC

Counseling
- Explain the benefits of KMC to the mother and the family members.
- Demonstrate the procedure to the mother gently with patience.
- Answer the questions as asked by the mother and the family members to remove anxiety.
- Allow the mother to interact with someone who have already practicing KMC for her baby.
- Discuss about the procedure to the mother-in-law husband or any other members of the family.

Mother's Clothing
Mother should wear front-open, light dress, as per local culture. Mother can wear sari-blouse, gown, shawl, etc.

Baby's Clothing

Baby should be dressed with front-open sleeveless shirt, cap, socks, nappy and hand gloves.

KMC Procedure

Kangaroo Positioning

- The baby should be placed between the mother's breast in an upright position.
- Baby's head should be turned to one side and in a slightly extended position which helps to keep the airway open and allow eye to eye contact between mother and baby.
- Baby's hip should be flexed and abducted in a frog-like position. The arms should also be flexed and placed on mother's chest.
- Baby's abdomen should be placed at the level of mother's epigastrium.

This position helps to reduce the occurrence of apnea, as mother's breathing and heartbeat stimulate the baby. Baby can be supported with a sling or binder or especially prepared KMC bag.

Monitoring during KMC

- During initial stage of KMC the baby should be monitored for airway, breathing, color and temperature. Hands and feet should be examined to assess the warmth. Airway must be kept clear with regular breathing, normal skin color and temperature.
- Baby's neck position should be neither too flexed nor too extended.

Feeding

- Mother needs help to breastfeed her baby during KMC. Holding the baby near the breast stimulates milk production and the kangaroo position makes the breastfeeding easier.
- Baby could be fed with paladai, spoon and tube depending upon the baby's condition.

Psychological Support to Mother

- Mother needs motivation to continue KMC.
- She should be encouraged to ask questions to remove anxieties.

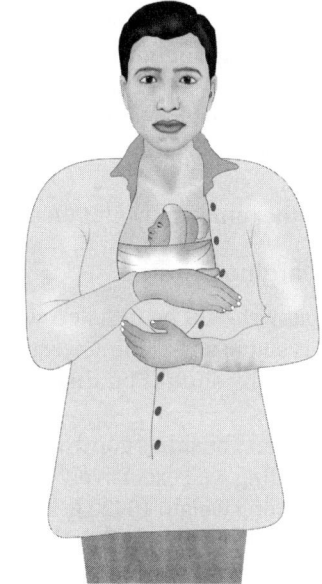

Fig. 9.2: Kangaroo mother care—father.

Privacy

Privacy should be maintained to avoid unnecessary exposure on the part of the mother which makes her nervous and demotivating.

Time of Initiation of KMC

- KMC should be initiated gradually with a smooth transition from conventional care to continuous KMC.
- KMC can be started as soon as the baby is stable in the neonatal care unit.

- Short KMC sessions can be initiated during recovery with ongoing medical treatment, i.e. IV fluid, oxygen therapy, etc.
- KMC can be provided while the baby is with gavage feeding.

Duration of KMC

- Duration of KMC should not be less than one hour to avoid frequent handling which may be stressful to the baby.
- Gradually the length of KMC sessions should be increased up to 24 hours a day. Interruption only can be done for changing of diapers.
- KMC should be continued in postnatal ward and home.
- It may not be possible for mother to provide KMC prolonged period in the beginning. Encourage her to increase the duration each time to provide KMC as long as possible.
- When mother is not available then other family members such as father, grandmother, aunty can provide KMC.

Can the Mother Continue KMC During Sleep and Resting?

- Mother can sleep with baby in KMC position in a reclined or semi-recumbent position about 15–30° from above the ground.
- A comfortable chair with adjustable back may be useful to provide KMC during sleep and rest at ward or home.
- Adjustable bed or several pillows or an ordinary bed can be used to maintain the position, which usually decreased the risk of apnea of the baby.
- Supporting garment can be used to carry the baby in kangaroo position during sleep and rest.
- Father and family members can provide KMC to relieve mother during and rest.

Discharging Criteria

The baby should be transferred from the neonatal care unit to the postnatal ward, when the baby is stable and gaining weight and the mother is confident to look after the baby.

The baby should be discharged from hospital when the baby is having the following conditions:

- General health is good and there is no evidence of infection and apnea.
- Feeding well exclusively with breast milk.
- Gaining weight 15–20 g/kg/day for at least three consecutive days.
- Maintaining normal body temperature satisfactorily for at least three consecutive days in room temperature.
- Mother and family members are confident to take care of the baby at home and would be able to come regularly for follow-up visits.
- Home environment should be suitable and congenial for continuation of KMC.

Discontinuation of KMC

- KMC can be continued until the baby gains weight around 2,500 g or reaches 40 weeks of postconception age.
- KMC can be discontinued if the baby starts wriggling to show discomfort or pulls limbs out, cries and fusses every time, when mother tries to put the baby back into skin contact.

- When mother and baby are comfortable, KMC can be continued as long as possible at health facility or at home.
- Mother can provide skin-to-skin contact occasionally after the baby bath and during cold nights.

Post-discharge follow-up
Each neonatal care unit should formulate its own policy for follow-up.
- In general, baby is followed up once or twice a week till 37–40 weeks of gestation or till the baby reaches 2.5–3 kg of weight.
- Thereafter a follow-up once in 2–4 weeks may be sufficient till 3 months of postconceptional age. After that 1–2 months during first year of life. The baby should gain adequate weight 15–20 g/kg/day up to 40 weeks of postconceptional age and 10 g/kg/day subsequently.
- More frequent visits should be made, if the baby is not growing well or the condition demands.

POINTS TO NOTE

As per WHO recommendations:
1. Kangaroo mother care is recommended for the routine care of newborns weighing 2,000 g or less at birth, and should be initiated in healthcare facilities as soon as the newborns are clinically stable.
2. Intermittent kangaroo mother care, rather than conventional care, is recommended for newborns weighing 2,000 g or less at birth, if continuous kangaroo mother care is not possible.

PRACTICE QUESTIONS

1. Define kangaroo mother care.
2. List down the benefits of KMC.
3. How do you explain the mother for KMC?

MULTIPLE CHOICE QUESTIONS

1. **Prevention of hypothermia in the community should focus on:**
   a. Kangaroo mother care
   b. Keeping the room warm (25-28° C)
   c. Ensure adequate breastfeeding
   d. All of the above
2. **What is kangaroo position?**
   a. The infant is placed in an upright position against bare chest and between her breasts
   b. The infant is placed with kangaroo toy
   c. The infant is placed horizontally to mother
   d. The infant is placed next to mother
3. **What is kangaroo nutrition?**
   a. Katori and spoon feed
   b. Breastfeeding on demand
   c. Hot milk
   d. Cold milk

ANSWER KEY

1. d   2. a   3. b

CHAPTER 10

Methods of Feeding

PRACTICE COMPETENCIES
On completion of the chapter, the students will be able to:
- Identify the impact of growth and development on feeding pattern.
- Describe techniques of various methods of feeding used in meeting nutritional requirements of children.
- Administer feeding to children in various developmental stages.
- Help and guide parents to meet nutritional needs of children in altered health status.
- Help the parents to practice correct feeding techniques.

ABSTRACT
Breastfeeding is the best way of feeding newborn infants. However, in many instances mothers are unable to breastfeed their newborn, especially when the baby is small for age or sick. Worldwide, only 34% of infants less than 6 months old are exclusively breastfed, with the figures ranging from 43.2% for the Southeast Asia region to 17.7% in Europe. Low prevalence of breastfeeding is a major problem across the globe, and alternative methods of enteral feeding (with bottle, gastric tube or cup) are in use to feed infants who are unable to breastfeed. Especially in under-resourced settings, bottle feeding has its own disadvantages namely risk of infection, nipple confusion in the infant, high cost, etc. Feeding infants by gastric tube needs proper training, and tubes are not readily available in all settings, especially in low income countries. This chapter contains technique of breastfeeding, bottle feeding, spoon/katori feeding, gavage feeding, gastrostomy feeding, gastrojejunostomy feeding.

Keywords: Methods of feeding, breastfeeding, bottle feeding, spoon/paladin/katori feeding, gavage feeding, intermittent indwelling, gastrostomy feeding, gastrojejunostomy feeding.

INTRODUCTION

Nutrition is vitally important in the maintenance of the body system throughout the life style. This is especially true during the years of growth and development. The illness and hospitalization has impact on nutritional intake of the child. Acute as well as chronic illness of childhood and hospitalization is a stress and emotional trauma. There may be restriction of food items in certain illness, e.g. nephritic syndrome, rheumatic fever, etc. thus, one of the important aspect of the pediatric nurse is to assist the child in meeting the fluid and nutritional requirement to maintain or improve the growth and development already achieved before the illness and avoid problems of severe depletion/under-nutrition/malnutrition.

PRINCIPLES OF FEEDING CHILDREN

- The neonatal reflexes such as sucking reflex and rooting reflex indicates newborn's ability and readiness to food. Sucking and swallowing reflex is coordinated at 34 weeks of gestation.
- The tongue retrusion reflex must not be mistaken for the infant's refusal food.
- The number of feedings decreases as the infant grows older.
- Infants need to satisfy their sucking urge.
- Feeding technique should faster growth and development.
- As the child grows, he gradually becomes independent in self-feeding.

BREASTFEEDING

Within few hour's of birth the mother should put the baby to her breast. For the first 48 hours, there is yellowish secretion from the breast called colostrums which is very rich in proteins and antibodies. So the baby should be breastfed according to the self-demand schedule. The baby should be fed at night also whenever, he is hungry. If the milk is adequate the baby will gradually make a 3 to 4 hourly schedule for himself. The demand schedule feeding facilitate meeting physiologic requirement promptly and the infant does not learn to associate prolonged crying and discomfort with feeding.

With this concept we shall now focus on procedure of breastfeeding.

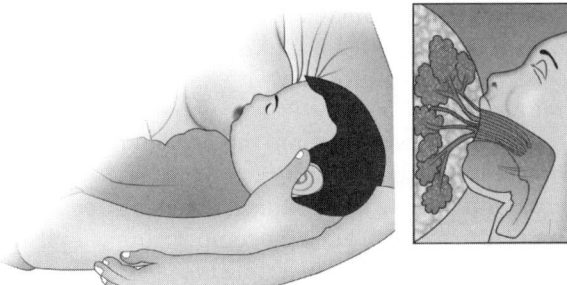

Fig. 10.1: Breastfeeding.

Procedure

- Encourage mothers to breastfeed rather than bottle-feed their infants.
- You should assist and reach the mother regarding technique of breastfeeding.
- Instruct mother to wash her hands before breastfeeding and clean breast with soap and water during bath.
- Encourage mother to feed the infant in sitting position (mother should be relaxed and comfortable).
- Place infant on mother's lap and infant's head should be higher than his abdomen.
- With hand press the areola (i.e. darkened area around nipple) into infant's mouth.
- Press breast away from infant's nose with 2 fingers.
- Use both breasts at each feeding, nurse infant for 5 minutes on each breast and then increase nursing time to 10 minutes.
- A feeding time of 15–20 minutes is usually enough.
- Burp infant by patting gently on the back or hold infant in upright position.
- Place infant on right sidelying position after feeding. Observe for abdominal distention and regurgitation feeding.

❖ When an infant is sick and unable to suck on the breast, it is important that mother empties her breasts with her hands.

Breastfeed infant according to the self-demand schedule:
❖ Promptly meets the physiological requirement.
❖ Infant does not learn to associate prolonged crying and discomfort with feeding.

BOTTLE FEEDING

Purpose

To provide nourishment to the child.

Equipment

❖ Sterile nipple and bottle
❖ Sterile formula or breast milk
❖ Clean cloth to cover bottle.

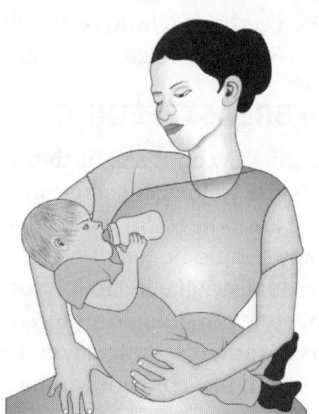

Fig. 10.2: Bottle feeding.

Procedure

❖ Infant should be awake and hungry. Change wet or soiled diaper.
❖ Prepare formula according to manufacture's instructions. Check formula for correct type and amount.
❖ Wash and rinse bottle, teat, cap thoroughly with water and boil for 15–20 minutes.
❖ Take required amount of boiled water into the bowl and add premeasured milk powder, stir it swiftly to prevent formation of lumps.
❖ Strain feed and pour into feeding bottle, attach teat to the feeding and cover it with cap.
❖ Wrap the bottle by a clean towel to keep the temperature of milk inside
❖ Check the temperature of the feed by inverting the feeding bottle over the visible veins of the wrist.
❖ Sit in a comfortable chair. Cradle the infant with one hand and arm, while supporting the infant against your body or lap.
❖ Let the infant root for the nipple by touching the corner of the infant's mouth opens, insert the nipple.
❖ Hold the bottle at an angle to completely fill the nipple with fluid.
❖ Never prop the bottle or leave the infant unattended during feeding.
❖ Handle the bottle carefully so as not to contaminate the nipple or fluid.
❖ Infant's feeding time will vary from 10–25 minutes.
❖ Position the infant. So eye contact can be established during feeding. Soothing and fondling can provide additional comfort to the infant.
❖ Burp the infant at least once during the feeding and at the end of the feeding.
❖ Place the baby in a sitting position in your lap, tilt slightly forward and gently rub or pat the back or abdomen.
❖ Place the infant in prone position on your shoulder and gently pat and rub the neck.
❖ Place the infant in a prone position or your lap and gently rub or pat the back.
❖ After final burping, change the infants wet or soiled diaper.
❖ Place the infant in the crib on the right side. This position aids in emptying the stomach and prevents regurgitation.

❖ Check the infant in a few minutes. If restless, pick infant up and burp. Note, if any spitting-up has occurred.

Nursing Alert

❖ When feeding a premature infant the infant will tiered more easily and fall asleep.
❖ Allow frequent rest periods, and use a soft nipple, so that less energy is needed to suck.
❖ To stimulate this infant to suck, the nurse can brush the infants cheek with her finger, place, the thumb or finger under the infant's chin or more the nipple slowly back and forth in the infant's mouth.
❖ Feeding time should not exceed 30 minutes.
❖ Keep the infant warm during feeding.

Replacement of Equipment

Wash, boil and dry the equipment used.

■ SPOON/PALADI/KATORI (CUP) FEEDING

Purpose

To provide nourishment to the child.

Indication

❖ To feed babies who are not able to suckle directly out the breast.
❖ Useful in most cases of cleft lip and palate.

Equipment

❖ Sterile formula milk or cow milk.
❖ Katori (cup), spoon or palada feeds.

Procedure

❖ A boiled or preferably autoclaved set should be used for each baby for every feed.
❖ The nurse or mother should wash her hands thoroughly before giving the feed.
❖ The baby should be well restrained and held comfortable on the lap, keeping the head elevated.
❖ For cup and spoon feeds, small quantities of milk should be poured through the angle of the mouth in small quantities at a time.
❖ Burp the baby after feeding.
❖ Do not use either method in crying babies.

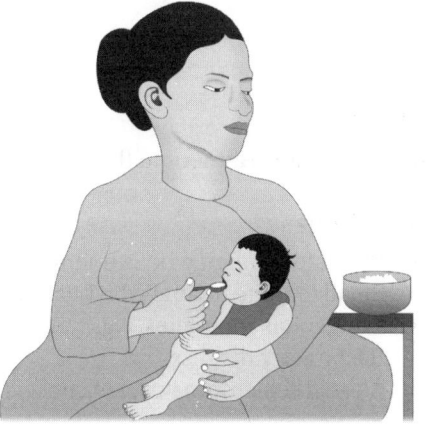

Fig. 10.3: Spoon or katori feeding.

Replacement of Equipment

Wash, boil and dry the equipment.

■ GAVAGE FEEDING

It is the administration of liquid nourishment through a tube passed via the nares/mouth, pharynx, esophagus into the stomach.

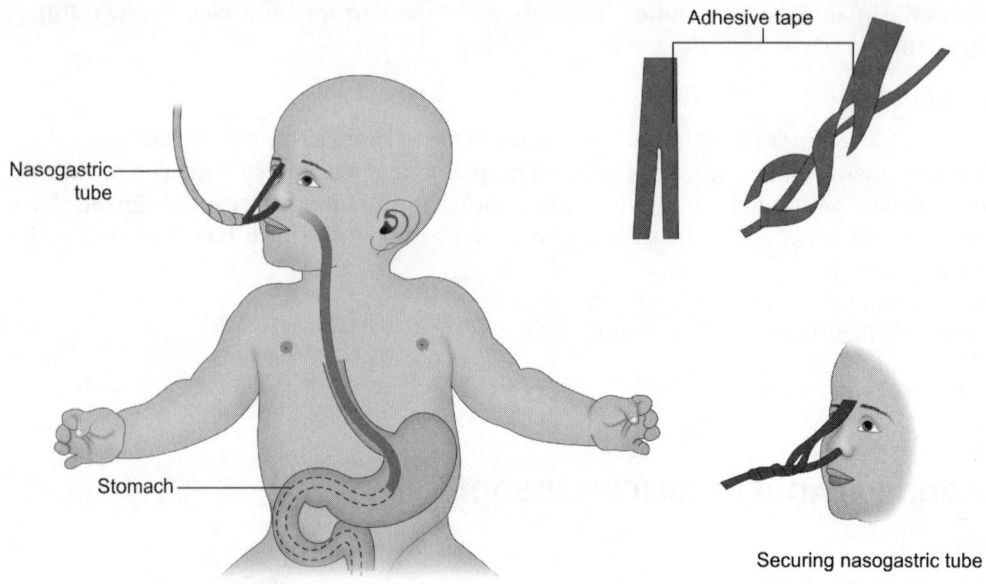

Fig. 10.4: Gavage feeding.

Purpose
To provide nourishment to the child.

Indications
- Premature infant who is unable to suck or swallow.
- Small for date infants who becomes fatigued with the effort of nursing.
- Congenital anomalies, e.g. cleft palate.
- Respiratory distress.
- Altered sensorium/level of consciousness.

Types of Tube Feeding
It may be intermittent or indwelling.

Intermittent: The feeding tube may be inserted and removed at each feeding.

Indwelling: The feeding tube is inserted and left taped securely in place for 24–72 hours.

Equipment
- Infant feeding tube
- Syringe 5 to 10 cc
- Stethoscope
- Reservoir
- Adhesive tape
- Sterile formula feed.

Procedure
- Explain the procedure to child and relative.

- ❖ Give recumbent position with his neck hyper flexed with a rolled towel placed under the neck. A restraint may be necessary to maintain position.
- ❖ Measure the tube by measuring from the bridge of the nose to umbilicus in infants and mark it.
- ❖ In older children, measure from the tip of the nose to the earlobe and then to the tip of the xiphoid process of sternum.
- ❖ Lubricate catheter with water.
- ❖ Insert the catheter with water.
- ❖ Insert the catheter through nares and/or mouth in case of nasogastric feeding. Slip the catheter into nostril and direct towards the occiput in a horizontal plane.
- ❖ In case of orogastric feeding pass the catheter through the mouth towards the back of throat.
- ❖ The passage of catheter may be synchronized with swallowing.
- ❖ Observe for vagal stimulation.
- ❖ Once the catheter has been inserted to premeasured length, tape the catheter to the patient's face.
- ❖ Test for correct position of the catheter in the stomach:
- ❖ Injection 0.5–1 mL air into the stomach through catheter. At the same time listen to the typical growling stomach sound with a stethoscope placed over the epigastric region.
- ❖ Withdraw injected air from the stomach.
- ❖ Place the infant in supine position or right sidelying with head and chest elevated.
- ❖ Aspirate stomach content.
- ❖ If more than half the previous feeding is obtained withhold the feeding.
- ❖ If small residual of formula is obtained, return it to stomach and subtract that amount from the total amount of formula to be given.
- ❖ Do not apply pressure.
- ❖ Elevate reservoir 15–20 cm above patients head.
- ❖ Feeding time should last approximately for 15–20 minutes.
  For infants—1 mL/min. Older children—5–10 mL/min.
- ❖ When the feeding is completed, irrigate the catheter with clear water.
- ❖ For intermittent feeding clamp the catheter and withdraw it.
- ❖ Burp the patient, place child on right side or on the abdomen.
- ❖ Observe for bradycardia, apnea, vomiting and abdominal distension, etc.
- ❖ Accurately describe and record procedure including time of feeding, type of gavage feeding, type and amount of feeding, fluid given, amount retained or vomited, how patient tolerated feeding and activity following feeding.

Nursing Alert

You have to be alert in observing the child before, during and after feeding for:
- ❖ Abdominal distension
- ❖ Vomiting or regurgitation
- ❖ Gastric residue 25–50% or more than that of the previous feed indicates
- ❖ Poor tolerance to enteral feeding.

Replacement of Equipment

Wash and dry the used equipment.

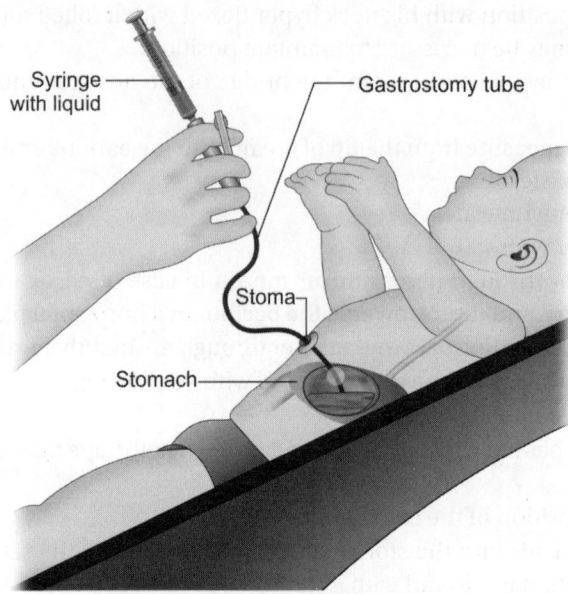

Fig. 10.5: Gastrostomy tube feeding.

GASTROSTOMY FEEDING

It is the administration of liquid nourishment through a tube directly inserted into stomach through the abdominal wall. A plain or Foley catheter is inserted through the abdominal wall into stomach while the child is under general anesthesia.

Purpose
- To feed a child who is unable to feed orally.
- To provide nourishment in child with congenital anamoly, e.g. trachea esophageal fistula;
- To decompress the stomach.

Equipment
- 20–50 cc syringe
- Sterile water
- Warm feeding formula
- Mackintosh and towel.

Procedure
- Place mackintosh and towel on child's abdomen.
- Attach tubing to 10–50 cc syringe.
- Hold child elevated.
- Elevate syringe to 10–20 cm
- Aspirate gently.
- Pour feed and allow flow them with the help of gravity.
- Don't apply pressure.
- Feed for 20–30 minutes.
- Irrigate with clear water.

- After feeds, the tube may be:
  - Left unclamped to provide constant decompression.
  - Elevated and covered with guage (to prevent gastric reflux, abdominal distension, regurgitation).
  - Clamped if patient is to be prepared for home care.
- Record types, amount of feed, child's activity.
- Keep child in fowlers position or turned right.
- The gastrostomy tube may be left opened and deviated to allow air to escape and decompress the stomach.
- The tube should be secured in place and avoid excessive traction.
- Keep the area/skin around gastrostomy clean and dry to prevent irritation and infection.

GASTROJEJUNAL FEEDING

- The physician inserts the nasojejunal tube (soft vinyl tube) through the nose into the jejunum (beyond the pylorus).
- Abdominal X-ray is taken to ensure placement of the tube.
- Place child always on the right side with thigh and hips deviated.
- Connect tube to the syringe or drip, using infusion pump. Give small feeds frequently.
- Do not aspirate the fluid.
- Record the procedures.

Precautions

- Check for abdominal distension by:
  - Measure abdominal girth 2–3 hourly
  - Palpate abdomen
  - Observe for movements in abdomen.
- Check stool for blood, pH and sugar to determine tolerance to feeds.
- Check vomiting of blood and report immediately.
- Ensure that child's head is elevated during and after feeds.
- Keep child always to the right side.
  Observe for cyanosis, regurgitation, bradycardia (due to vagal reflex).

CONCLUSION

Till now we discussed about introduction, principles of feeding, breastfeeding and procedure of breastfeeding, bottle feeding, spoon feeding and gavage feeding purposes, indications, equipment and procedure discussed.

> **POINTS TO NOTE**
>
> When beginning enteral feedings, monitor the patient for feeding tolerance. **Assess the abdomen by auscultating for bowel sounds and palpating for rigidity, distention, and tenderness.** Know that patients who complain of fullness or nausea after a feeding starts may have higher a gastric residual volume (GRV).

PRACTICE QUESTIONS

1. What are the indications for gavage feeding?

2. What is a gastrostomy feeding?
3. What is a gastrojejunal feeding?

MULTIPLE CHOICE QUESTIONS

1. BFHI stands for:
   a. Breast friendly hospital initiative
   b. Breastfeeding health initiative
   c. Breast friendly health initiative
   d. Baby friendly hospital initiative
2. How do enteral and parenteral nutrition differ?
   a. Enteral is administered via a vein; parenteral via the ilium.
   b. Enteral is administered via a blood vessel; parenteral via the mouth.
   c. Parenteral is administered via GI tract; enteral via a site outside the GI tract.
   d. Enteral is administered via the GI tract; parenteral via a site outside the GI tract.
3. Complications of a tube feeding into the stomach include:
   a. Regurgitation
   b. Aspiration pneumonia
   c. Gastric atrophy
   d. a and b

ANSWER KEY

1. d			2. d			3. d

CHAPTER 11

Drug Administration

PRACTICE COMPETENCIES

On completion of the chapter, the students will be able to:
- Administer the drug correctly and restore patient's health.
- Understand fundamentals of drug administration:
  – Routes
  – Dosage calculations
  – Techniques for injection
  – Seven rights
  – Patient education

ABSTRACT

The administration of medicines has always been an integral part of nursing care, but when caring for children it involves several problem areas. The responsibility of the child nurse in ensuring that the correct medication is safely and appropriately administered to the correct child is a huge undertaking which requires many different skills. Children are particularly risk from medication for a number of reasons. Their immature bodies systems make them less able to absorb metabolize and excrete drugs. Their age, weight and surface area varies widely making standardize dosages impossible. In addition, many children dislike taking medication, so the nurse has to be able to find an acceptable method of administration for each individual child to promote compliance. This may be further aided by the nurse's knowledge of alternative preparations available for each medication. Although it is mostly the doctor's responsibility to prescribe appropriate medication, the nurse who will be administering the prescription should have an understanding of the appropriate dosage, route of administration, desired action, possible side effects and contraindications of each medication to be given. The nurse will also need to be able to explain most of these aspects to the child and family and ensure continued acceptance of the regimen. This chapter contains oral, intravenous medications, intramuscular medications, fluid calculations for IV infusions, exchange transfusion, total parenteral nutrition.

Keywords: Drug administration to children, five rights, young's rule, Clark's rule, ventrogluteal site, vastus lateralis, dorsogluteal, exchange transfusion, total parenteral nutrition.

ORAL ADMINISTRATION OF MEDICATIONS TO CHILDREN

Administering to pediatric patients is more specialized skill, they need for accuracy in preparing and giving drugs to children is even greater than with adult patients. Since, the pediatric dose is often relatively small in comparison with the adult dose, a slight increase in the amount of a drug administered represents a greater proportional error, as there exist a narrow margin between therapeutic level and toxic level in some drugs.

The responsibility of a nurse is important because the child is unable to communicate verbally any signs of distress that indicate over dosage, side effects or allergic reaction.

Safety Measures

It is essential to revise the five rights before administration of medication to the pediatric group they are:
  i. The right patient
  ii. The right drug
  iii. The right dose
  iv. The right route
  v. The right time.

The sixth right added recently is the right of the parents and children to know "the drug they are receiving its action and side effect, thus reducing the chances of misuse as they would be likely to use it unsafely if they were not given the information.

For example, if the child was receiving tablet eptoin for convulsion and the mother had not noticed the convulsion which her child was having as they were a mild nature. She may find that after this particular medication the baby sleeps and she may administer it when the baby is irritable or crying to make the child sleep thinking the baby will have peaceful sleep and this itself can be harmful.

Possible Errors in Drug Administration

There can be various reasons for errors in administering drugs:
  i. Poor communication of intention by the prescriber.
  ii. Failure to keep an established routine when administering therapy.
  iii. Lack of understanding of the objectives of therapy.
  iv. Failure of the nurse to recognize that the medical officers and pharmacy departments may make errors.
  v. Poor concentration or constant interruption.
  vi. Ignoring the need for an experienced person to double check the drug, the dose, identification of the patient and any previously administered preparation.
  vii. Failure to calculate to one's own satisfaction.
  viii. Failure to learn appropriate pediatric doses of commonly used medications.
  ix. Lack of knowledge regarding drug interaction and side effects.
  x. Inadequate security of drug storage.
  xi. Failure to record administered doses.

If you are in doubt, do not give the medication, however, no medication should be omitted without the medical officer's order.

Oral Route

1. Pediatric medications are prepared as tablets, powders.
2. It is earlier to persuade older children to swallow capsules.
3. It is essential to remember that children can be easily persuaded to have bitter medications if they are assured of a reward in the form of a chocolate or sweets, if permitted.

4. They can be made acceptable if given along with fruits flavored syrups but should not be mixed with food as the child may develop aversion to particular food, if mixed with the medicine.
5. Capsules should not be opened and administered as the powder is unpalatable.
6. If the child cannot swallow open the capsule and mix the powder with honey or sugar and other sweetened syrups.

Purposes

To safely and effectively administer the drugs to the patient by mouth.

> **POINTS TO NOTE**
>
> ➤ Liquid forms are safer to swallow to avoid aspiration.
> ➤ When mixing drug with palatable flavoring and such as syrup/honey, use only small amounts.
> ➤ Calculate the pediatric dose (or) amount needed carefully.
> ➤ Do not use drug which is discovered or
> ➤ Do not administer contaminated drugs (drugs fallen on the floor).
> ➤ Nurses should try to be aware of a medicine taste as that they can answer questioning by the child.
> ➤ Caution must be exercised to prevent aspiration when giving medication to children. So give to infants in small amounts to avoid choking.
> ➤ If children are placed in a sitting position they are learn likely to aspirate the medications than if lying on their backs.

Administration of Medicine by Mouth

For Infants (Fig. 11.1)

Take the medicine in a dropper syringes or in a tea spoon.

* Hold the infant in her mother's lap.
* Medicines are generally administered before feeding unless contraindicated. Children head and shoulder should be raised and the chin should be depressed with thumb to open the mouth.
* The dropper (or) the spoon should be placed on the middle of the tongue and slowly dropped in the tongue.
* The thumb be released and the child should be allowed to swallow.

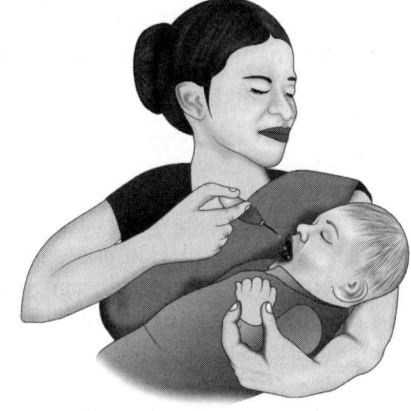

Fig. 11.1: Infants oral drug administration.

For Toddlers (Fig. 11.2)

The medicine should be taken in a measuring cup (or) in a teaspoon. The child head and shoulder be raised medicine cup should be held to the mouth and medicine should be released slowly.

Pre-school Age Children

When children are old enough to take a tablet they should be taught to place the tablet at the back of the tongue.

The emphasis should be given on swallowing fluids with the tablet. After swallowing the medicine, children's chin should be always raised.

Equipment

- Medicines card
- Medication tray
- Disposable medication cups
- Oral medication, e.g. tablets, syrup, etc.
- Medicine measures
- Glass of water, juice or preferred fluid
- Milliliter measures
- 1 mL syringe
- 5 mL spoon, plastic dropper
- Motor and piston
- Paper towels
- Toy appropriate to the age.

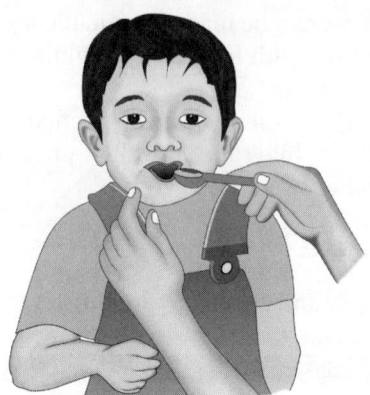

Fig. 11.2: Toddler oral drug administration.

Steps of Procedure

Assess for any contraindications to client receiving oral medications. Is client able to swallow, is client suffering from nausea (or) vomiting, is client has current gastrointestinal surgery.

- Does client need gastric suction?
- Determine client's preference for fluids
- Prepare the needed equipment
- Check accuracy and completeness of each medication card form of printout with physicians written medication and time for administration.

Prepare Drug

a. Wash hands.
b. Arrange medication tray and cups in medicine room. Prepare medication for one client at a time. Keep medication cards for each client together.
c. Select stock supply. Compare label of medication card.
d. Calculate current drug dosage, time, double check calculation.
e. To prepare tablet (or) capsules from bottle, pour required number into bottle cap and transfer medications to medication cup. Do not touch medicines with finger. Extra capsules may be removed to bottle.
f. All tablets given to child at one time may be placed in one cup except for those requiring pre-administration assessment.
g. If the client has difficulty in swallowing, grind tablet in motor and piston.

Prepare Liquids

- Remove bottle cap from container and place cap upside down
- Hold bottle with lable against palm of hand while pouring.
- Had medication cup at eye level and fill to derived levels/scale.

Administrating Medication

a. Take medication to clients at correct time.

b. Identify client by comparing name on card printout from (or) with name (or) patients identification bracelet. Ask patient to state his full name.
c. Perform necessary pre-administration for specific medication.
d. Explain purpose of each medication and its action to client (or) parents. Allow them to ask any questions.
e. Assist patient to sitting/lateral position.
f. After full glass of water (or) juice drugs to be swallowed.
g. For sublingual administration drugs, client have to place medication under tongue and allow it dissolve.
h. Record actual time, each drug administered on medication record (or) computer include initials and signature.

After Care of Equipment

- Dispose all solid supplies.
- Cups, spoons, droppers should be washed with soap and water and make them dry and replace in cupboard.
- Keep the client unit neat and tidy.
- Return in 30 minutes to evaluate the client's response to medications.

Calculation for Administration of Medication

Many formulas are used to determine a dose of a drug to be given to a child.

1. **Young's rule**:
   Which applies to children 1–12 years of age

   $$\text{Child's dose} = \frac{\text{Child age (in years)}}{\text{Child age} + 12} \times \text{Adult dose}$$

   Example: A child aged 10 years, suffering from tuberculosis requires to be given injection streptomycin intramuscularly. Calculate the dose.

   $$\text{Child's dose} = \frac{10}{10+12} \times 1000 \text{ mg}$$
   $$= \frac{10}{22} \times 1000 \text{ mg}$$
   $$= \frac{10000}{22}$$
   $$= 454 \text{ mg}$$

2. **Clark's rule:** Uses the children weight to calculate the appropriate dose and assumes that the adult dose is based on 150 lb person.

   $$\text{Child dose} = \frac{\text{Weight of child (pounds) in lb}}{150 \text{ pounds}} \times \text{Adult dose}$$

   1 lb = 454 g
   1 kg = 2.2 lb
   1000 gm = 2.2 lb

Example: A child weighing 20 lbs requires IM streptomycin. Adult dose is 1000 mg.

$$= \frac{20}{150} \times 1000 \text{ mg}$$

$$= \frac{2}{15} \times 1000 \text{ mg}$$

$$= 133 \text{ mg}$$

3. **Surface area:** Surface area is determined with a nanogram

$$\text{Child dose} = \frac{\text{Surface area in square meter}}{1.73} \times \text{Adult dose}$$

4. **Fried's rule:** Applies to a child younger than 1 year old age. The rule assumes that an adult dose should be appropriate for a child who is 12 years.

$$\text{Child dose} = \frac{\text{Infant age (in months)}}{150} \times \text{Adult dose}$$

INTRAMUSCULAR DRUG ADMINISTRATION

Definition

It is a process of injection of medication into the muscle tissue of the body with syringe and needle.

Purpose

- To administer drugs when quick action is required.
- To administer drugs when patient is not able to swallow and retain as in psychiatric or unconscious patients.
- To administer drugs which are inactivated by gastric enzymes or which irritates the gastric mucosa.
- To administer oil suspended drugs, e.g. paracetamol.

POINTS TO NOTE

While Selecting the IM Injections
- Be very careful when selecting IM injection sites.
- Children can be unpredictable and uncooperative.
- Distracting the child with conversation or a toy may reduce pain perception.
- Give injection quickly and do not fight with the child.
- Use strict aseptic techniques.
- Do not use any drug which is discolored or has rudiments.
- Multiple dose vial should be replaced in medicine cupboard or refrigerator as directed in the label.
- Calculate the dose (or) amount needed carefully.

Selection of Sites

1. Ventrogluteal
2. Deltoid muscle
3. Vastus lateralis site
4. Dorsogluteal.

Intramuscular Injection Sites

Intramuscular injection sites and their landmarks
1. **Ventrogluteal site:** Is the most comfortable and safest for IM injections. This site is not close to any major blood vessels or nerves. The landmarks for this site include the greater trochanter, anterior superior iliac spine and iliac crest. With the patient on their side place the palm of your hand on the greater trochanter, the index finger on the anterior superior iliac spine and the middle finger pointing toward the iliac crest **(Fig. 11.3)**.

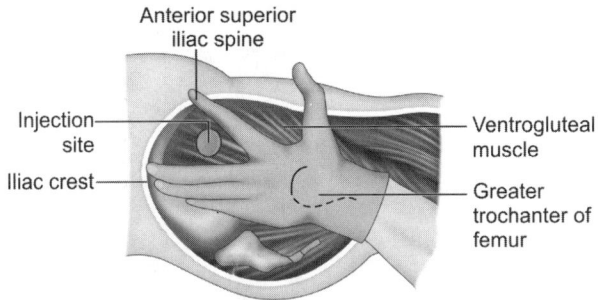

Fig.11.3: IM injection—ventrogluteal site.
(*Source:* http://intramuscularinjectionsim.blogspot.com)

2. **Deltoid site:** This site is most common for small volumes. To inject into this site you must first locate the acromion process, place a finger on the process and measure 3-finger breadths down. The injection is given into the fullest part of the deltoid **(Fig. 11.4)**.

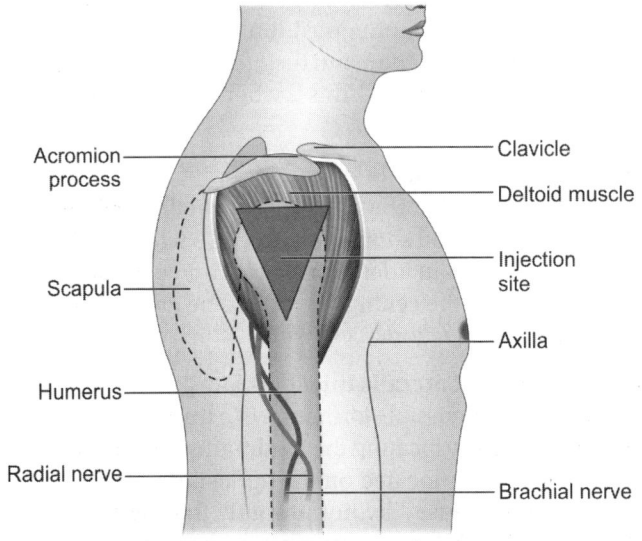

Fig. 11.4: IM injection—deltoid site.
(*Source*: http://intramuscularinjectionsim.blogspot.com)

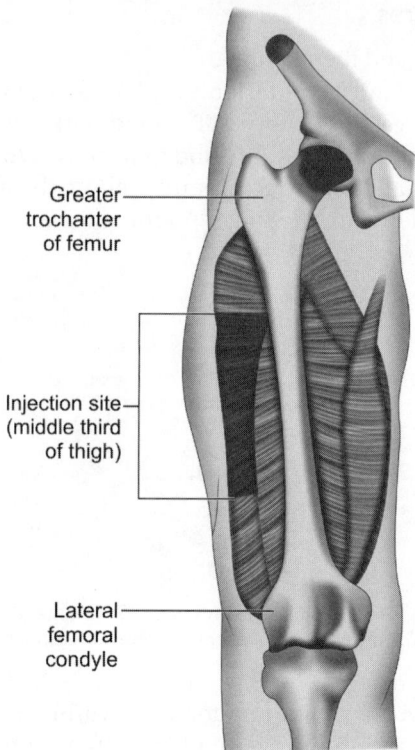

Fig. 11.5: IM injection—vastus lateralis site.
(*Source*: http://intramuscularinjectionsim.blogspot.com)

3. **Vastus lateralis:** Is located on the lateral aspect of the thigh, it is the number one site for newborns and infants who have not developed any of the gluteal muscles or the deltoid muscle. Have patient assume a supine position, divide the thigh into thirds. Place one hand next to the head of the trochanter and the other hand just above the patella. The area between your hands is the middle third; this is where the injection is given into the thickest portion of the muscle **(Fig. 11.5)**.

Advantages of the Vastus Lateralis Injection Site
Main advantage of this site is that the muscle is normally well developed even in infants and children. The amount of fluid should not exceed 2.0 mL for children older than 1 year. Fluid should not exceed 1.0 mL in infants. It is best to give this injection lying flat or on the side with the side pointing at the ceiling. It can also be given while sitting own, especially handy, if you are giving the injection to yourself.

Disadvantages of the Vastus Lateralis Injection Site
Some advantages include the possible formation of a thrombosis in the femoral artery. This is only possible by not properly locating the landmarks associated with the vastus lateralis injection. The femoral artery is located on the opposite side of the injection site. Another possible injury that can be caused by not properly finding landmarks is damage to the sciatic nerve. Also possible to hit the sciatic nerve by using to long of a needle and injecting to far back. The vastus lateralis injection is more painful than the deltoid or ventrogluteal injection sites.

4. **Dorsogluteal site:** This site is never used in infants and small children. Because of the proximity to the sciatic nerve, it is only used as a last resort in adults. The landmarks for this site are the posterior superior iliac spine and the greater trochanter. An imaginary line is drawn between the two landmarks. Find the center of the line and move one inch above the line **(Fig. 11.6)**.

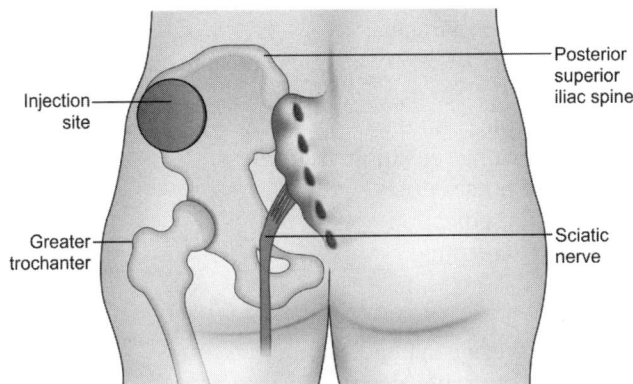

Fig. 11.6: IM injection—dorsogluteal site.
(*Source*: http://intramuscularinjectionsim.blogspot.com)

Equipment

A tray containing
- 1–2 mL syringe
- 25 to 27 gauze needle
- ½ inch length for child
- 5/8 inch for newborn
- Cotton swabs in a container
- Antiseptic or spirit solution
- Disposable gloves
- Medication ample or vial
- Medicine card.

Procedure
- Identify the child
- Obtain medical history and history of allergies.
- Wash hands
- Prepare needed equipment and supplies
- Check medication orders
- Prepare correct dose from ampule or vial check carefully.
- If IM injection, change the needle while drawing the medicine from vial.
- Use disposable syringes.
- Once again identify the client.
- Explain procedure to client parents, proceed calm and confident manner.
- Close the room curtains or use bed side screen.
- Select appropriate site, inspect skin over sites for inflammation and bruising rotate sites.
- If injections are given frequently rotate the sites.

- Assist the child for comfortable position depending upon the site of injection.
- Relocate the site anatomical land marks.
- Cleanse the site with cotton swab at center of site and rotate out ward in circular direction for about 5 cm.
- Position nondominant hand at proper anatomical land marks and spread skin tightly. Inject needle quickly at 90° angle in the muscle. If clients muscle mass is small, grasp body of muscle between thumb and finger.
- Withdraw needle while apply, keep swab above the site.
- Massage site gently
- Assist client for comfortable position
- Observe site for pain, burning sensation, numbness.
- Record the procedure in nurses notes
- Evaluate the response to medication
- Replace the articles after cleaning.

Care of Equipment and Child

- Discard the needle and syringe in needle container.
- Discard the swabs and disposable gloves.
- Wash and replace the equipment.
- Replace the remaining equipment and medication in cupboard.

FLUID CALCULATION FOR IV INFUSION

Introduction

Water is the largest single component of the body comprising approximately 75% of total body weight in the term newborn total body water (TBW) falls during early infancy to about 60% of body weight by 4 to 6 months of age. A more gradual reduction in TBW then occurs approaching adult values of 50 to 60% at puberty.

Water distribution into two major compartments in the body, the intracellular and extracellular fluid spaces (ICF and ECF, respectively). Both of these compartments also undergo age dependent changes.

Maintenance Therapy

Maintenance fluid requirements are the quality of fluid and electrolytes necessary to achieve zero water and electrolyte balance water loss occurs from two main sources:
1. Insensible (evaporative)
2. Urine

Approximately two-thirds of evaporative fluid losses occur through the skin, with the remainder being lost through the respiratory tract. Infants and children on mechanical ventilators or in mist tents do not lose water through their respiratory tract and actually receive water while inspiring humidified air. On the other hand, hyperventilation or hyperthermia will increase insensible losses. Under normal conditions, insensible losses comprise 30 to 40% of maintenance fluid requirements. Evaporative water loss increases by approximately 12% per degree of fever above 38°C. The factors known to influence insensible water losses are hyperthermia, increased activity, hyperventilation, radiant warmers and phototherapy.

Body Fluids

Stable internal environment is maintained by the balance of body water and electrolytes disturbances in the fluid and electrolytes balance is very common problem usually found in association with several disease conditions. Growing children are more susceptible to disturbances of fluid and electrolyte balance during their illnesses correction of imbalance and maintenance of fluid and electrolyte balance are the prime importance for the management of any disease conditions.

Water is the largest component of human body. Total Body Water (TBW) in full-term neonates is approximately 73 to 80% of body weight and gradually reduces to 60% by one to two years of age.

Total body water consists of two compartments—intracellular fluid (ICF) and extracellular fluid (ECF) and two minor compartments—transcellular fluid (TCF) and slowly exchangeable fluid (SEF) compartments. ICF volume represents 35 to 40% of body weight and is the sum total of fluids from the cells in different locations, ECF volume represents 20 to 25% of body weight and consists plasma water and interstitial water. TCF volume represents about 2% of body weight; it's most important components being gastrointestinal secretions, urine in kidney and lower urinary tract, CSF, aqueous, humor and synovial, pleural and peritoneal fluids. SEF volume represents 8 to 10% of body weight and is contained in bones, dense connective tissues and cartilages.

Sodium and chloride are the principal electrolytes in the ECF, while potassium and phosphates are the principal electrolytes in the ICF.

Hypotonic Solutions

It provides more water than electrolytes diluting the ECF. Osmosis then produces a movement of water from the ECF to the ICF. For example 0.45% NaCl.

Isotonic Solutions

Administration of an isotonic solution expands only the ECF. There is no net loss or gain from the ICF. An isotonic solution is the ideal fluid replacement from a patient with an ECF volume deficit. For example, 0.9% NaCl, RL. These solutions have sodium concentration somewhat higher than plasma and chloride concentration.

Hypertonic Solutions

These solutions initially raise the osmolality of ECF and expand it. It is useful in the treatment of hypovolemia and hyponatremia. For example, 10% dextrose solutions, 5% DNS.

Management of Dehydration

In severe dehydration and shock rapid expansion of intravascular volume is required to maintain vital functions. This is achieved by rapid intravenous infusion of 100–120 mL/kg of isotonic iso-osmotic solution. Ringer lactate or normal saline (or) plasma.

Dehydration

It is the fluid imbalance due to excessive loss of body water. Dehydration can be hypotonic, isotonic or hypertonic. The common type is isotonic dehydration with proportion loss of water and solutes from ECF. The ICF volume remains intact as there is no redistribution of fluid.

In hypotonic dehydration, the depletion of solutes in ECF is much more than the water losses. Hypotonicity of ECF leads to shift of water from ECF to ICF causing further contraction of ECF and shock.

In hypertonic dehydration, excess loss of water proportionate to the solutes causing movement of water from the cells in the ICF-leading to intracellular dehydration.

Electrolyte Imbalance

Hyponatremia is termed when serum sodium level is less than 130 mEq/L. It occurs due to water retention, sodium loss or both.

Management

Administering 3% solution of sodium chloride (saline), 10 mL/kg body weight at the rate of 1 mL per minute intravenously to correct the sodium deficit. Calculated extra sodium should be administered slowly in 24 to 48 hours.

Hypernatremia

When serum sodium is more than 150 mEq/L. It results from deficit of water with respect to sodium stores due to water loss in diarrhea, vomiting, dieresis, burns or excessive sodium intake.

Management

Hypernatremia should be treated promptly with rapid intravenous infusion of ringer lactate or saline to correct hypovolemia.

Hypokalemia

The serum potassium level is less than 3.5 mEq/L.

Management

Slow administration of potassium over 24–28 hours. Potassium infusion should be given using infusion pump at the rate of 0.3 to 0.35 mEq/kg/h till the ECG become normal. Infusion rate should not exceed 0.6 mEq/kg/h. Infusion fluid should not contain more than 40 mEq/L of potassium. Higher rates and concentrations may cause cardiac depression. Potassium should be administered only when urinary flow is established.

Hyperkalemia

Serum potassium level is more than 5.5 mEq/L.

Management

Mild hyperkalemia (5.5 to 6 mEq/L) is managed by stopping the potassium intake. Moderate hyperkalemia (6 to 8 mEq/L) is managed with glucose-insulin infusion or sodium-bicarbonate infusion and additional supportive measures along with discontinuation of potassium intake.

Burns Management

Fluid replacement is done promptly on the basis of TBSA burnt and body weight of the child. The Parkland formula is most commonly used.

Parkland formula: (4 mL/kg body wt × % of body surface area) + maintenance requirement of 1500 mL/m²
- Of the total 50% is given within the first 8 hours.
- Remaining over next 16 hours.
- Ringers lactate is preferred on 1st day. Subsequently fluids may be given as N/2 in 5% dextrose.
- Fluids should be reduced to 50% after the 1st day.
- Colloids can be administered if the serum albumin levels are less than 2 g/dL or fluid requirement is in excess of 300 mL/m²/h.

In case of very sick child, parental route is used. Intravenous fluid therapy refers to the infusion of fluid directly in to venous system which may be accomplished through the use of needle, cannula, or venous cut-down.

Purpose
- To restore fluid
- To reduce electrolyte deficits.

Maintenance requirements of fluid and electrolytes:
For infants and older children fluid requirement in 24 hours are:
- Up to 10 kg—1000 mL
- 10-20 kg—1000 mL + 50 mL/kg increase in body weight beyond 10 kg
- 20-30 kg—1500 mL + 20 mL/kg increase in body weight above 20 kg
- 30-40 kg —60 mL/kg/day

Maintenance of electrolyte requirement is:
Sodium	3 mmol/kg/day
Potassium	2 mmol/kg/day
Chloride	3 mmol/kg/day

Example:
Calculation of fluid requirement in 24 hours for a child weighing 12 kg:
10-20 kg: 1000 + 50 mL/kg increase in body weight beyond 10 kg.
12 kg: 1000 + 50 × 2 = 1100 mL (child is 2 kg more than 10 kg).
1100 mL is fluid requirement

Calculation of flow rate:
The calculation of rate of flow of fluids is main responsibility to facilitate administration of correct amount of fluid in right duration of time.
The formula to compute the flow rate is:

$$\frac{\text{Volume of solution}}{\text{Time intervals in minutes}} \times \text{Drops factor} = \frac{\text{Drops}}{\text{Minutes}}$$

Drop factor for microdrip set = 60
Volume of solution—125 mL
Drop factor—60
Time interval in minutes—60 × 60

$$= \frac{125 \times 60}{6 \times 60} = 20.83$$

The rate of flow to be regulated is 20–21 drops/min.

Veins used for infusion in newborn and infancy

Scalp veins—frontal, superficial temporal vein, umbilical veins—(during first few days of life). Superficial veins—of the hands, wrist, arm and foot

Older children: On the basis of accessibility of veins. For right handed children left hand is preferred.

Nursing management:
- During parenteral fluid therapy, clinical and biochemical indicators of water and electrolytes status should be monitored closely.
- The pulse rate, blood pressure, capillary refill time and sensorium should be monitored.
- In take and output chart should be maintained.
- Laboratory tests should be done daily to adjust intake of water and electrolytes.
- Body weight should be recorded daily.

EXCHANGE TRANSFUSION

Introduction

Since the introduction of intensive phototherapy and immunoglobulin infusion for isoimmune hemolytic jaundice, exchange transfusions are performed in rare instances in the neonatal intensive care unit, and only after careful consideration. The procedure is utilized for the management of hyperbilirubinemia and hemolytic disease of the newborn, when other methods of treatment have been ineffective.

Aim

To modify abnormal values of the circulating bloods composition, by removing one or more components whilst maintaining a close to constant blood volume.

Points to Remember

1. The procedure is streamlined. Never rushed, and the infant's wellbeing is monitored and supported accordingly to promote immediate and long-term outcomes.
2. Asepsis is maintained throughout procedure.
3. Parents are fully informed of procedure and signed consent for blood products is obtained on the blood transfusion form.
4. Supportive strategies are implemented post-procedure to assist therapeutic efficacy.

Indications for Exchange Transfusion

- Hyperbilirubinemia—to lower serum bilirubin (SBR) levels and prevent kernicterus
- Rhesus/ABO incompatibility—removal of red blood cells with antibodies or free circulating antigens to reduce degree of red cell destruction
- Severe anemia—replace volume with that containing a higher red blood cell mass
- Hydrops fetalis—to regulate blood volume and allay potential heart failure
- Other rare indications—hyperkalemia, drug toxicity, disseminate intravascular coagulation (DIC).

Exchange Transfusion Formulae

The volume required is dependent on the reason for exchange and is determined by the consultant.

1. Single volume exchange (anemia with volume overload)
   Preterm/term infant—80–100 mL/kg
   Extremely preterm (< 28 weeks) infant—100–120 mL/kg

$$\text{Volume exchanged (mL)} = \frac{\text{Wt (kg)} \times \text{Blood volume} \times (\text{Hb desired} - \text{Hb initial})}{\text{Hb of red blood cells} - \text{Hb initial}}$$

2. Double volume exchange (for hyperbilirubinemia)
   Preterm/term infant—80–100 mL/kg × 2
   Extremely preterm (< 28 weeks) infant—100–120 mL/kg × 2

Pre-exchange Requirements

Staffing

- The exchange transfusion should ideally be performed in the intensive care nursery.
- It must always be supervised by an experienced senior medical staff member and an experienced senior nurse. These two clinical members must carry out the exchange from beginning until completion.
- Attach a "Do not disturb during procedure" sign at bedside.

Ordering Blood

- Use current bare weight or birth weight (whichever is greater) for calculations.
- Calculate volume of blood products required in accordance with relevant formula and in accordance with the indication for exchange transfusion.
- Request appropriately cross-matched blood products (packed red blood cells and FFP) from hematology indicating reason for exchange transfusion
  - Specify total volume required for exchange including priming of lines
  - Donor blood should be CMV negative and irradiated
  - Request most freshly available blood; to promote count of viable RBC and to minimize risk of hyperkalemia and acidosis.

Consent

- Informed parental consent for procedure must be attained prior to commencement
- Signed consent should be obtained on blood transfusion form for blood products as per unit guidelines.

Monitoring Equipment

- Nurse infant on open care bed with servo controlled radiant heater, ensure temperature probe secured to infant
- Cardio-respiratory monitor applied to infant
- Pulse oximeter applied
- ABG and BSL available.

Resuscitation Equipment

- Check infant's resuscitation equipment connected and in working order
- Ensure resuscitation trolley checked, stocked and in close proximity.

Nursing Management

- ❖ Infant should be made nil by mouth with a size 8 orogastric tube in situ. Any gastric contents must be aspirated and discarded and the orogastric tube must remain on free drainage.
- ❖ Ensure availability of separate IV line for maintenance of fluids and medications
- ❖ Ensure that the infant is safe and settled using non-pharmacological means (e.g. nesting, sucrose, pacifier)
- ❖ Phototherapy should preferably be continued during the exchange transfusion
- ❖ Record baseline observations, including;
  - Heart rate
  - Temperature
  - Respirations
  - Blood pressure
  - Oxygen saturations
  - Infant's color, tone, and behavior
  - Urine output/urinalysis.

Initial Steps

- ❖ Confirm correct patient, check patient identification labels on infant
- ❖ Undertake set-up in a sterile manner
- ❖ Follow the neonatal intensive care unit (NICU) guidelines for insertion of UVC and UAC (optimal for monitoring and sampling, necessary for isovolumetric method) using appropriate set up
- ❖ Check blood products as per hospital policy
- ❖ Set up two sterile trolleys for second sterile procedure (using equipment from exchange transfusion box);
  - One for exchange procedure
  - One for line set up
- ❖ Determine need for using FFP/4% albumin by checking Hct of packed cells to be used. Determine required volume of FFP/4% albumin to be infused.

Exchange Transfusion Equipment Box

- ❖ 50 mL Syringe—2
- ❖ 21-guage needle—2
- ❖ Adult blood filter—3
- ❖ Albumin filter—2
- ❖ Intravenous giving set—3
- ❖ Intravenous extension line (for blood warmer)
- ❖ Exchange transfusion pack (containing blood waste disposal system)
- ❖ 3 way taps—5
- ❖ 5 mL syringes—2
- ❖ 10 mL syringes—2
- ❖ Small sterile plastic drape
- ❖ Large sterile drape
- ❖ Small sterile fenestrated drape
- ❖ EDTA, heparin and coagulation tubes
- ❖ Blood gas syringes
- ❖ Heparin ampoules (50 IU in 5 mL)

- ❖ Normal saline (10 mL) ampoules
- ❖ Calcium gluconate ampoules
- ❖ Exchange transfusion recording chart

Additional Equipment Required

- ❖ Sterile gown pack
- ❖ Appropriate sized sterile gloves
- ❖ Blood warmer (set 37 degrees)
- ❖ Infusion pump (adult settings/capable of volumes up to 500 mL/h)(necessary for isovolumetric method only).

Exchange Transfusion Methods

1. Push–pull Method (Fig. 11.7)

This method requires reliable venous access-preferably via a centrally placed umbilical venous catheter. This is a one person method where blood is slowly withdrawn, at a predetermined aliquot following which donor blood is replaced slowly through manual infusion of an aliquot of matching volumes. This process is attended by the medical officer, whilst the nurse monitors and records volumes in/out and vital signs.

The procedure takes 90–120 minutes. The volume in/volume out balance should not exceed 5% of infant's blood volume. Thumb rule: 5 mL aliquots for a preterm baby (< 2,000 g); 10 mL for a term baby (or > 2,000 g). Calculate the actual time per aliquot.

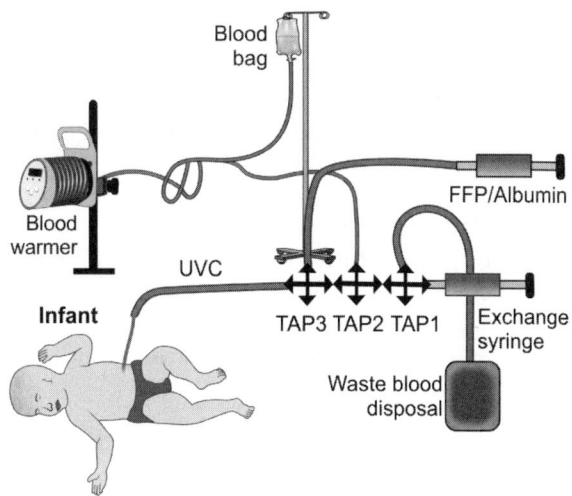

Fig. 11.7: Push-pull method.

Steps

- ❖ Connect 2 three-way taps and a syringe (size appropriate to pre-determined aliquot volumes) in sequence.
  Note: You may require a third three-way tap (tap 3) for infusion of FFP/Albumin
- ❖ Connect the filtered line from blood pack to the proximal three-way tap (tap 1—closer to the infant)
- ❖ Attach the line to the waste bag to the distal three-way tap (tap 2—closer to the syringe) for closed disposal of withdrawn blood
- ❖ Prime the set-up system from blood pack and ensure set-up free of air bubbles
- ❖ Set up blood line within the blood warmer at set temperature of 37 degrees
- ❖ Connect set-up to primary lumen of umbilical venous catheter-ensure tap 1 turned off to blood pack and tap 2 turned off to waste disposal bag
- ❖ Withdrawn first aliquot slowly, announce volume, (X–mL) 'out', nurse records, attain baseline blood samples from this volume, including ;

- Rhesus group, direct Coombs'
- SBR
- UEC and Ca^+
- Arterial blood gas
- FBC
- Newborn screening test (NBST) (if less than 48 hours of age)
- Ensure extra samples kept on 'hold' (Heparin, EDTA and plain)
❖ Fill syringe for replacement from blood pack via tap 1. Infuse the desired amount and announce volume (X-mL) "in", nurse records. The following out is sent to the disposal bag via tap 2.
❖ Volumes 'in' and 'out' are repeated sequentially (approximately 1 minute for each action) and recorded each time by the nurse on flow sheet including running totals
❖ The nurse announces the running total every 100 mL
❖ Vital signs must be recorded at 5 minute intervals from baseline, including;
- Heart rate
- Temperature
- Respirations
- Non-invasive blood pressure every 15 minutes
- Oxygen saturations
- Infant's color, tone, and behavior
- Blood warmer temperature
❖ Gently agitate the blood bag every 10–15 minutes to prevent setting of red blood cells
❖ Check ABG every 30 minutes (or more frequently if required), including ionized Ca^+, BSL and K^+
❖ Attend formal blood tests at midway point of exchange, including;
- EUC
- Ca^+
- FBC
❖ Continue process until the pre-calculated volume to be exchanged is achieved
❖ End in exact balance (or positive balance if indicated by Hemoglobin level)
❖ Collect last out sample for testing as described in the section on post-exchange care.

2. Isovolumetric Method
(Fig. 11.8)

The isovolumetric method of exchange transfusion requires an arterial access (peripheral or preferably umbilical arterial) and venous access (preferably umbilical venous). It can be a two person method where blood is slowly withdrawn, at pre-determined aliquots with concurrent manual replacement of donor blood by the second person using the same aliquot size.

Preferably, it is a one person procedure where blood is slowly

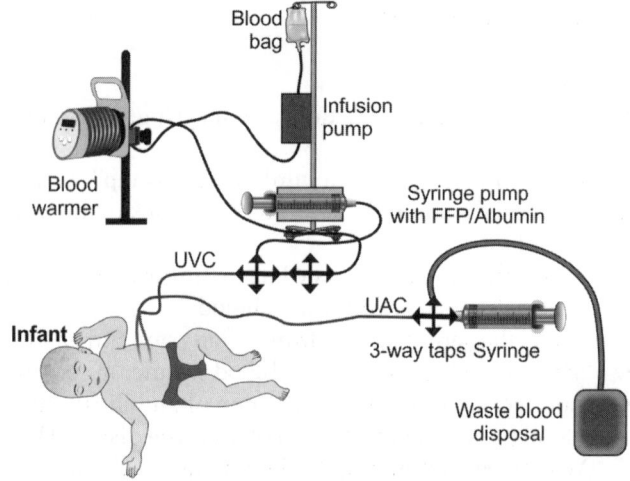

Fig. 11.8: Isovolumetric method.

withdrawn manually at a constant rate over a fixed period, and in lieu of manual replacement of volumes, donor blood is continuously infused in coordination with the infant's blood that is withdrawn, via mechanical pumps. This removal process is attended by the medical officer whilst the nurse is responsible for the set up and monitoring of the infusing blood, recording of the blood volumes in/out, and monitoring and recording of infant's vital signs. This process generally takes up to 60–90 minutes to complete.

Key Points to Consider with Exchange Transfusions

- BSL tends to rise due to the preservative in the blood bag and should settle without requiring treatment (see post-exchange care)
- Occasionally, Ca^+ correction may be required at the midway point, or in event of unexplained arrhythmias
- If FFP/albumin required, infuse via syringe pump to complete volume over the exchange period for the isovolumetric method. For push-pull method of exchange, infuse one aliquot of FFP/albumin after every 5 aliquots of packed cells. Calculate aliquot size of FFP/albumin as follows:

$$\frac{\text{Total FFP / Albumin required}}{[\text{Exchange volume} / (5 \times \text{aliquot volume for exchange})]}$$

- Monitor the infant continuously, slowly the rate of exchange, temporarily pausing the procedure or curtailing it a warranted by the infant's condition
- If the exchange has to stop completely if or when the infant's condition warrants, the exchange is over despite the point of procedure.

Post Exchange Care

The last out specimen must be sent for follow-up testing including;
- SBR
- EUC/Ca^+
- Coagulation studies
- ABG
- BSL
- FBC

These bloods should be repeated again at 4–6 hours post exchange and then as per consultant ***particularly SBR levels**.

The infant must be kept NBM for a minimum of 4 hours post exchange (to decrease the risk of NEC) after which feeding may be cautiously re-initiated.

Monitor BSL's closely for a minimum of 6 hours for rebound hypoglycemia (as banked blood is preserved in dextrose, it triggers and increase in insulin production leading to increased glucose metabolism).

The infant must remain in a level three setting for 48 hours post exchange.

Monitor infant for abnormal signs and symptoms and possible complications including thrombocytopenia, bleeding, signs of infection, feed intolerance or abdominal distension.

High intensity phototherapy needs to be continued and reviewed in relation to SBR results.

Once discharged the infant must be followed up in NICU follow up clinics to monitor anemia, growth and development and assess neurological outcomes.

Complications, Prevention and Management

1. **Hypothermia:** If baby's skin temperature falls below 36°C
   Prevention and Management: Confirm placement of temperature probe and take axilla reading. Confirm blood warmer is at 37°C turn up the servo control or isolette and slow the exchange.
2. **Hyperglycemia:** Donor blood is preserved in dextrose
   Prevention and Management: Blood glucose levels can be elevated during the exchange and generally resolve without intervention.
3. **Hypoglycemia:** May occur during and shortly after the exchange
   Prevention and Management: If baby's reagent strip blood glucose is less than 2.5 mmol/L give slow push of 2 mL/kg of 10% dextrose (via peripheral line or flush catheter dead space before and after dextrose injection). Repeat screening blood glucose level on next cycle. Continue to monitor glucose levels.
4. **Hyperkalemia:** Unlikely to happen with red blood cells less than 5 days old but is more likely to happen with a sick preterm infant refer to hyperkalemia protocol.
   Prevention and Management: If K^+ > 6.0 mmol/L give calcium gluconate if Ca < 2.0 mmol/L and recheck K^+ frequently. Stop exchange if K^+ > 7.0 mmol/L and treat until K^+ < 6.0 and then restart exchange. Peaked T waves/widened QRS/VEBs can be seen with hyperkalemia.
5. **Hypocalcemia:** This is rare with the preservative anticoagulants used now rarely need treating.
   Prevention and Management: If Ca^{++} drops to < 1.5 mmol/L then flush catheter dead space with normal saline and give urgent correction: 0.23–0.46 mmol/kg (1–2 mL/kg of calcium gluconate 10%) by slow IV injection of diluted solution over 10 minutes. Do not give into a peripheral vein. Prolonged QT interval can be seen with hypocalcemia.
6. **Metabolic acidosis:** Mild metabolic acidosis is common and usually does not need treating. Correct hyperkalemia/hypocalcemia before giving H_2CO_3.
   Prevention and Management: If baby's base excess falls below minus 10 mmol/L then flush catheter dead space with normal saline, and half correct with 4.2% sodium bicarbonate (mmol of bicarbonate = [body weight × base excess × 0.3]/2). If acidosis worsens or persists, then consider stopping exchange.
7. **Thrombocytopenia:** Store red cells are platelet depleted, so the platelet count will tend to fall during the exchange transfusion. This rarely needs intervention.
   Prevention and Management: If the platelet count falls to < 50,000 consider stopping exchange and arrange a platelet transfusion through a peripheral vein.
8. **Air Embolus:**
   Prevention and Management: Ensure lines are set up and primed correctly. Observe lines for presence of air during exchange and ensure 3-way taps are closed to the infant when filling or expelling contents of syringe.
9. **Anemia/polycythemia:**
   Prevention and Management: Ensure HCT of RBCs/FFP infusion is kept consistent throughout procedure. Gently agitate burette at frequent intervals to prevent separation of red cells and FFP.
10. **Necrotizing Enterocolitis:** Ensure the UVC is in correct position.
    Prevention and Management: Perform isovolumetric exchange transfusion or use small aliquots if single lumen technique used.

TOTAL PARENTERAL NUTRITION

Definition

Total parenteral nutrition is the administration of highly concentrated, hypertonic nutrient solution via intravenous route.

Goal

- Preventing infection
- Maintaining the parenteral nutrition system
- Preventing metabolic electrolyte fluid balance complications.
- Assessing the client's readiness for parenteral nutrition
  Or
  Discharge planning for parenteral nutrition.

Purposes

- To restore the fluid volume that is lost from the body due to hemorrhage, vomiting, diarrhea, drainage, etc.
- To meet the patient's basic requirements for calories, water, minerals and vitamins.
- To prevent and treat shock and collapse.
- To supply the body with adequate amounts of fluids, electrolyte amounts if by mouth or oral intake is contraindicated or impracticable.
- To administer medicines.

Indications

- To save the patients in life-threatening situation, e.g. Patient having hemorrhage, shock, extensive burns, etc.
- To supply fluids and nutrients to the patients who may have nothing by mouth or who are unable to ingest oral liquids owing to prolonged nausea, vomiting, diarrhea, peritonitis, paralytic items. fistulas, etc.
- To supply fluids and nutrients to the patients who are unable to digest or absorb a diet administered by mouth or through the nasal tube, e.g. patients who do not have anatomically intact intestinal tract or patient with septicemia, etc.
- To dilute toxins in case of toxemia or septicemia.
- To administer medicines that are destroyed by gastric juice or that will not be absorbed by the gastrointestinal track, administered orally.
- Preoperative malnutrition, e.g. BMI < 18 or 20% weight loss.
- Postoperative complications delaying enteral feeding. For example, paralytic ileus items, obstruction, short bowel syndrome, fistula, peritoneal sepsis.
- Acute or chronic GI inflammation which is not responding to treatment, e.g. chronic disease, ulcerative colitis, severe gastroenteritis.
- Malabsorption, e.g. in cancer and cancer chemotherapy or radiotherapy, where there inflammation of the mucosa.

Contraindications

- Patients with severe renal disease, adrenal insufficient.
- Hyperpotassemia.
- In a severe liver disease, isolyte–G should not be used, because ammonia may not be converted into urea.

Instructions

- Follow strict aseptic technique.
- Verify the physician's order, name of solution, route, time, name of client, etc.
- Maintain rate of flow.
- Watch for side effects.
- Observe rate of flow, needle site.
- Urinary output, amount of fluid.
- Observe potency of IV tube.
- Maintain intake output chart.
- Observe five rights rule. The right patient, the right medicine, right dose, right time, right amount.
- Check the expiry date of the fluid.
- Shake the fluid and look for the suspended articles, cloudy and discolorization.
- Check working condition of infusion set.
- Select proper site.
- Never allow the bottle to empty completely to prevent the entry air into the tissue.

Equipment

- IV pole/IV stand
- Adhesive or non-allergenic tape
- Clean gloves
- Tourniquet
- Antiseptic swab
- Intravenous catheter or butterfly needle
- Arm split
- Towel or pad
- Electronic infusion device pump
- Intravenous solution
- Intravenous set
- Paper bag or kidney tray
- Mackintosh
- Sterile forceps in jar
- IV line filters.

Preparation of Articles

A Tray Containing

1. IV solution (sterile and clear) in required number of bottles for a day
2. Sterile IV tubing with attached drip chamber and clamp
3. Sterile butterfly or scalp vein needle with a protective cap on needle
4. Sterile syringes (2 or 5 mL) with needle no. 20 and 22
5. Sterile transfer forceps in jar
6. Sterile cotton swabs and gauze piece in sterile container
7. Methylated sprit container
8. Kidney tray and paper bag
9. Bowl with water
10. Tourniquet
11. Adhesive plaster with scissors

12. Covered arm splint with roller bandages
13. Mackintosh and towel
14. IV pole.

Procedure

Steps of Procedure

1. Wash hands
2. Prepare the IV solution:
    a. Carefully remove the bottle seal, clean the top with spirit swab insert drip set
    b. Close the screw clamp
    c. Hang the bottle on the IV pole about 18 – 24 inches high
    d. Connect the butterfly or needle to the IV tube
    e. Open the clamp and flush the IV fluid into the kidney tray the air removed.
3. Prepare few strips of adhesive tape and keep ready for use
4. Prepare the vein puncture site:
    a. Place the extremity in a dependent position (lower than patient's heart)
    b. Apply a tourniquet firmly 6–8 inches proximal to the vein puncture site
    c. Massage or stroke the vein distal to the knot and in the direction of the venous flow (towards the heart)
    d. Encourage the patient to clench and unclench the fist rapidly
    e. Lightly tap the vein finger trips
    f. If the veins are not visible by the above steps, remove the tourniquet and apply heat to entire extremity for 10–15 minutes. Then apply tourniquet.
    g. Clean the area with spirit swab
    h. Dry the area with a sterile dry swab.
5. Insert the needle into the vein:
    a. Grasp the arm distally to the point of entry of the needle. Place left thumb one inch below the expected point of entry. Pull the skin tightly
    b. Holding the needle at a 30° angle with the level up. Once the needle enters the skin lower the angle of the needle
    c. When back flow of blood occurs into the needle and tubing, insert the needle further up into the vein about ¾ to 1 inch
    d. Release the tourniquet and open the clamp to allow the fluid to run in.
6. Secure the needle and tubing in place:
    a. Securing the scalp vein needle either by the 'H' method or by criss-cross method. Apply two strips of adhesive tape to the wing as needle parallel to the needle
    b. Secure the scalp vein tubing to the skin by forming a loop
    c. Secure the IV tubing to the skin
    d. Cover entry site with sterile gauze piece
    e. Use arm board to immobilize the nearest joint.

Solutions Used

1. Nutrient solutions:
    For example, dextrose, 5%, 10%, 20%, 25%, 50%, etc.
2. Electrolyte solution available in isotonic, hypotonic and hypertonic concentration:
    For example, normal saline, Dextrose saline, Lactated Ringer solution, 1/6 molar sodium lactate solution, etc.

3. Alkalinizing and acidifying solutions:
   For example, sodium lactate solution, Sodium bicarbonate, Potassium chloride, etc.
4. Blood volume expanders: These are plasma substitutes and contain large molecular substance which will not escape through the vessel walls and tend to prevent the circulating fluid from leaking in the tissues.
   For example, dextran, lomodex, hemocele, etc.

After Care of the Equipment

- Maintain the specific rate of flow throughout the procedure.
- Remove the Mackintosh and towel.
- Make the client comfortable in bed.
- Instruct the client not move the hand or part which is equipped with needle.
- Collect all articles.
- Clean the articles with cold water and then with warm soapy water and rinse them thoroughly with clean water. Dry them and replace in their proper places.
- Record the procedure with date and time:
  a. Type of fluid administered
  b. Concentration of solution
  c. Amount of fluid
  d. Rate of flow
  e. Any medicine added to the infusion
  f. Any reaction noticed.
- Teach the family members to observe and report:
  a. The fluid chamber is not dripping
  b. Bottle of fluid nearly empty
  c. Back flow of blood
  d. Disconnection of needle or tube
  e. Increase pain or discomfort
  f. Swelling
  g. Side effects like chills, restlessness, fever, redness, etc.
- Inform to the next shift staff about general condition of the client.
- Clamp the infusion before removing old fluid bottle.
- When fluid is completed, to discontinue it:
  a. Clamp the infusion-loosen adhesive tape.
  b. Take the sterile cotton and withdraw the needle while applying pressure over punctured area
  c. Apply small sterile dressing
  d. Discard bottle and set as desired.
- Record and report the condition of the client.

Complications

1. Circulatory overload means that IV compartment contains more fluid than the normal.
2. Infiltration is the escape of fluid into the subcutaneous tissues due to dislodgement of needle.
3. Damage to the walls of blood vessels and extravasations of blood (hematoma).
4. Thrombophlebitis—mechanical trauma to the veins or chemical irritation to the veins.

5. Pyrogenic reactions—symptoms generally appear in 30 minutes after IV started. Characteristics are fever, chills, nausea, vomiting and circulatory collapse.
6. Air embolism
7. Infection at the needle site.
8. Allergic reaction
9. Serum hepatitis—attributed to improperly disinfected syringes and needles.
10. Osmotic dieresis
11. Nerve damage.

> **POINTS TO NOTE**
> - The nurse is responsible for interpreting the prescription accurately, recording that the drug has been given and observing the patient's response.
> - The nurse must also be aware that some drugs, even if stopped before discharge, may still exert an action or cause side-effects.

PRACTICE QUESTIONS

1. What are the five rights for drug administration?
2. What are the sites for IM injection?
3. Parkland formula for fluid replacement _____
4. What do you mean by exchange transfusion?
5. Write short notes on total parental nutrition.

MULTIPLE CHOICE QUESTIONS

1. The nurse is giving instructions to a mother with a child receiving a liquid oral iron supplement. The nurse tells the mother to:
   a. Take it with meals
   b. Mix it with food
   c. Mix it with milk
   d. Administer it using a straw
2. Regarding prescription instructions, nurses should:
   a. Give the patient website addresses where he or she can learn more about the drug
   b. Explain what the medication is and does, as well as its potential side effects
   c. Tell the patient to read the detailed sheet that accompanies the medication
   d. Do nothing, it just confuses the patient
3. Which area of medication administration is most commonly neglected and is frequently the subject of investigations by professional nursing regulatory bodies?
   a. Record keeping
   b. Dosage calculations
   c. Routes of administration
   d. Drug given to the wrong patient

ANSWER KEY

1. d   2. b   3. a

CHAPTER 12

Pediatric Drug Calculation

PRACTICE COMPETENCIES
On completion of the chapter, the students will be able to:
- Understand the need for accuracy in preparing and administrating medication to children is greater than that of an adult.
- Carry out appropriate drug calculation to avoid greater error.

ABSTRACT
In pediatric practice medication, dosages are calculated based on the child's weight. For making the dosage much more precise it is important that the child's most recent weight in kilograms is entered into the health information system so that drug dosage calculations are accurate.

Keywords: Dosage, volume, percentage, ratio.

METRIC UNITS

1 gram (g) = 1,000 milligrams (mg)
1 milligram (mg) = 1,000 micrograms (µg)
1 microgram (µg) = 1,000 nanograms (ng)
1 liter (L) = 1,000 milliliters (mL)

Answer the following decimal unit questions:

1. 4 g = how many mgs?
2. 1,575 µgs = how many mgs?
3. 750 mg = how many g?
4. 0.025 L = how many mL?
5. 0.25 µg = how many nanograms?
6. 350 mL = convert into liters?
7. 0.03 mg = how many µgs?

Answers

1. 4,000 mg
2. 1.575 mg

3. 0.750 g (0.75 g)
4. 25 mL
5. 250 nanograms
6. 0.35 L
7. 30 µg

Solutions

1. 4 g × 1,000 mg = 4,000 mg
2. 1,575 µg =
   1 mg = 1,000 µg
   $1{,}575 \text{ µg} = \dfrac{1{,}575}{1{,}000} = 1.575 \text{ mg}$
3. 750 mg = how many grams
   1 gram = 1,000 mg
   $750 \text{ mg} = \dfrac{750}{1{,}000} = 0.75 \text{ g}$
4. 0.025 L = how many mL
   1 liter (L) = 1,000 milliliters (mL)
   0.025 L = 0.025 × 1,000 = 25 mL
5. 0.25 µg = how many nanograms
   1 µg = 1,000 nanograms
   0.25 µg = 0.25 × 1,000 = 250 nanograms
6. 350 mL convert into liters
   1 L = 1,000 mL
   $350 \text{ mL} = \dfrac{350}{1{,}000} = 0.35 \text{ L}$
7. 0.03 mg = how many µg?
   1 mg = 1,000 µg
   0.03 mg = 0.03 × 1,000 = 30 µg.

■ DOSAGE CALCULATIONS

Many pediatric medication doses are calculated by the child's body weight, i.e., mg/kg or µg/kg, etc. The prescribing doctor should work this out and prescribe the dose required.

For example:
Dose required is 4 mg/kg
The child weighs 5 kg = 5 × 4 = 20 mg

Answer the Following Questions

1. A baby requires cefotaxime. The dosage is 50 mg/kg, the baby weighs 2.4 kg. What dose is required?
2. A 4-month-old is pyrexial and needs an anti-pyrexial drug. Paracetamol is effective, the dosage is 15 mg/kg and the child weighs 7.9 kg. What is the dose required?
3. An 11-year-old needs fluconazole. The dosage is 12 mg/kg and the child weighs 26 kg. What is the dose required?
4. You need to give a drug for a child weighing 4 kg. The dosage is 450 µg/kg. What is the dose required?
4a. How many mgs this?

Answers

1. 120 mg
2. 118.5 mg
3. 312 mg
4. 1,800 µg

4a. 1.8 mg

Solutions

1. 50 mg/kg × 2.4 kg = 120 mg
2. 15 mL/kg × 7.9 kg = 118.5 mg
3. 12 mg/kg × 26 kg = 312 mg
4. 4 kg × 450 µg/kg = 1,800 µg

4a. $\dfrac{1,800}{1,000} = 1.8$ mg

■ VOLUME OF DRUG TO GIVE

Once the medication dosage is prescribed, the volume of drug to be administered needs to be worked out. Often the drug you need to give is a fraction of the concentration stated on the label. There is a straight forward formula for working this out which can be used for the majority of calculations:

$$\text{Volume needed} = \frac{\text{What you want}}{\text{What you have got}} \times \text{The volume it is in}$$

Example: A child requires paracetamol as pain relief. The dosage is prescribed as 180 mg. The paracetamol comes as oral suspension 120 mg is 5 mL.

180 mg = What you want
120 mg = What you got
5 mL = Volume it is in

$$\frac{180}{120} \times 5 = 7.5 \text{ mL}$$

The child needs 7.5 mL of the paracetamol liquid.

Answer the Following Questions

1. Ibuprofen 130 mg is to be given orally for relief. The stock mixture contains 100 mg in 5 mL. What is the volume to be given?
2. A dose 208 mg of flucloxacillin is prescribed. The mixture available is 250 mg in 5 mL. Calculate the volume required?
3. Prescribed is oral alcohol free phenobarbitone 45 mg. It is available as 50 mg/mL, what is the volume required?
4. Metronidazole comes as 500 mg in 100 mL bag. The child is prescribed 75 mg I/V. What is the drug volume required?
5. 200 µg is prescribed and the drug comes as 5 mg in 5 mL. What volume is required?
6. 0.5 mg is required for a postoperative patients. The IV drug is available as 250 µg per mL. What is the volume required?

Answers

1. 6.5 mL
2. 4.1 mL
3. 0.9 mL
4. 15 mL
5. 0.2 mL
6. 2 mL

Solutions

$$\text{Volume needed} = \frac{\text{What you want}}{\text{What you have got}} \times \text{The volume it is in}$$

1. $\dfrac{130 \text{ mg}}{100 \text{ mg}} \times 5 \text{ mL} = 6.5 \text{ mL}$

2. $\dfrac{208 \text{ mg}}{250 \text{ mg}} \times 5 \text{ mL} = 4.1 \text{ mL}$

3. $\dfrac{45 \text{ mg}}{50 \text{ mg}} \times 1 \text{ mL} = 0.9 \text{ mL}$

4. $\dfrac{75 \text{ mg}}{500 \text{ mg}} \times 100 \text{ mL} = 15 \text{ mL}$

5. $\dfrac{200 \text{ µg}}{5 \text{ mg}} \times 1000 \times 5 \text{ mL} = 0.2 \text{ mL}$

6. 0.5 mg = 0.5 × 1,000 = 500 µg
   Available 250 µg/mL
   $\dfrac{500 \text{ µg}}{250 \text{ µg}} \times 1 = 2 \text{ mL}$

■ PERCENTAGE CALCULATIONS

Drug calculations are not always measured by mg or µg per mL. Drug dosages can also be prescribed in % (w/v).

% means the number of grams dissolved in 100 mL of solution, i.e., 1 % (w/v) = 1 g in 100 mL.

Example:
1. Glucose 5% (w/v) means that 5 g of glucose is contained in 100 mL solution.
2. A child is prescribed 5 g of mannitol; you have a 20% (w/v) solution. How many mL do you need?
   20% (w/v) = 20 g in 100 mL.
   5 ÷ 20 × 100 mL = 25 mL

Answer the Following Questions

1. What volume of 20% (w/v) potassium chloride injection contains 3 g of potassium chloride?

2. Potassium chloride 2 g is prescribed. It is to be added to a 1 liter bag of sodium chloride 0.9%. The ampoules are 20% (w/v). What volume do you add to the bag?
3. What concentration in mg/mL is 8.4% (w/v) sodium bicarbonate?
4. What concentration in µg/mL is 4.2% (w/v) lidocaine ?

Answers

1. 15 mL
2. 10 mL
3. 84 mg/mL
4. 42,000 µg

Solutions

1. 20% (w/v) KCl = 20 g in 100 mL
   3 g = ?
   $\dfrac{3}{20} \times 100 = 15$ mL

2. Ampoules are 20% (w/v) =
   20 g in 100 mL
   2 g = ?
   $\dfrac{2}{20} \times 100 = 10$ mL

3. $NaHCO_3$ = mg/mL
   8.4% w/v = 8.4
   8.4 mg in 100 mL = 8.4 x 100 = 8.4 mg

4. Lidocaine = µg/mL = 4.2% (w/v)
   4.2% (w/v) = 4.2 mg
   4.2 mg in 100 mL = 42 mg
   42 × 1,000 = 42,000 µg

■ RATIO CALCULATION

Ratio calculations are essential for measuring the concentration of drugs such as adrenaline. It is stated as 1 in 100, 1 in 10,000, etc.

> One in something concentrations means grams in mL, i.e.,
> 1 in 100 means 1 g in 100 mL
> 1 in 1,000 means 1 g in 1000 mL
> 1 in 10,000 means 1 g in 10,000 mL

Example: Give 1 mg of adrenaline using:
1 in 10,000 injection
1 in 10,000 = 1 g in 10,000 mL
 = 1,000 mg in 10,000 mL
What you want = 1 mg
What you got = 1,000 mg
Volume it is in = 10,000 mL
1 ÷ 1,000 × 10,000 = 10 mL

Chapter 12: Pediatric Drug Calculation | 109

Answer the Following Questions

1. Give 5 mg of adrenaline using 1 in 1,000 injection.
2. Give 0.5 mg of adrenaline using 1 in 10,000 injection.
3. A newborn weighing 2 kg requires 30 µg/kg of 1 in 10,000 of adrenaline.
4. A child weighing 12 kg requires 10 µg/kg of 1 in 10,000 of adrenaline.
5. A child weighing 19 kg requires 100 µg/kg of 1 in 1,000 of adrenaline.

Answers

1. 5 mL
2. 5 mL
3. 0.6 mL
4. 1.2 mL
5. 1.9 mL

Solutions

$$\frac{\text{What you want}}{\text{What you got}} \times \text{Volume it is in}$$

1. 1 in 1,000 = 1 g in 1,000 mL
   = 1,000 mg in 1,000 mL
   What you want = 5 mg
   What you got = 1,000 mg
   Volume in it is 1,000 mL
   $$\frac{5}{1,000} \times 1,000 = 5 \text{ mL}$$

2. 1 in 10,000 mL = 1 g in 10,000 mL
   = 1,000 mg in 10,000 mL
   What you want = 0.5 mg
   What you got = 1,000 mg
   Volume in it is = 10,000 mL
   $$\frac{0.5}{1,000} \times 10,000 = 5 \text{ mL}$$

3. 1 in 10,000 = 1 g in 10,000 mL
   = 1,000 mg in 10,000 mL
   = 1,000,000 µg in 10,000 mL
   Newborn weight = 2 kg
   Requires = 30 µg/kg
   = 30 × 2 = 60 µg
   What you want = 60 µg
   What you have = 1,000,000 µg
   Volume in it is = 10,000 mL
   $$\frac{60}{1,000,000} \times 10,000 = 0.6 \text{ mL}$$

4. 1 in 10,000 = 1 g in 10,000 mL
   = 1,000 mg in 10,000 mL
   = 1,000,000 µg in 10,000 mL
   Child weight = 12 kg
   Requires = 10 µg/kg
   = 12 × 10
   = 120 µg/kg

   $\dfrac{120}{1,000,000} \times 10,000 = 1.2$ mL

5. 1 in 1,000 = 1 g in 1,000 mL
   = 1,000 mg in 1,000 mL
   = 1,000,000 µg in 1,000 mL
   Child weight = 19 kg
   Requires = 100 µg/kg
   = 19 × 100 µg
   = 1,900 µg

   $\dfrac{1,900 \text{ µg}}{1,000,000} \times 1,000 = 1.9$ mL

POINTS TO NOTE

- There are wide variations in the actual weight of a child of a given age compared to the average weight for a child of that age. Consequently dosages are usually calculated according to body weight. In more complex situations dosages are based on body surface area, for example in chemotherapy.
- Body surface area can be determined using the body weight and height of a child. When dealing with an infant (a child aged less than 1 year) body weight and length are used.
- Body surface area determines the loss of fluid from the body by evaporation. This fluid loss is critical in the case of some medications and this is when body surface area is used in a calculation, rather than weight.
- The prescription should specify whether to use weight or body surface area.

PRACTICE QUESTIONS

1. 2 g = how many mg?
   2,000 mg
2. 250 mL = convert into liters
   0.25 L
3. 500 mg = how many grams?
   0.50 g
4. A 10-year-old child needs fluconazole. The dosage is 10 mg/kg and the child weighs 25 kg. What is the dose required?
   250 mg

MULTIPLE CHOICE QUESTIONS

1. Your patient needs 2,000 mL of saline IV over 4 hours for a patient with hypovolemia. How many milliliters per hour will you set on a controller?
   a. 500 mL/hr
   b. 250 mL/hr

c. 5000 mL/hr
d. 50 mL/hr

Solution : Total infusion volume (mL) = 2,000 mL
Total infusion time = 4 hours

Computation:

$$\frac{2,000 \text{ mL}}{4 \text{ hours}} = 500 \text{ mL/hour}$$

2. A patient is ordered to receive 1,000 mL of NSS to be administered at 125 mL/hour. How many hours will pass before you change the IV bag?
   a. 4 hours
   b. 12 hours
   c. 8 hours
   d. 10 hours

Solution: Total volume to infuse = 1,000 mL, Volume infused per hour = 125 mL/hour

Calculation:

$$\frac{1,000 \text{ mL}}{125 \text{ mL/ hours}} = 8 \text{ hours}$$

ANSWER KEY

1. a   2. c

CHAPTER 13

Oral Rehydration Therapy (ORT)

PRACTICE COMPETENCIES
On completion of the chapter, the students will be able to:
- Assess severity of dehydration as well as prescribe and supervise oral rehydration therapy to treat the following nursing diagnosis: fluid imbalance, less than body requirements, related to diarrhea.
- Prevent dehydration.
- Prevent morbidity and mortality due to acute diarrheal diseases.

ABSTRACT
Diarrheal disease is one of the leading causes of worldwide morbidity and mortality, especially in children. It causes loss of body fluid, which may lead to severe dehydration, electrolyte imbalance, shock and even to death. The mortality rate from acute diarrhea has decreased over the last few decades. This decline, especially in developing countries is largely due to the implementation of the standard World Health Organization-oral rehydration solution (WHO-ORS). However, the use of standard ORS has been limited by its inability to reduce fecal volume or diarrhea duration. ORT is the giving of fluid by mouth to prevent and/or correct the dehydration that is a result of diarrhea. As soon as diarrhea begins, treatment using home remedies to prevent dehydration must be started. If adults or children have not been given extra drinks, or if in spite of this dehydration does occur, they must be treated with a special drink made with oral rehydration salts (ORS).

Keywords: Oral rehydration therapy, diarrhea, children, dehydration.

DEFINITION
Oral rehydration therapy (ORT) is a type of fluid replacement used to prevent and treat dehydration, especially that due to diarrhea. ORT is an effective alternative to intravenous therapy. It involves drinking water with modest amounts of sugar and salts, specially sodium and potassium. Oral rehydration therapy can also be given by a nasogastric tube.

RECOMMENDED HOME FLUIDS
- Breast milk
- Cow milk
- Cereal based gruel
- Soup
- Yogurt

- Whey
- Rice water
- Fresh fruit juice
- Plain water with food

Components

1. Sodium chloride 2.6 g/L
2. Glucose anhydrous 13.5 g/L
3. Potassium chloride 1.5 g/L
4. Tri-sodium citrate dihydrate 2.9 g/L.

■ HOW TO PREPARE ORS?

- Wash your hands with soap and water
- Measure 1 liter of clean water. It is best to boil and cool the water before use but if this is not possible use clean drinking water available
- Pour all the powder from one packet of ORS into a clean container
- Pour the water into the container. Mix well with a clean spoon until the powder is dissolved
- Taste the solution so that you would know its taste like salt
- Then give the child frequent small sips out of a cup or spoon. If the child vomits, wait for 5–10 minutes, then continue giving ORS slowly
- Mix fresh ORS each day in a clean container. Keep the container covered.

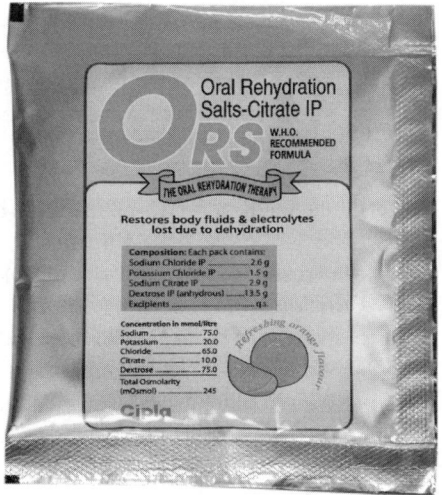

Fig. 13.1: Oral rehydration salts packet.

Standard protocol for oral replacement therapy in levels of dehydration:

- **Mild dehydration (standard replacement)**
  - Total ORS: 50 mL/kg over 4 hours by syringe, spoon or cup
  - Give 1 mL/kg of ORS by syringe every 5 minutes for 4 hours or
  - Give 3 mL/kg of ORS every 15 minutes for 4 hours
- **Moderate dehydration (accelerated replacement)**
  - Total ORS: 100 mL/kg over 4 hours or WHO age and weight specific recommendations
    - Weight <5 kg (age <4 months): 200–400 mL in 4 hours (50–100 mL/h or 2–3 oz/h)
    - Weight 5–8 kg (age 5–12 months): 400–600 mL in 4 hours (100–150 mL/h or 3–5 oz/h)
    - Weight 8–11 kg (age 12–24 months): 600–800 mL in 4 hours (150–200 mL/h or 5–7 oz/h)
    - Weight 11–16 kg (age 2–5 years): 800–1,200 mL in 4 hours (200–300 mL/h or 7–10 oz/h)
    - Weight 16 to 30 kg (age 5 to 15 years): 1,200–2,200 mL in 4 hours (300–550 mL/h or 10–18 oz/h)
    - Weight >30 kg (age >15 years): 2200–4000 mL in 4 hours (550–1000 mL/h or 18–33 oz/h)
  - *Infant example: 200–400 mL in 4 hours*
  - Give >50 mL (~2 oz) per hour of ORS
  - Give 5–10 mL (1–2 tsp) every 5 minutes

Toddler example (age 2): 600-800 mL in 4 hours
- Give >150 mL (5 oz) per hour of ORS
- Give 15-30 mL (0.5-1 oz or 1-2 tbs) every 5-10 minutes

Preschool child example (age 4): 800-1200 mL in 4 hours
- Give >200 mL (~7 oz) per hour of ORS
- Give 30-45 mL (1-1.5 oz or 2-3 tbs) every 5-10 minutes

❖ Severe dehydration failing oral rehydration with reassessment every 1-2 hours (WHO protocol)
  - Caution, this WHO protocol is very high volume (adjust per clinical situation, illness severity)
  - Age <12 months: LR 30 mL/kg IV over 1 hour, then 70 mL/kg IV over 5 hours
  - Age >12 months: LR 30 mL/kg IV over 30 min, then 70 mL/kg IV over 2.5 hours

❖ Ongoing losses (added replacement per stool or emesis)
  - Method 1: Give an additional 10 mL/kg per stool or 2 mL/kg per emesis, or
  - Method 2: Give an additional one-half to one cup ORS per stool (older children)
  - Method 3: Replace for each episode of diarrhea or vomiting
    - Age <2 years or weight <22 pounds: Give 60-120 mL (2-4 oz)
    - Age 2-10 years or weight >22 pounds: Give 120-240 mL (4-8 oz)
    - Age >10 years may drink as much as they wish up to 20 mL/kg/hour total
    - Vomiting
  - Pause feeding for 30-60 minutes if vomiting occurs
  - Give 5-10 mL every 5 minutes
  - May resume above diarrheal replacement after no Vomiting for 30-60 minutes
  - Consider Ondansetron (Zofran) 4 mg ODT tablets
    - Weight 8-15 kg (17-33 lb): Ondansetron 2 mg (half tab)
    - Weight 15-30 kg (33-66 lb): Ondansetron 4 mg (one tab)
    - Weight >30 kg (>66 lb): Ondansetron 4-8 mg (4 mg is typically sufficient)

Management

a. Assess the degree of dehydration, mild 5%, moderate 10%, severe 15%
b. Investigation is needed in sever and complicated cases
c. Withdrawal of feeding may delay the recovery
d. Breastfeeding should be continued
e. ORS for children under two, quarter to half following each loose bowel movement and older children a half to full cup. In addition, adding zinc supplements.
   - ORS should be begun at the beginning of diarrhea in order to prevent dehydration.
   - Infants may be given one teaspoon every 1-2 minutes (we can use either dropper or a syringe).
   - Older children should take frequent sips of a cup.
   - Uses of ORS decreases the risk of death from diarrhea by about 93%.
f. IV fluids is indicated in sever type.
g. Antibiotic according to general stool examination.

Clinical Assessment of Dehydration

❖ Mild dehydration:
  - Lose body weight 5%
  - Thirst

- Dry mouth
- Decrease urine output
❖ Moderate dehydration:
  - Lose of body weight 10%
  - We will find two or more of the following features:
    - Restlessness (irritability).
    - Sunken eyes.
    - Thirsty and drinks eagerly.
❖ Severe dehydration:
  - Lose of body weight 15%
  - We will find two or more of the following features:
    - Abnormally sleepy (lethargic).
    - Sunken eyes.
    - Drinking poorly or not at all.
    - Pinch test (skin turgor): The skin fold is visible for longer than 2 seconds.

Additional signs of severe dehydration include:
❖ Circulatory collapse (weak rapid pulse and hypotension and blue extremities)
❖ Rapid breathing (air hunger)
❖ Sunken anterior fontanelles

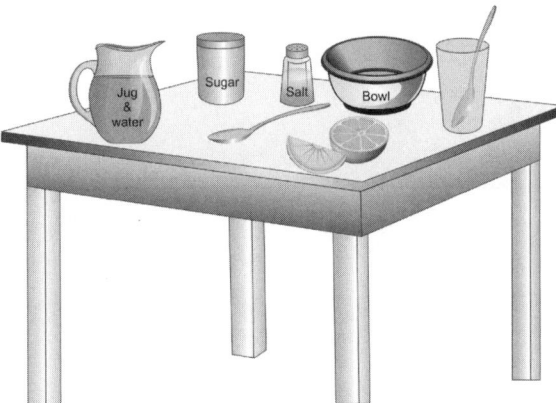

Fig. 13.2: ORS preparation at home.

If ORS packet is not available at home:
❖ Wash hands
❖ Take 250 mL water in a glass (take boiled and cooled water if clean and chlorinated water is not available).
❖ Add 1 pinch of salt made up of two fingers and thumb into it. Stir it well with spoon.
❖ After adding salt in water taste it, it should be like tears, if it is not, discard it and make it again.
❖ Then add 1 spoon of sugar by leveling it with the finger.
❖ Add 2 drops of lemon into it and stir it well with spoon.
❖ After mixing it properly stain it with strainer in another glass.
❖ Give the preparation to the child as per the requirement.
❖ Use its within 24 hours. Discard if it is not consumed within 24 hours.

Chapter 13: Oral Rehydration Therapy (ORT)

> **POINTS TO NOTE**
> - Oral rehydration therapy (ORT) is an effective form of treatment for dehydration caused by gastroenteritis.
> - ORT is an effective alternative to intravenous therapy and can be given in a range of settings.
> - Oral rehydration solution (ORS) can be bought in stores in a pre-mixed bottle or packaged powder.
> - ORS should be given in small, frequent amounts.
> - If your child's dehydration or sickness does not improve with ORT, take them to the hospital for assessment.

■ MULTIPLE CHOICE QUESTIONS

1. Following are the contents of ORS, *except:*
   a. Sodium chloride
   b. Sugar
   c. Potassium chloride
   d. Calcium carbonate
2. A freshly prepared ORS should not be used after:
   a. 24 hours
   b. 12 hours
   c. 6 hours
   d. 4 hours
3. Oral rehydration solution (ORS) is used to treat:
   a. Jaundice
   b. Diarrhea
   c. Typhoid
   d. Plague

ANSWER KEY

1. d   2. a   3. b

CHAPTER 14

Empowering Parents on Prevention of Malnutrition in Children

PRACTICE COMPETENCIES
On completion of the chapter, the students will be able to:
- Teach about nutritional requirements, and plan an eating program that includes high-calorie, high-protein foods and supplements and reflects her food preferences.
- Encourage small, frequent meals. Encourage to keep a food intake diary. Teach strategies to reduce risks for infection.
- Educate patients about the nutritional content of food and how to make healthy choices.
- Address patient nutritional needs by conducting screenings, performing assessments and administering interventions.

ABSTRACT
Addressing malnutrition requires enhanced knowledge on good nutrition and care practices for parents and caregivers, focusing on both prevention and treatment of cases. They also promote the use of locally-available foods with rich nutrient contents, for complementary feeding, following the six months of exclusive breastfeeding. Consequently, uptake and practice of information on prevention of malnutrition will reduce childhood morbidity and mortality related to malnutrition and infectious diseases. With increased knowledge and optimal care, malnutrition can be prevented or rapidly managed, for every child.

Keywords: Parents, feeding, weaning, child.

All parents should know how to prevent malnutrition from recurring. Before the child is discharged, ensure that the parents or care givers understand the causes of malnutrition and how to prevent its recurrence, including correct feeding and continuing to stimulate the child's mental and emotional development. They must also know how to treat or obtain treatment for, diarrhea and other infections and understand the importance of regular treatment for intestinal parasites. The parents have much to learn; teaching them should not be left until a few days before the child is discharged.

The mother should spend as much time as possible at the nutrition rehabilitation center with her child. This may be facilitated by providing the mother with money for transportation and meals. The mother, in turn, should help prepare her child's food and feed and look after her child. A rotation of mothers may also be organized to help with general activities on the ward, including play, cooking, feeding, bathing and changing the children, under supervision. This will enable each mother to learn how to care for her child at home; she will also feel that she is contributing to the work of the center. Teaching of mothers should include regular sessions at which important parenting skills are demonstrated and practiced. Each mother should be taught the play activities that are appropriate for her child, so that she and others in the family can continue to make toys and play with the child after discharge.

The staff must be friendly and treat the mothers as partners in the care of the children. A mother should never be scolded, blamed for her child's problems, humiliated or made to feel unwelcome. Moreover, helping, teaching, counseling and befriending the mother are an essential part of the long-term treatment of the child.

■ TEACHING MOTHERS/PARENTS: FEEDING AND WEANING

Weaning is a process by which food other than breast milk is introduced gradually into the baby's diet first to complement the breast milk and then to replace it with thicker feeds.

Weaning practices are vulnerable to social pressures. Majority of nutritional problems in rural areas are due to faulty weaning practices.

When to Start?
a. Child is above 6 months of age
b. Child weighs 7 kg

What to Give?

There are many weaning foods advised and available. Commercially available Frex, Ceralac, etc., have the advantage of palatability, convenience of preparation and fortification with vitamins and minerals. The disadvantage is the cost and improper use. Many mothers add a measure Farex to bottle of milk. This practice defeats the whole purpose of weaning. Mother gets the satisfaction of giving Farex but the child doesn't get the advantage of getting Farex. So Farex should not be used as a drink, it is to be given in form of a paste.

The ideal advice would be to take:
1. 2 tsp. cooked rice,
2. 2 tsp. cooked dal,
3. 2 tsp. cooked vegetables (before adding chili and spices).
4. A piece of roti.

Ground it to prepare a paste like *chutney*. It is to be given initially twice a day, then thrice a day and then quantity is increased gradually. For a malnourished or a child above 1 year age still not weaned, 2 tsp of groundnut powder and 2 tsp of milk powder is to be added.

This preparation overcomes the social, cultural, financial and nutritional restraints of successful weaning. There will not be any protein gap or food gap.

As a rule after 1 year, child should be offered full family diet.

Problems of Weaning: With Child

Infections, malnutrition and refusal to accept food are major problems. Proper weaning advice can prevent infections and malnutrition. If a child doesn't accept food, following are the possibilities.

1. As yet he does not know it is a food. Within weeks of starting it, child will develop a liking.
2. He doesn't like taste or appearance of particular preparation
3. Child is being forced or rushed through a feed

4. Food is too hot
5. He wants to drink first
6. He is not hungry
7. He is uncomfortable due to heat, cold or a wet napkin
8. He wants his favorite cup or dish
9. He wants to feed himself.

Problems with Parent

Parents just do not know that child needs food. The religious ceremony required for starting food is many times postponed. Either parents don't get time or there is no motivation to perform the ceremony. "starting food ceremony should be performed in sixth months".

CONCLUSION

Exclusively breastfeeding for first six months, timely and adequate supplementation, maintaining breast milk long enough to ensure its replacement by a safe and nutritious diet and discouraging a bottle are therefore extremely important measures to ensure a healthy start in life.

POINTS TO NOTE

- Breastfeeding within the first hour of life, is vital to the survival of children.
- Exclusive breastfeeding in the first six months of life makes children healthier.
- Solid foods and mother's milk after six months of age help infants grow quickly and strong.
- The right foods-in quantity and quality-fed frequently from 6 to 24 months ensure optimal growth and development.
- Good hygiene and clean hands keep young children healthy and strong.
- Iron and vitamin A supplementation and deworming protect young children from diseases and anemia.
- Nutritious foods given frequently during and after illness are necessary for the child's recovery.
- Life-saving food and care given at the right time save severely—undernourished children.
- Improving the nutrition of adolescent girls today secures the nutrition of children tomorrow.
- Better nutrition, particularly during pregnancy and lactation is essential to women's health.

PRACTICE QUESTION

1. Prepare health education plan for weaning an infant.

MULTIPLE CHOICE QUESTIONS

1. Which of the following is essential to include in a malnutrition care plan?
   a. Patient preferences
   b. Treatment goals
   c. Prescribed treatment or intervention
   d. All of the above
2. Which of the following is true regarding a nutrition assessment?
   a. All admitted patients should receive a nutrition assessment
   b. The assessment should utilize a standardized tool
   c. The assessment should be led by a nurse or nurse practitioner
   d. Limited patient/family caregiver involvement should be required

3. How soon should the implementation of a malnutrition care plan begin once a patient is diagnosed as malnourished or at risk for malnutrition?
   a. Within 48 hours following creation of the malnutrition care plan
   b. Within 24 hours following creation of the malnutrition care plan
   c. Immediately following creation of the malnutrition care plan
   d. Within 12 hours following creation of the malnutrition care plan

ANSWER KEY

1. d   2. b   3. c

CHAPTER 15

Empowering Parents on Immunization

PRACTICE COMPETENCIES
On completion of the chapter, the students will be able to:
- Educate parents about early childhood vaccination on vaccination status and improve parental knowledge, attitudes and intention to vaccinate.
- Perform Immunization as per the universal immunization program (UIP).
- Prevent communicable diseases and improve the survival of children by vaccinating the children.

ABSTRACT
The ultimate goal of immunization is to reduce the incidence of vaccine preventable diseases by attaining high levels of routine immunization coverage with potent vaccines administered at the appropriate ages and at the right intervals. Knowledge of mothers needs to be enhanced by educating through healthcare provider. They should have adequate knowledge and positive attitude towards immunization

Keywords: Immunization, vaccine, children.

INTRODUCTION

Immunization is the process by which an individual's immune system becomes fortified against an agent.

DO'S AND DON'TS DURING IMMUNIZATION

Difference between do's and don'ts during immunization is summarized in **Table 15.1**.

Table 15.1: Difference between do's and don'ts during immunization.

Do's	Don'ts
• DO attempt to feed a whole-foods diet free of processed foods and white sugar for your child. Preferably always, but definitely the weeks prior to scheduled vaccination. • DO administer the chosen vaccines apart from each other. Give as few together as possible (I'm not talking injection, I'm talking vaccine). Limit the use of 'live' viruses given together. • DO ask the nurse to pull the shot from the vials in front of you. BE SURE if they are multi-dose vials, that she SHAKES it well before pulling it up (This disperses the preservatives throughout the vial so it doesn't all end up in your kids body).	• DO NOT give a fever-reducer before or after vaccination, simply to comfort your child's pain or reduce a low-grade fever. The vaccine doesn't work as well when this is done. • DO NOT give your child a vaccine that they have previously reacted too. If you've given them together and aren't sure which one caused the reaction, proceed very cautiously. There is a reason they reacted to it and often subsequent reactions are more severe.

Do's	Don'ts
• DO give your child Vacci Shield prior to vaccination. This combination supplement will help support and fortify your child's immune system. • DO proceed very carefully if your child shows signs of a compromised immune system, chronic problems such as asthma, eczema, allergies, developmental delays or constant infections. • DO proceed very carefully if your child was born via C-section and not breastfed. Their beneficial gut-flora may be compromised.	• DO NOT get ANY vaccine for your child while they are sick. It does not matter what the office may say.

IMMUNIZATION SCHEDULE, SOURCE—WHO 2013

Vaccine	When to give	Dose	Route	Site
For pregnant women				
TT-1	Early in pregnancy	0.5 mL	IM	Upper arm
TT-2	4 weeks after TT-1	0.5 mL	IM	Upper arm
TT-booster	If received 2 doses in pregnancy within the last 3 years	0.5 mL	IM	Upper arm
For infants				
BCG	At birth	0.5 mL until 1 month of age	Intradermal	Left upper arm
Hepatitis-B	At birth within 24 hours	0.5 mL	IM	Anterolateral of mid-thigh
OPV-0	At birth within 15 days	2 drops	Oral	Oral
OPV-1, 2, 3	At 6,10,14 weeks	2 drops	Oral	Oral
DPT-1, 2, 3	At 6,10,14 weeks	0.5 mL	IM	Anterolateral of mid-thigh
Hepatitis-B 1, 2, 3	At 6,10,14 weeks	0.5 mL	IM	Anterolateral of mid-thigh
Pentavalent-****1, 2, 3	At 6,10,14 weeks	0.5 mL	IM	Anterolateral of mid-thigh
Measles-1	9–12 months	0.5 mL	Subcutaneous	Right upper arm
JE-1 **	At completed 12 months	0.5 mL	Subcutaneous	Left upper arm
Vitamin-A 1st dose	At 9 completed months with measles	1 mL (1 lakh IU)	Oral	Oral
For children				
DPT-1st booster	16–24 months	0.5 mL	IM	Anterolateral of mid-thigh
Measles- 2nd dose	16–24 months	0.5 mL	Subcutaneous	Right upper arm
OPV booster	16–24 months	2 drops	Oral	Oral
JE**	16–24 months	0.5 mL	Subcutaneous	Left upper arm
Vitamin-A *** dose (2nd -9th dose)	16 months then one dose every 6 months up to 5 years	2 mL (IU)	Oral	Oral
DPT-booster-2	5–6 years	0.5 mL	IM	Upper arm
TT	10–16 years	0.5 mL	IM	Upper arm

Note:
* Give TT-2 doses or Booster dose before 36 weeks of pregnancy. However, give these events if more than 36 weeks have passed. Give TT to a woman in labor, if she has not previously received TT.
** JE vaccine is introduced in selected endemic districts after the campaign.
*** The 2nd dose to 9th doses of vitamin A can be administered to children 1-5 years old during biannual rounds in collaboration with ICDS.
**** Pentavalent vaccine is introduced in place of DPT and Hep-B 1, 2, and 3 in selected states.

POINTS TO NOTE

- Parents can hold their child during vaccinations in recommended ways, which may reduce the child's stress and help healthcare professionals more easily administer shots.
- Prepare for your child's doctor vaccine visit and know what to do to support your child during and after your child is vaccinated.
- Help your child see vaccines as a good thing. Never threaten your child with shots by saying, "If you misbehave I will have the nurse give you a shot." Instead, remind children that vaccines can keep them healthy.
- Be honest with your child. Explain that shots can pinch or sting, but that it won't hurt for long.

PRACTICE QUESTIONS

1. What are the do's and don'ts during immunization?
2. Prepare health education plan on immunization schedule.

MULTIPLE CHOICE QUESTIONS

1. The vaccine which is administered as nasal spray is:
   a. Influenza
   b. Measles
   c. Poliomyelitis
   d. Rubella
2. Which of the following vaccine is a combined vaccine?
   a. MMR
   b. Smallpox vaccine
   c. Chickenpox vaccine
   d. Rotavirus vaccine
3. Pentavalent vaccine protects against:
   a. DPT, measles, rubella
   b. DPT, polio, hepatitis B
   c. DPT, polio, hepatitis A
   d. DPT, *Haemophilus influenzae*–B, hepatitis B

ANSWER KEY

1. a   2. a   3. d

CHAPTER 16

Urine Specimen Collection

PRACTICE COMPETENCIES
On completion of the chapter, the students will be able to:
- Perform the correct method of sample collection to ensure there is no contamination from external contact.
- Communicate effectively with patience and clear explanations to support children of all ages and their parents to cooperate with the task in hand.

ABSTRACT
Urinalysis, in which the components of urine are identified, is part of every client assessment at the beginning and during an illness. Clean urine samples are necessary to accurately diagnose several diseases in infants, especially urinary tract infections (UTIs). A wide range of clinical interventions for urine collection is described in the literature, including noninvasive and invasive methods. The most common noninvasive technique is urine collection using sterile bags, which is associated with significant patient discomfort and contamination of samples. Obtaining a clean catch urine sample is the recommended method for urine collection in children, who are able to cooperate. This chapter contains urine specimen collection from male and female children.

Keywords: Urine specimen collection, morning specimen, 24 hours urine specimen, clean catch urine specimen, test tube method.

DEFINITION

The urine specimen collection is a procedure used to obtain a sample of urine from a patient for diagnostic tests.

Purpose

The purpose of obtaining a urine sample is to test for any abnormalities that may be present, such as bacteria, ketones, or drugs.
- To determine the presence of microorganisms.
- To determine the type of organisms.
- The antibiotic which the organisms are sensitive.
- To assess progress.

GENERAL PRINCIPLES

1. Before collection of specimen
   a. The requested examination and the nature of specimen to be collected should be confirmed from doctors laboratory form.

b. Proper specimen container should be chosen.
   c. Label with required particulars should be attached, i.e.
      - Name
      - Registered number
      - Age
      - Unit
      - Ward
      - Name of the specimen and test to be done
      - Date and time of collection send.
2. During collection of specimen
   a. Routine specimen should be collected during laboratory working hours to prevent deterioration.
   b. For sterile specimen; to prevent contamination of specimen use straight container.
3. After collection specimen
   a. Date and time of collection should be entered on the form.
   b. The completed label should be attached to the body and not the lid of the container and upright position should be maintained.
   c. The written laboratory report should be attached to the record and informed the doctor.

Precautions

The skin of the genital area should be cleansed with a mild disinfectant to prevent contamination of the urine specimen or irritation of the delicate membranes of the area.

Types of Urine Specimen

Over the course of a 24-hour period, the composition and concentration of urine changes continuously. For this reason, various types of specimen may be collected, including:
- First morning specimen
- Single random specimen
- Timed short-term specimen
- Timed long-term specimen: 12 or 24 hours
- Catheterized specimen or specimen from an indwelling catheter
- Clean-catch (midstream) specimen for urine culture and cytological analyses.

First Morning Specimen

The first voided morning specimen is particularly valuable because it is more concentrated and abnormalities are easier to detect. An early morning specimen is also relatively free of dietary influences and changes due to physical activity.

Single Random Specimen

Single random specimen may be taken at any time of the day or night.

Timed Specimen

Timed specimen range from short-term 2-hours collections to 24-hours collections.

A 24-hour Urine Specimen

A 24-hour urine specimen is an extremely important diagnostic test because it reveals how the kidney adjusts to changing physiologic needs over a long period. Substances excreted by the

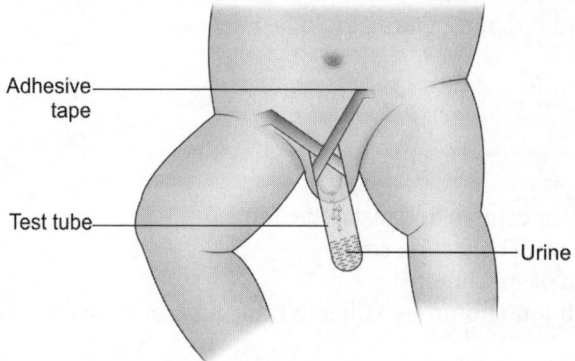

Fig. 16.1: Urine specimen collection—male infant.

kidney are not excreted at the same rate or in the same amounts during different periods of day and night; therefore, a random urine specimen does not accurately represent the processes taking place over a 24-hour period. However, a 24-hour urine specimen is useful only when all the patient's urine is collected for 24 hours. Even if just one sample is discarded, the results will be inaccurate. The nurse must ensure that the patient and all assistive personnel understand the importance of saving all the urine. To begin the 24-hour collection, the person first voids and discards the urine already present in the bladder.

All urine starting with the next voiding is collected for the next 24 hours and put into a large collection bottle. To prevent breakdown of urinary components, the collection has a preservative added to it or is refrigerated.

Bladder Catheterization

Bladder catheterization is employed when a specimen is urgently needed for or when the child is unable to avoid or otherwise to provide an adequate specimen.

Indwelling catheter will be placed in the bladder through urethra and collect the specimen.

Clean-Catch Urine Specimen

The term clean-catch specimen or midstream specimen traditionally refers to a urine sample obtained for culture after the urethral meatus is cleaned and the first few milliliters of urine is voided before the urine specimen collected.

Equipment needed for procedure:
- One clean tray containing
- Computer printed labels that have the patient's name and hospital ID number
- A bottle of hexachlorophene 3% (known as pHisoHex, a sudsing antibacterial skin cleanser)
- Sterile gauze sponges (4 × 4)
- Sterile water
- Sterile collection bottle
- Non-sterile gloves
- Mackintosh
- K-basin with paper.

IN ELDER CHILDREN

- ❖ Gather the necessary articles needed for the collection of urine specimen.
- ❖ Use visible aids if available to assist the client to understand the midstream collection technique.
- ❖ Explain to the client that urine specimen is required give the reason and explain the method of collecting the specimen.

For Male Child

- ❖ Give some sterile cloths along with the collection cup
- ❖ Explain child to wash their hands thoroughly, and wash the genital area and then wipe the head of penis with the cloths.
- ❖ Hold the specimen cup in one hand but be sure not to touch the inside of the cup or you will possibly contaminate the sample.
- ❖ Begin to urinate into the toilet. After a few seconds, without stopping the urine flow, collect the urine into the cup to the fill line.
- ❖ Then finish voiding the remainder of your urine into the toilet.
- ❖ Place the cap tightly on top of the specimen cup, and return the cup to your healthcare provider or lab assistant.

For Female Child

- ❖ Wash your hands thoroughly.
- ❖ Then sit on the toilet seat with your knees as far apart as is comfortable.
- ❖ Using one of the sterile cloths, cleanse the inner labia, wiping from front to back.
- ❖ Hold the specimen cup in one hand without touching the inside of the cup, and with the other hand, separate the lips of the labia as you begin to urinate.
- ❖ Urinate for a few seconds, and then collect urine into the specimen cup up to the fill line.
- ❖ Finish voiding the rest of your urine into the toilet.
- ❖ Replace the cap on top of the specimen cup, and return the cup to your healthcare provider or lab assistant.

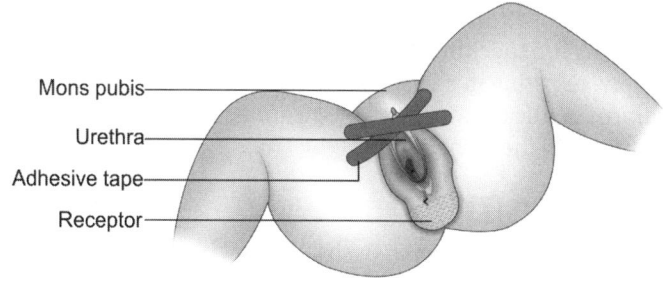

Fig. 16.2: Urine specimen collection—female infant.

IN AN INFANT

a. Collect the equipment
b. Explain the procedure to the mother
c. Cut a small thin strip of adhesive and line rim of test tube.

Test tube method of collecting urine from male infant:
- To use a test tube to collect urine, line the edges of the test tube with adhesive tape.
- Insert the penis in the tube and secure the adhesive tape to the pubis.
- The infant's legs should be restrained for safety.
- Place the infant in Fowler's position to aid the flow of urine by gravity.
- Remove the test tube by peeling the adhesive from the skin.
- Transfer the urine to a specimen bottle, label it and sent it to the laboratory.
- This method should be used only when plastic disposable urine collectors are not available.

Fixing the test tube by inserting the penis into the tube and stick the adhesive tape in cross over manner.

For Female Baby
- Take a square piece of adhesive cut an inch at four corner. Make a hole the center of the adhesive piece to pass and fix the container.
- Clean perineum with soap and water with clean towel or pad or clean the perineum with antiseptic lotion and dry it.
- Separate the labia majora, identify urethra and place the container over urethra.
- Fix adhesive superiorly over mons pubis inferiorly over perineum and laterally over the side of thighs.
- Restrain infant's legs for safety, if necessary.
- When child voids, remove the container gently and empty urine into specimen bottle.
- Label the bottle and send to laboratory.
- Record it in child's case sheet.

A piece of adhesive tape sticks over mons pubis, perineum, laterally over the sides of thighs with center hole to fix container.

Other two methods of urine collection:
- Collecting from diaper by squeezing technique
- Collecting from diaper by withdrawing with syringe.

Complications

If there is a delay in sending the specimen for testing, some organisms present in the urine may die while others multiply, resulting in a false reading.

Patients should inform medical staff of any medications currently being taken as elements of the drugs may be present in the urine.

NURSING RESPONSIBILITY
- Before feeding the baby, the collection bag should attach.
- Check for every 15 minutes to see baby has passed urine.
- Should not apply too tight nappy.
- Should not leave bag on baby for more than one hour.
- Should be discontinued if skin develops any symptoms of allergy.
- Discarding the bag by folding the two surfaces together and seal it.
- Put the label and send to lab within 30 minutes.

Chapter 16: Urine Specimen Collection

> **POINTS TO NOTE**
> - Throughout the preparation and during the procedure, someone should be available to catch some urine as the child may pass urine at any time during the process.
> - Do not collect samples from the drainage bag as these are likely to be stale and contaminated.

■ PRACTICE QUESTIONS

1. What are the general principles of urine specimen collection?
2. How do you collect a 24 hours urine collection?
3. How do you collect urine specimen in a female child?

■ MULTIPLE CHOICE QUESTIONS

1. The commonest cause of enuresis in children is:
   a. Urinary tract infection
   b. Spina bifida
   c. Psychological stress
   d. Diabetes mellitus
2. Which of these has the highest concentration in the urine?
   a. Glucose
   b. Sodium
   c. Uric acid
   d. Phosphate

ANSWER KEY

1. c   2. b

CHAPTER 17

Restraints

PRACTICE COMPETENCY

On completion of the chapter, the students will be able to:
- Assess and determine the need of a client to be restrained or secluded and they also assess the appropriateness of the type of restraint/safety device that is used in context with the client's current condition and behaviors; they assess and reassess the client in a regular and ongoing basis.

ABSTRACT

The terms 'restraint', 'therapeutic holding', 'clinical holding', 'holding' and 'immobilization' are all used when referring to restricting a child's movement. The Joint Commission on the Accreditation of Health Care Organizations (JCAHO, 2002), defines restraint as any physical or chemical method that restrict a person's movement, physical activity, or normal access to his or her body. Restraint is used to carry out a procedure, to which the child objects and usually involves preventing a child from moving for a period of time to prohibit interference with equipment or a procedure. This chapter contains jacket restraint, mummy restraint, elbow restraint, abdominal restraint and mitts.

Keywords: Hazards of restraints, mitts, abdominal restraint, extremity restraint, elbow restraint, mummy restraint, jacket restraint, restraints.

All infants and children's have physiologic and psychological needs to be mobile, prolonged immobility of children may result in physiological loss of muscular strength and flexibility. It also affect the physiological functioning of the body such as influencing the respiratory volume and peripheral circulation.

Psychologically long periods of restraints may result in the child's inability to develop motor and sensory contact with the surrounding environment. Restraints are necessary part of nursing children, but it must be the last resort.

DEFINITION

Restraints is a means of limiting physical movement of the child to facilitate examination, do a procedure or to prevent injury to the child.

Purposes

- To maintain safety of the child
- To facilitate physical examination and diagnostic procedures
- To allow healing of a part due to immobilization.

Precautions

- ❖ Restraints must be applied correctly to avoid circulating impairment and skin irritation.
- ❖ Adequately pad the restraint to protect the skin.
- ❖ Place the child in correct body alignment.
- ❖ Tie all restraints to the bed frames and not to side rails.
- ❖ Release restraints every 2–3 hours.
- ❖ Observe the child when restraints are released to avoid injury.

TYPES OF RESTRAINTS

Commonly used restraints for children include jacket restraint, mummy restraint, elbow restraint, extremity restraint, abdominal restraint, and crib with dome.

Jacket Restraint

It can be used to help the child remain flat in bed in a supine position to prevent the child falling from height.

The jacket is put on with the strings in the back, so that the child cannot reach them.

The main danger of the jacket restraint is that of strangulation through pressure of restraint that has supplied out of place and encircled a child's neck.

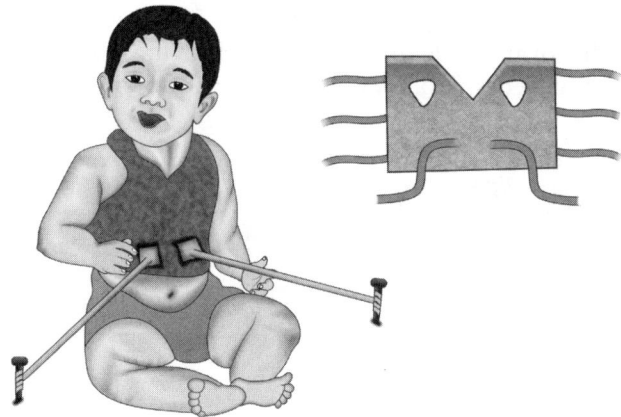

Fig. 17.1: Jacket restraint.
(*Source:* www.google.com)

Mummy Restraint

When the infant or small child requires short-term restraints for examination or treatment that involves the head and neck, when jugular venous puncture is to be done, when a scalp vein needle is to be inserted and during the gastric lavage and gavage is done.

Procedure

- ❖ A blanket or sheet is opened on the bed or crib with one corner folded to the center.
- ❖ The infant is placed on the blanket with the shoulders at the fold and feet toward the opposite corner.
- ❖ With the infants right arm straight down against the body, the right side of the blanket is pulled firmly across the infants right shoulder and chest and secured beneath the left side of the body.

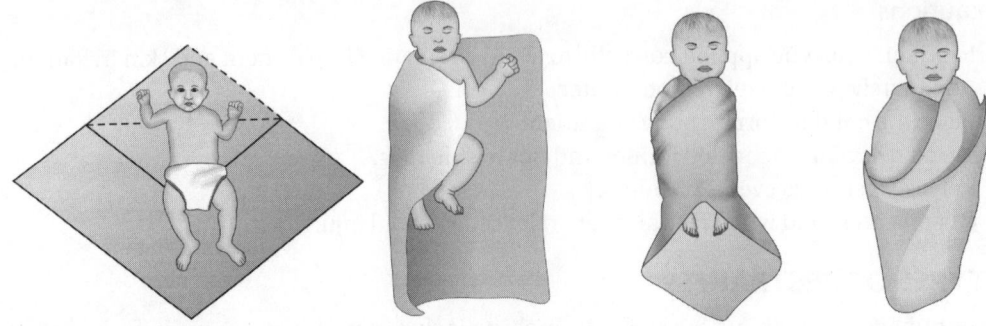

Fig. 17.2: Mummy restraint.

- The left arm is placed straight against the infant's side, and the left side of the blanket is brought across the shoulder and chest and locked beneath the infant's body on the right side.
- The lower corner is folded and brought over the body and tucked or fastened securely with safety pins.
- Safety pins can be used to fasten the blanket in place at any step in the process.

Modified Mummy Restraint

To modify the mummy restraint for chest examination, the folded edge of the blanket is brought over the body and each arm and under the back, after which the loose edge is folded over and secured at a point below the chest to allow visualization and access to the chest.

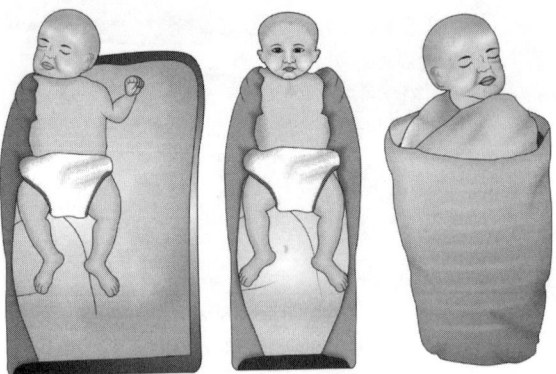

Fig. 17.3: Modified mummy restraint.

Elbow Restraint

Purpose

- This is used to hold the elbow in an extended position, so that the infant cannot reach the face.
- It is used in the head and facial surgeries, cleft palate repair, skin disorders (eczema) or scalp vein needle is in place.

Equipment

A piece of material with pockets to insert the tongue depressors.

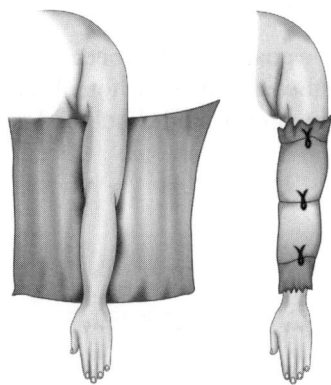

Fig. 17.4: Elbow restraint.

Procedure

- Insert tongue depressor into pockets.
- Pad arm with gown/cotton and wrap restraint around the arm.
- Pin it securely.
- Do not rub child's axilla or wrist.

Extremity Restraint

This may be used to immobilize one or more extremities. Clove hitch restraint is one type of extremity restraint.

Equipment

- 3–4 feet length of gauze folded lengthwise
- Padding material.

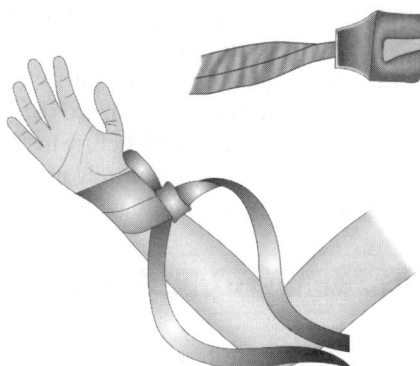

Fig. 17.5: Extremity restraint.

Procedure

- To apply the restraint, spread the gauze strip out on the bed with one end toward the nearer side of the bed.
- In the middle of the strip make a figure of eight.
- Place the gauze padding around the infant's wrist or ankle as necessary.
- Place the circles of the restraint around the padding on the extremity.
- Tie the ends of the gauze to the frame of the crib.
- Care must be taken to prevent the cutting of circulation.

Abdominal Restraint

It helps to hold the child in a supine position on the bed. It should be applied with precautions, so that respiratory movements of the abdomen are not inhibited. The strip of material is wider and has only one wide flap for fastening around child's abdomen.

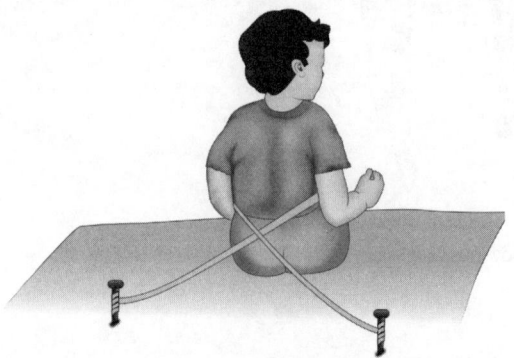

Fig. 17.6: Abdominal restraint.

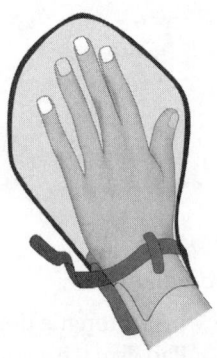

Fig. 17.7: Mitts restraint.

Mitts Restraint

Mitts are used for infants to prevent self-injury by hands in case of burns, facial injury or operations, eczema of the face or body. Mitten can be made wrapping the child's hands in gauze or with a little bag putting over the baby's hand and tie it on at the wrist.

HAZARDS OF RESTRAINTS

- ❖ Inappropriate use of restraints may cause injury to the brachial plexus, sore or gangrene, exhaustion and loss of energy, dislike for the hospital and health team members, etc.
- ❖ Prolonged immobility of children may result in physiologic loss of muscular strength and flexibility which influence the respiratory volume and peripheral circulation.
- ❖ Long periods of restraints may result psychological hazards and inability to develop motor and psychosocial skills in children. They may be difficulty in developing own body image.
- ❖ The nurse should use restraint only when it is absolutely necessary, remembering that all infants and children have physiologic and psychologic needs to be mobile.

POINTS TO NOTE

- ➤ Keep your child as comfortable as possible.
- ➤ Check your child's vital signs (temperature, pulse, breath, and blood pressure).
- ➤ Make sure your child is getting enough to eat and drink.
- ➤ Help your child go to the washroom when needed.

PRACTICE QUESTIONS

1. Define restraint.
2. What is a mummy restraint?
3. What do you mean by mitts restraint?
4. What are the hazards of restraints?

MULTIPLE CHOICE QUESTIONS

1. **General points for use of restraints:**
   a. Select appropriate, safe and comfortable restraint
   b. Restraint should be tight as possible
   c. Sufficient padding must be used for extremity restraint
   d. Restraint should not be very tight
2. **A 10-month-old child is recovering from a cleft lip repair, and the provider has determined the child would benefit from restraints postoperatively. Which kind of restraints would the nurse most likely apply to this child?**
   a. Jacket restraint
   b. Elbow restraint
   c. None, unless the child demonstrated being uncooperative
   d. Mummy restraint

ANSWER KEY

1. b   2. b

CHAPTER 18

Play Needs for Different Age Groups

PRACTICE COMPETENCIES

On completion of the chapter, the students will be able to:
- Select play material for different age groups.
- Utilize appropriate play material that helps physical, mental, emotional, and spiritual aspects of child along with social relationships.

ABSTRACT

Playing is integral to children's enjoyment for their lives, their health and their development. Children and young people, disabled and nondisabled: whatever their age, culture, ethnicity, or social and economic background, need and want to play indoors and outdoors, in whatever way they can. Through playing, children are creating their own culture, developing their own abilities, exploring their creativity and learning about themselves, other people and the world around them. Children need and want to stretch and challenge themselves when they play. Play provision and play space that is stimulating and exciting allows children to encounter and learn about risk. This helps them to build confidence, learn skills and develop resilience at their own pace. This chapter contains importance of play, functions of play, and types of play as per stages of development, types of play according to socialization, toy safety and selection of play materials for different age groups, therapeutic play during bed side care.

Keywords: Socioeffective play, sense pleasure play, play needs for children, skill play, dramatizing play, onlooker play, parallel play, solitary play, associative play, cooperative play, toys for different age group, therapeutic play.

INTRODUCTION

Play is a natural and most easily available outlet for children's expressions of needs and feelings. It is the necessary stimulation for optimal development and support for their natural curiosity.

Spontaneous play evolves from children's need for self-expression, mastery in the environment and integration of past and current experiences. Young children play with exhilaration and total enjoyment. A play is important for the children's physical, psychosocial and intellectual development.

Importance of Play

Through the medium of play, children learn what no one can teach them. They learn about their world and how to deal with this environment of objects, time, space, structure and people. They learn about themselves operating within the environment—what they can do, how to relate to things and situations and how to adopt themselves to the demands society makes on them. Play is the work of the child. In play, children continually practice the complicated, stressful processes of living, communicating and achieving satisfactory relationship with others.

FUNCTIONS OF PLAY

I. **Sensorimotor development:** Sensorimotor activity is a major component of play at all ages is the predominant form is infancy. Active play is essential for muscle development and serves as a useful purpose for the release of surplus energy
   - Infants gain impressions of themselves and their world through, tactile, auditory, visual and kinesthetic stimulation
   - Toddlers and preschoolers revel in body movements and explore things in space
   - Very young children, incorporate or modify the motions into increasingly complex and coordinated activities such as races, games, bicycle riding, etc.

II. **Intellectual development:** Through exploration and manipulation children learn colors, shapes, sizes, textures and the significates of objects.
   - They learn the significance of numbers and how to use them. They learn to associate words with objects
   - Activities such as puzzles and games help them develop problem solving skills
   - Books, stories and films expand knowledge and provide enjoyment as well
   - Play helps children comprehend the world in which they live and distinguish between fantasy and reality.

III. **Socialization:** From very infancy children show interest in pleasure in the company of others
   - Apart from their initial contact with their mother, by playing with other children, they learn to establish social relationships
   - They learn to give and take more from critical peers than from tolerant elders
   - They learn the sex role, that the society expects them to fulfill
   - Closely associated with socialization, is development of moral values and ethics
   - Children learn right from wrong.

IV. **Creativity:** In no other situation, there is more opportunity to be creative than play
   - Children can experiment and try out their ideas in play through every medium at their disposal
   - Creativity is stifled by pressure towards confirmity
   - Creativity is primarily a product of solitary activity yet, it is enhanced in group settings while listening to others ideas.

V. **Self-awareness:**
   - Beginning with active exploration of their bodies and awareness of themselves as separate from mother, the process of self-identity is facilitated through play activities
   - Children learn who they are and their place in the world
   - They regulate their own behavior and compare their behavior with that of others
   - They test their own abilities.

VI. **Therapeutic value:** Play is therapeutic at any age
   - It gives relief from tension and stress of the society and environment
   - Children are able to experiment and test fears and can assume and vicariously master the roles they are unable to perform in reality

- Children reveal much about themselves in play
- Through out the play, children need the acceptance of adults and their presence to help them control aggression and to channel their destructive tendencies.

VII. **Moral value:**
- Although children learn at home and at school, the behaviors in culture, interaction with peers during play contributes significantly to their moral training
- Children learn to be less tolerant of violations than adults, so, they confirm to the standards to stay in a group.

DEVELOPMENT ROLE OF PLAY

From the developmental point of view, patterns of children's play can be categorized according to content and social character.

At each stage in development a new behavior predominates.

Types of play according to the:
A. **Content of play:** The content of play involves primarily the physical aspects of play, although social relationships cannot be ignored. The content of play follows the directional trend of the simple to the complex.
B. **Socioeffective play:** Infant takes pleasure in relationship with people infant learns to provoke parental emotions and responses with behaviors as smiling, cooing or initiating games and activities to adults ways like talk, touch, nuzzle, etc.
C. **Sense pleasure play:**
   - Sense pleasure play is a non-social stimulating experience that originates from within
   - Objects in environment:
     - The light and color
     - Tastes and odors
     - Textures and consistencies, attract child attention, stimulates their senses and give pleasure
   - Pleasurable experiences are derived from handling raw materials (water, sand, food), from body motions (swinging, bouncing, rocking), from uses of senses and abilities (smelling, humming).
D. **Skill play:** After infants develop ability to grasp and manipulate they demonstrate and exercise their newly acquired skills by skill play, repeating action over and over again.
E. **Unoccupied behavior:** Children here are not playful but focus their attention momentarily on anything that strikes their interest.

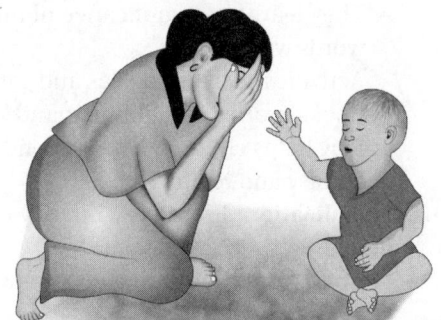

Fig. 18.1: Socioeffective play.

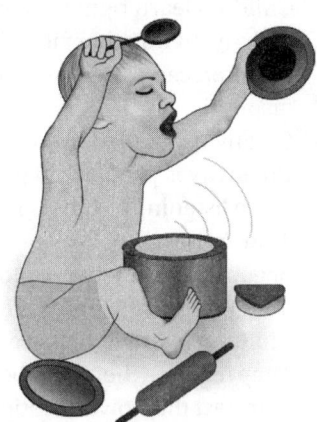

Fig. 18.2: Sense pleasure play.

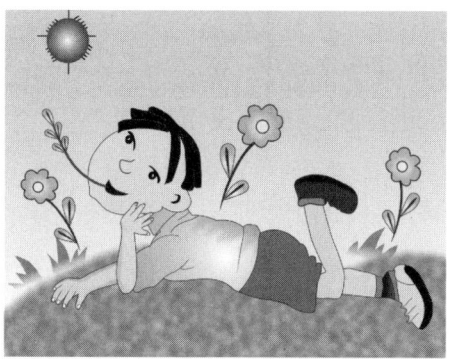

Fig. 18.3: Unoccupied play.

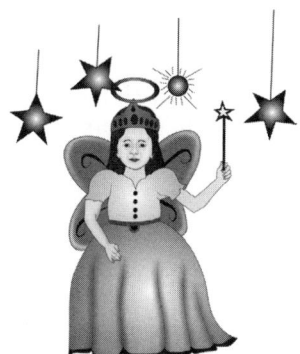

Fig. 18.4: Dramatic play.

Children day dream, fiddle with clothes or objects, or walk aimlessly.

The role differs from that of onlookers, who actively observe the activity of others.

F. **Dramating or pretend play:**
   - In children's process of identification, one of the vital elements is dramatic play, symbolic or pretend play
   - It begins in late infancy (11 to 13 months) and continues into preschool child
   - After they invest with situations and people with meanings, they can pretend and fantasize almost anything
   - By acting out events of daily life, children learn and practice the roles and identities of members of family and society
   - Toddler practices imitative, simple, dramatic plays like using a telephone, driving a car, rocking a doll, etc.
   - Older children work out elaborate themes, act out stories and compose plays.
G. **Games:** All girls and boys participate in sports during adolescents for fun. They learn to complete on same teams or against each other.

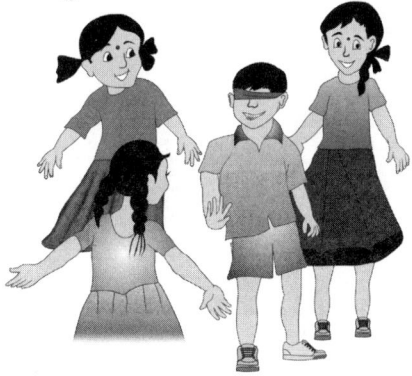

Fig. 18.5: Games in children.

■ TYPES OF PLAY ACCORDING TO SOCIALIZATION

The play interactions of infancy are between the child and an adult. Children continue to enjoy the company of an adult but are increasingly able to play alone. Through continued interaction, with peers and the growth of conceptual abilities and social skills, children are able to increase participation with others in the following types of play.

I. Onlooker Play

- Children watch other children's play but do not enter play activity
- There is an active interest in observing the interactions of others, but there is no movement towards participation. For example, watching an older sibling bounce the ball.

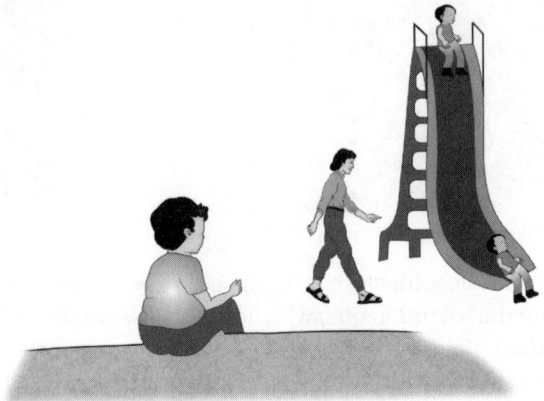

Fig. 18.6: Onlooker play.

II. Parallel Play

- Children play independently, but among other children
- They play with toys around them just as the toys with which other children around are playing
- They play beside, but not with other children
- There is no group association
- It is the characteristic play of toddlers, but may occur in other groups also
- Children working on creative craft with each person separately working on individual project engage in parallel play.

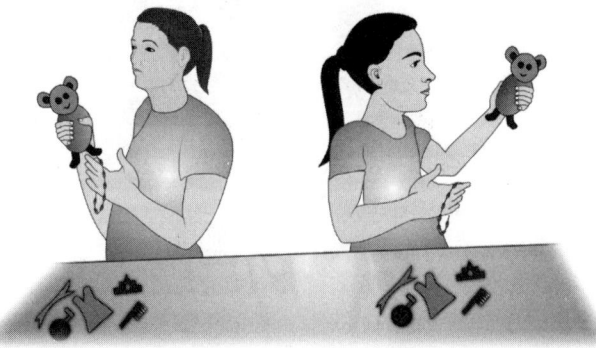

Fig. 18.7: Parallel play.

III. Solitary Play

- Children play alone with toys different from those used by other children in the same area
- They enjoy the presence of other children but make no effort to get closer to speak to them
- Their interest is centered on their own activity.

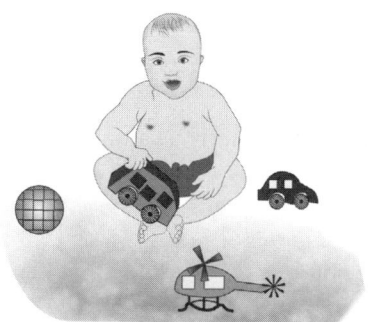
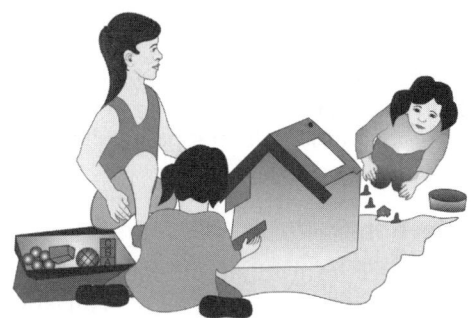

Fig. 18.8: Solitary play. **Fig. 18.9:** Associative play.

Associative Play

- Children play together and are engaged in similar or even identical activity, but there is no organization, division of labor, leadership or mutual goal
- Children borrow and lend play materials follow each other with wagons or tricycles
- Children act according to his/her own wish, e.g. two children with dolls borrowing articles of clothing from each other and engage in similar conversation, but neither controls others activities
- If one child initiates an activity, the entire group will follow the activity.

Cooperative Play

Cooperative play is organized and children play in a group with other children
- They discuss and plan activities for accomplishing an end
- For example, to make something:
  - To attain a competitive goal
  - To dramatize situation of adult or group life or, to play formal games
  - The group is loosely form but there is a marked sense of belonging
- Attainment of goal requires organization of activities, division of labor and playing roles
- Leader-follower relationship is established and activity is maintained by one or two members who assign roles to others
- One child will supplement others function to complete the goal.

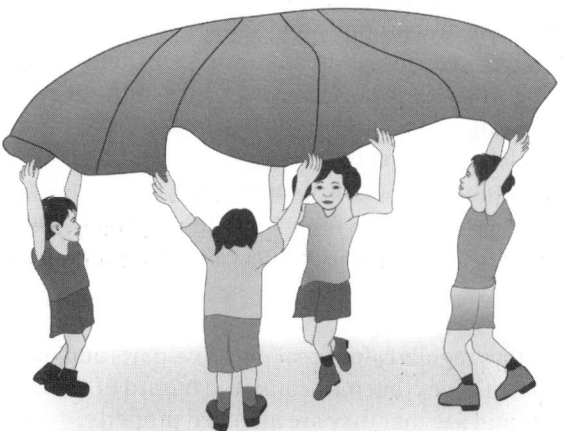

Fig. 18.10: Cooperative play.

TOY SAFETY

Selection of toys and play equipment is a joint effort between parents and children, but evaluating their safety is the responsibility of the adults.

As government did not pass policies and inspect the toy making properly, evaluating their safety must be careful.

Selection

- Select the toys that suit skills, abilities and interests of the child
- Select toys for specific age (as on label) that are safe.
- Toys good for one age group may not be safe for another.
  For example, for infants avoid toys with strings or cords that are 7" or longer as they may cause strangulation.
- For infants, toddlers and children who put objects in mouth. Avoid small parts that may pose fatal chocking or aspiration.
- For children less than 5 years avoid arrows or darts.
- For children younger than 8 years avoid electric joys with heating elements.
- Check for "flame retardant" or "flame resistant" labels.
- Select toys durable for rough play
- Look for tightly secured eyes, nose or any small parts
- Select light-weight toys, so that they may not harm, if they fall on children.
- Look for toys with smooth-rounded edges.
- Avoid toys with sharp points
- Avoid toys with shooting or throwing objects that can damage eyes.
- Arrows or darts which make loud noise and cause hearing damage.
- Check toy instructions for clarity.

Supervision

- Maintain safe play environment
- Remove and discard plastic toy wrappings immediately
- Remove large toys, bumper pads and boxes as children may use them for climbing.
- Set 'ground rules' to play
- Supervise young children closely during play
- Teach children how to use toys properly and safely
- Instruct older children to keep toys away from younger siblings or friends
- Keep children playing with toys away from stairs, hills traffic or swimming pools
- Insist children on wearing helmet during cycling or skating
- Instruct children on electrical safety
- Instruct the child to unplug the electrical toy properly
- Teach children use of safe utensils as under few circumstances they may cause injuries.
  For example, scissors, knives, needles, heating elements, loops, long strings or card.

Maintenance

- Inspect old and new toys regularly for breaking loose parts and potential hazards.
- Look for jagged or sharp edges that may cause the hazard of chocking.
- Check movable parts and see that they are attached properly.
- Maintain toys in good repair without rest, weak seams spinters or sharp edges.
- Sand sharp edges till they are smooth.

- Use only paint labeled "non-toxic".
- Check electrical cards and plugs for cracked and fraying parts.

Storage
- Provide a safe place for children to store toys.
- Select a toy-chest that is well ventilated and free of self-locking that could not trap a child inside and that has a lid designed not to pinch a child's finger or fall on child's head.
- Play things of elder children should be placed in high shelves out of reach for younger ones.

■ SELECTION OF PLAY MATERIALS FOR DIFFERENT AGE GROUPS

Infancy
Play during infancy represents the various social modalities observing during cognitive development. The activity in infancy revolves around their own body. Their body parts are the primary objects of play and pleasure.

    1 month—Independent play, quieting attitude
    2 months—Smile
    3 months—Squeal
    4 months—Loud laugh for toys, food
    6 month-1 year—Involves sensorimotor skills
    6 months—Extension of arms to be picked up
    7 months—Cough to make presence known
    10 months—Pull parent's clothes
    12 months—Calls by name.

Play Magnifies Infant's Visual, Auditory, Tactile and Kinetic Stimulation

Birth to 6 Months

Nursery mobiles, unbreakable mirrors, See through crib bumpers, Colored sheets	Visual stimulation
Music boxes, musical mobiles, crib dangle bells, small handled clear rattle	Auditory stimulation
Stuffed animals, soft clothes, soft or furry quilt, soft mobiles	Tactile stimulation
Rocking crib/cradle, weighted or suction toy, infant swing	Kinetic stimulation

6–12 Months

Various colored boxes, nested boxes or cups books with rhymes and bright pictures, strings of big beads, simple take apart toys, large ball, cups and spoon, large puzzles, jack-in-the box	Visual stimulation

Rattles of different sizes, shapes, tones and bright colors, squeaky animals and dolls, records with light rhythmic music } Auditory stimulation

Soft different texture animals and dolls, sponge toys, floating toys, squeeze toys, teething toys, books with textures, object like fur and zipper. } Tactile stimulation

Activity box for crib, push toys, pull toys, wind–up swings } Kinetic stimulation

Toddler

Play magnifies the toddler's physical and psychosocial development. Interactions with people becomes increasingly important.

- ❖ The toddler inspects the toy, talks to the toy, tests its strength and disability and invents several uses for it.
- ❖ Toys for boys: Trucks, carriages, trailers, men and logs.
- ❖ Toys for girls: Dolls, doll houses, dishes, cooking utensils, child-size furniture, dress-up clothes.
- ❖ Other plays: Push-pull toys,

Straddle trucks or cycles,
Small gym and slide,
Balls of various sizes. } For energetic toddlers

Rocking houses
Finger paints
Thick crayons, } For creative toddlers

Chalk, blackboard,
Paper and puzzle
Interlocking blocks

Age—appropriate tape players
Talking dolls and animals
Toy telephones
Children TV programs } For music lovers

Preschooler

Preschoolers enjoy associative play.

Their play includes,
- ❖ Jumping
- ❖ Running
- ❖ Climbing
- ❖ Tricycles
- ❖ Scooter trucks
- ❖ Wagons
- ❖ Gym and sports equipment
} For physical development

- ❖ Sand boxes
- ❖ Wading pools
- ❖ Winter sleds
- ❖ House/hold items like broom sticks, sand, etc.
- ❖ Easy construction sets
- ❖ Large blocks of various sizes and shapes
- ❖ Counting frame
- ❖ Alphabet frame
- ❖ Alphabet or numerical flash cards   } For fine-motor development
- ❖ Paints
- ❖ Crayons
- ❖ Simple carpentry tools
- ❖ Musical toys
- ❖ Illustrated books
- ❖ Simple sewing
- ❖ Handicraft sets
- ❖ Large puzzles and clay
- ❖ Electronic games and computer programs are especially valuable in helping children learn basic skills, such as letters and simple works.
- ❖ Toys that help in self-expression:
  - Dress up clothes
  - Dolls
  - Housekeeping toys
  - Doll houses
  - Playstore toys
  - Telephones
  - Farm houses
  - Village sets
  - Trains
  - Cars
  - Planes
  - Hand puppets
  - Doctor and nurse kits
  - Television
  - Video tapes.

School-age Child

Play taken on new dimensions that reflect a new stage of development in the school years. Their play includes:

- ❖ **Rules and rituals:** Childhood is full of chants and taunts such as "ringa-ringa roses", "eeeny, meeny, miney, mo", etc.
- ❖ **Team play:** All team games and sports with a referee so as to learn game properly.
- ❖ **Quite games and activities:** Board, card, computer games books, sewing, cooking, carpentry, gardening and creative activities like painting, music and art.
- ❖ **Athletic:** Skills like swimming, horse riding, dancing, skating, etc.

THERAPEUTIC PLAY DURING BEDSIDE CARE

Story telling: Before age 5 years story with themes about people who shut their eyes. Cover their ears, or left at door steps or thing that are missing or change appearance. Ages 5-10 years: Stories with themes about making things that last acquiring a skill that is competitive with others pleasing adults, other than parents.

Water play during bath: Blowing soap bubbles, filling and squeezing a both sponge, bathing a doll, playing with boats to bubble bath, washing clothes, sponge objects and other toys.

Television: Telling about programs, commercials, etc., use of closed circuit TV to present health teachings films and to provide lessons in finger charts.

Needle play: Handling empty syringe, IV tubing, etc., and pretending to give short to a dull, stuffed animal, parents or nurse. The nurse can demonstrate the method of giving on injection by drawing up the solution or water and squirting a bit into the air.

Art: Drawing with crayons on blank paper followed by discussing of what is drawn.

SUMMARY

Through this lesson we are able to acquire knowledge on play, importance of play, development in play activities, types of play and toy selection with different age groups and therapeutic use for play.

CONCLUSION

After going through this lesson, we can choose the kind of play to be adopted with different age groups, the toys to be selected, the care of toys, their maintenance and usage can be understood.

POINTS TO NOTE

There is no substitute for being with the children when they are playing. Supervision is as important as any other safety measure. Avoid impulse buying of toys because of ads in the mass media.

PRACTICE QUESTIONS

1. What are the functions of play?
2. How do you select toys for different age group children?
3. What is a therapeutic play?

MULTIPLE CHOICE QUESTIONS

1. The parents of a two-year-old boy arrive at a hospital for a visit. The child is in the play room when the parents arrive. When the parents enter the play room, the child does not readily approach the parents. The nurse interprets this behavior as indicating that:
   a. The child is withdrawn
   b. The child is self-centered
   c. The child has adjusted to the hospitalized setting
   d. This is a normal pattern

2. A nurse is preparing to care for a five-year-old who has been placed in traction following a fracture of the femur. The nurse plans care, knowing that, which of the following is the most appropriate activity for this child?
   a. Large picture books
   b. A radio
   c. Crayons and coloring book
   d. A sports video

ANSWER KEY

1. d   2. c

CHAPTER 19

Care of Child with Phototherapy

PRACTICE COMPETENCY

On completion of the chapter, the students will be able to:
- Provide nursing care to the patients on phototherapy.

ABSTRACT

Phototherapy is the use of visible light for the treatment of hyperbilirubinemia in the newborn. This is relatively common therapy lowers the serum bilirubin level by transforming bilirubin into water soluble isomers that can be eliminated without conjugation in the liver. The dose of phototherapy is a key factor in how quickly it works; dose in turn is determined by the wavelength of the light, the intensity of the light (irradiance), the distance between the light and the baby and the body surface area exposed to the light. Proper nursing care enhances the effectiveness of phototherapy and minimizes complications. Care giver responsibilities include ensuring effective irradiance delivery, maximizing skin exposure, providing eye protection, and eye care, careful attention to thermoregulation, maintaining adequate hydration, promoting elimination, and supporting parent: infant interaction.

Keywords: Phototherapy, jaundice, premature infants, serum bilirubin level, fluorescent tube lights, irradiation, phototherapy unit.

Purpose

To reduce serum bilirubin level.

Equipment

- Phototherapy machine with white and blue light
- Diaper to close the genitalia of the baby
- Eye bandage or pads to prevent eye damage of the baby.

Indications

- When there is an abnormal rise in the bilirubin level which may be due to physiological or pathological jaundice or any other problem.
- In severely bruised premature infants and who are likely to develop dangerous levels of bilirubin.
- In hemolytic disease of the newborn, phototherapy is used while the rise in the serum bilirubin level is plotted and while waiting for exchange transfusion. In such cases, phototherapy is started immediately at birth.

Contraindications

Do not give phototherapy for conjugated jaundice.

Set up of Phototherapy Unit

Phototherapy generally consists of four to eight cool white, day bright, or special blue fluorescent tube lights covered by a plastic shield and placed about 18 inches or 45 cm away from the baby. The spectrum of light at 420–460 nm is the most effective. The energy output in this spectrum should be checked periodically to ensure efficiency. The efficiency of phototherapy depends on energy output of the spectrum and on the surface area of the infant exposed to those lights. Though, blue lights are the most effective, they are not widely used because they mask the clinical signs of cyanosis and color change in the infant. White light permits better visual monitoring. The plastic shield absorbs ultraviolet irradiation. A photo reaction occurs in the very outer layers (to 2 mm) of the skin. Once phototherapy has been initiated, serum levels of bilirubin must be monitored frequently (every 4–12 hours).

Place the infant naked under the lights with shielding over the eyes. A small cloth may be placed for scrotum protection in male babies. The infant's position should be changed frequently. This permits maximal skin exposure to the lights. Make sure that baby is 18 inches or 45 cm away from light.

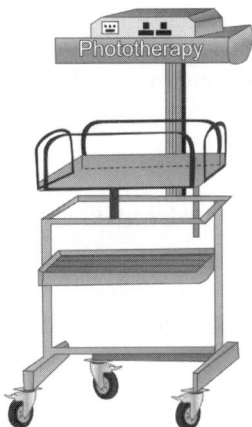

Fig. 19.1: Phototherapy unit.

Nurses Role

Check the lights of phototherapy unit before use and place it in a proper place.

Eye Care

Because of the potential for eye damage, the eyes should be covered while phototherapy is in use. Cover the eyes with pads without placing excessive pressure on the eyes and be carefully positioned to avoid occluding the nares. To permit evaluation of the infants eyes, eye patches should be removed every 4 hours and changed every 8 hours. The patches should be removed during feedings and parental visits.

Temperature: Monitor the infants temperature frequently.

Fluid Requirement for Low Birth Weight Babies

- ❖ The low birth weight babies are classified according to birth weight are:

- <1,000 g
- 1,000–1,500 g
- >1,500 g

❖ Baby with birth weight <1,000 g requires 100 mL/kg on the 1st day and daily increases 15 mL per kg till day 7 and onwards.
❖ Baby with birth weight 1,000–1,500 g requires 80 mL/kg on the 1st day and with daily increment of 15 mL per kg till day 7 onwards.
❖ Baby with birth weight >1,500 g requires 60 mL/kg on the 1st day and with daily increment of 15 mL per kg till day 7 onwards.

General Guidelines for Fluid Therapy

❖ On the first day fluid requirement range from 60–100 mL/kg (The difference between the three categories being 20 mL/kg each)
❖ The daily increment in all groups is around 15 mL per kg till day 7.
❖ Extra 20–30 mL/kg fluid should be added for infants nursed under a radiant warmer. For those receiving phototherapy, add extra 10 to 15 mL/kg fluid.
❖ However, fluid therapy of every baby should be individualized.

Parental Explanations

The treatment of phototherapy can be very disturbing to parents. Reassurance and support are vital especially for the lactating mother who may question her ability to adequately feed her infant. The lights should be turned off and eye patches removed during visits, so that normal parent infant interaction can occur.

Complications of Phototherapy

Insensible water loss: There is increased insensible water loss in infants undergoing phototherapy.

Gastrointestinal effects: Phototherapy is associated with watery diarrhea and increased fecal water loss. The diarrhea may be caused by increased bile salts and unconjugated bilirubin in the bowel due to decreased out transit time.

Decreased in serum calcium levels in preterm infants have been described with phototherapy.

Retinal damage: It has been described in animals whose eyes have been exposed to phototherapy.

Skin: Exposure to wave lengths in the 360–400 nm range may cause erythema and increased skin blood flow.

Bronze baby syndrome: Phototherapy should not be used in infants with liver disease or obstructive jaundice.

Cell damage: It effects in tissue culture cells exposed to phototherapy have been seen. These include mutation, and DNA strand brakes. Hence, it may be wise to shield the scrotum during phototherapy.

Phototherapy upsets the usual maternal infant interaction.

POINTS TO NOTE

During phototherapy neonates require ongoing monitoring of: adequacy of hydration (urine output) and nutrition (weight gain) temperature. Clinical improvement in jaundice.

PRACTICE QUESTIONS
1. What are the indications of phototherapy?
2. How do you calculate fluid requirement for a low birth weight baby who is on phototherapy?
3. What are the complications of phototherapy?

MULTIPLE CHOICE QUESTIONS
1. Neonatal jaundice or neonatal hyperbilirubinemia is also known as:
    a. Icterus neonatorum
    b. Neonatorum palsy
    c. Hypobilirubinemia
    d. Hyponatremia
2. What is the mechanism action of phototherapy?
    a. It converts bilirubin into albumin
    b. It converts unconjugated bilirubin into more soluble form of bilirubin
    c. It inhibits bilirubin formation
    d. It provides coolness
3. Complication of phototherapy in a neonate include, *except*:
    a. Retinal damage
    b. Bronze baby syndrome
    c. Hyperthermia
    d. Hypothermia

ANSWER KEY
1. a   2. b   3. d

CHAPTER 20

Care of the Child in Incubator

PRACTICE COMPETENCIES
On completion of the chapter, the students will be able to:
- Assist in the maintenance of thermoneutral ambient temperature.
- Promote desired humidity and oxygenation.
- Observe sick neonates.
- Isolate newborn babies from infections, unfavorable external environment.

ABSTRACT
Newborn babies take time to accustom to the external environment especially, if they are premature and low birth weight. As they are on risk to develop hypoxia, hypothermia and other many associated adverse conditions, need special care and attention. The term incubation has derived from a Latin word "incubare", that means "lie on". Incubation is the process of providing an environment to keep them warm and suitable for their development as birds sit on their egg to hatch them. Similarly, incubator is an apparatus used to care the premature, low birth weight, and very sick babies in thermoneutral environment.

Keywords: Incubator, servo control probe, thermostat knob, thermoregulation, preterm infants, low birth weight infants, neutral thermal environment, humidification, radiant warmer.

Purpose
- To provide isolation
- To maintain optimal body temperature and humidity
- To administer oxygen.

Equipment
The parts of the incubator are:
1. **Indicator light:** Two white lights on the control panel. One white light indicates power is on and the other indicates the air circulation system is operating.
2. **Temperature indicator meter:** Provides continuous readings of the infants temperature when the probe is affixed to skin.
3. **Thermostat knob:** Maintain the incubator temperature at the desired level.
4. **Servo control probe:** The probe is secured to the midline of the abdomen, halfway between the umbilicus and the xiphoid.

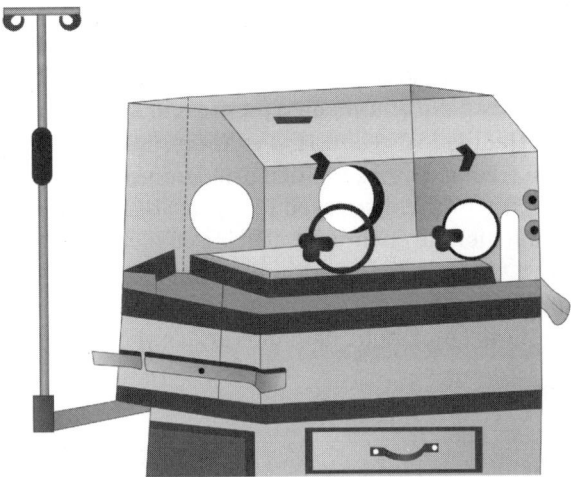

Fig. 20.1: Incubator.

5. **Thermometer:** The thermometer inside the incubator indicates the temperature of the incubator.
6. **Control point adjust button:** The temperature control point of the infant servo control unit in fixed at 97°F.
7. **Oxygen inlet:** The tube attached to the source of oxygen flow should be connected at this oxygen inlet.
8. **Humidity chamber:** It should be filled with sterile distilled water. High humidity aids in relieving respiratory difficulty. Add 0.8–2.5 mL of 1: 10,000 solution of silver nitrate per liter of water to inhibit the growth of microorganism.
9. **Port holes:** It can be opened and closed by turning a metal ring. One port hole door is located at the foot end of incubator through which contaminated lines and other articles may be removed.
10. **Weighting facility:** The vent at top portion of the Plexiglas hood is used to facilitate weighting of the infant.
11. **Heater output monitor:** Provides information regarding the amount of heat generated by the incubator warmer to keep the infant homeothermic.

THERMOREGULATION

Introduction

- Thermoregulation is the means by which the neonate's body temperature is maintained by balancing heat generation and heat loss in a changing environment.
- Normal temperature range is 36.5–37.5°C.
- Temperature regulation is poor in the newborn for several reasons:
  - The ratio of large body surface to body mass.
  - Limited ability to generate heat from muscular movements.
  - Limited subcutaneous fat and brown fat.
  - Mechanism of heat loss:
    - **Convection:** Heat is lost to air or fluid around the infant that is cooler than infants temperature. For example, Air draft on infant from open door in delivery room.

- **Radiation:** Heat is lost to solid objects near infants that are cooler than infant's temperature. For example, windows to the outside not covered by drapers.
- **Conduction:** Heat is lost to cold surfaces or to object with which the infant has contact. For example, X-ray plate or unheated mattress or scale.
- **Evaporation:** Heat is lost when H_2O evaporates from the infant's skin surface or respiratory tract. For example, infant if dried immediately after birth.

Prevention of heat loss in the distressed infant is absolutely essential for survival and maintaining a Neutral thermal environment. It is a challenging aspect of neonatal intensive care nursing care.

Neutral thermal environment is the temperature range in which body temperature can be maintained with minimal metabolic demands and oxygen consumption.

Incubator Indications

- ❖ Preterm infants.
- ❖ Low birth weight infants.

Purpose

To use the overhead radiant warmer or the servo mechanism controlled incubator to help the newborn achieve and maintain a stable body temperature that is within normal limits.

Maintenance of Temperature

The incubator temperature should be such as it will maintain the axillaries temperature of the body between 35°C–37°C. This temperatures will be changed according NTE range and the age of the infant.

Incubators (Isolettes)

- ❖ Standard closed incubators also known as Isolettes' are used to provide a warm and humidified climate for neonates and assist them in controlling their body temperature.
- ❖ Convectively warmed incubators are single or double layered plastic walled chambers that rest on a base.
- ❖ A small insulated mattress rests on the base. A system of fans that force filtered room air over heating elements and fans that can be filled with H_2O rests below the base.
- ❖ Warm air and humidity will be within the enclosed chamber.
- ❖ Utilizing various thermostats and regulators, one can manipulate the internal temperature of the incubator to deliver on environment that assists the infant in maintaining a normal body temperature.

■ THE NEUTRAL THERMAL ENVIRONMENT (NTE)

The normal range body temperature for newborns is generally accepted to be 36.2°C to 37°C through narrower ranges have been accepted.

Setting of the incubator temperature is based on the concept of neutral thermal environment or NTE. NTE is the ideal thermal environment in which a neonate is placed that allows him or her to maintain a normal body temperature while expending a minimal amount of energy to maintain basic life sustaining metabolic process. These guidelines are based on the neonate's birth weight and chronological age and are utilized to adjust the interior temperature.

Neutral Thermal Environment by Infant Age

NTE under 1200 grams

0–24 hours	34.0–35.4°C
24–96 hours	34.0–35.0°C
4–12 days	33.0–34.0°C
12–14 days	32.6–34.0°C
2–3 weeks	32.2–34.0°C
3–4 weeks	31.6–33.6°C
5–6 weeks	30.6–32.2°C

NTE 1200–1500 grams

0–6 hours	33.9–34.4°C
6–12 hours	33.5–34.4°C
12–24 hours	33.3–34.3°C
48–96 hours	33.0–34.0°C
4–12 days	33.0–34.0°C
12–14 days	32.6–34.0°C
2–3 weeks	32.2–34°C
3–4 weeks	31.6–33.6°C
5–6 weeks	30.6–32.3°C

NTE 1500–2500 grams

0–6 hours	32.8–33.8°C
6–12 hours	32.2–33.8°C
24–36 hours	31.6–33.8°C
48–72 hours	31.2–33.4°C
72–96 hours	31.1–33.2°C
4–14 days	31.0–33.2°C
2–3 weeks	30.5–33.0°C
3–4 weeks	30.0–32.7°C
4–5 weeks	29.5–32.2°C
5–6 weeks	29.0–31.8°C

NTE over 2500 grams

0–6 hours	32.0–33.8°C
6–12 hours	31.4–33.8°C
24–36 hours	30.7–33.5°C
48–72 hours	30.4–33.2°C
72–96 hours	29.8–32.8°C
8–10 days	29.0–31.8°C
10–12 days	29.0–31.4°C
10–14 days	29.0–30.8°C

- ❖ NTE parameters may need to be altered for infants who cannot maintain their temperature between 36.3°C and 36.8°C. For example, infants who may need special consideration are infants who are small or large for gestational age, infants at risk for sepsis, any infant greater than 6 weeks of age who may have a neurologic impairment affected by temperature regulation.
- ❖ The single walled incubator is used most commonly.
- ❖ The double walled incubator is a recent development that adds a second wall of Plexiglas around the chamber.
- ❖ The double walls of the incubator are separated by air, several centimeters thick. It is believed that which this design radiant and convection heat lost by the infant will be reduced further.
- ❖ Interior incubator temperature should be monitored every 30–60 minutes when the heater output is controlled manually.
- ❖ Isolates equipped with a servo control utilize a small temperature probe that is placed on the infants abdomen.
- ❖ This probe measures the abdominal skin temperature and is attached to a thermo regulating device inside the isolate.
- ❖ A control point, the desired skin temperature is set by the nurse and subsequently the heater output will be regulated automatically and normally ranges between 36°C to 37°C
- ❖ Servo control automatically to maintain the neonate's temperature at the selected point.

Disadvantages

- ❖ One disadvantage of the servo control method that it does not allow for the monitoring of alterations in body temperature that can be an indication of an illness or change in the infants states.
- ❖ An infant who is septic may become hypothermic but may not display this sign because of the automatic adjustment mode by the servo control unit to maintain the present control point.
- ❖ The hypothermic infant will require an overhead heater output to maintain the body temperature at the designated point.
- ❖ The servo control temperature probe attachment must be monitored also to ensure a secure attachment to the infant's skin.
- ❖ A partially or completely dislodged temperature probe will affect the heater output mechanism.
- ❖ A dislodged probe can seriously overheat the neonate.

Humidification

Usually 60–70% humidification required:
- ❖ Although most isolates are equipped, i.e. supplemental humidification systems, not all infants benefit from this.
- ❖ Some infants, however, will benefit from the humidity if they are stressed by the neutral conditions.
- ❖ Other literature suggests that only infants under 1,500 g will require additional humidity, i.e., in the incubator.
- ❖ The primary reason not to add additional humidity to the incubator is that pseudomonas and similar organisms may proliferate in the H_2O reservoir and contaminate the air inside the incubator.

- Use sterile H_2O inside the incubator. The H_2O need to be drained every 48 hours and refilled with fresh sterile H_2O.
- The entre incubator is changed every 7 days.

Incubator Child Care Activities

- The heated environment of the incubator is lost when it is opened to provide care for neonate.
- Care activities should be organized to minimize the number of entries mode into the incubator.
- Incubators cool rapidly when they are opened, there by stressing the neonate. One helpful adjunct in maintaining a constant environmental temperature, i.e., in the incubator is to utilize flexible plastic sleeves on all particles.
- The critically ill neonate who requires numerous interventions, i.e. multiple entries into the incubator requires close temperature monitoring and additional protection.
- These additional protective measures may include the temporary use of a radiant warmer or a heating lamp or swaddling or covering.
- Placing stockinet hot over the infants head will help the infant maintain body heat.
- The incubator should be prewarmed, before placing the child in the incubator. Temperature should be set to 36°C.
- After an additional 15 minutes, i.e., a response the temperature may be increased to 38°C.
- Many incubators may sound an alarm at 38°C because of the presence of internal safety thermostat.
- Swaddling the infant or adding a radiant warmer over the incubator may be necessary.
- Because of incubator size, the use of this device is for the relatively small infant. Additional interventions to help infants maintain their body temperature include the use of Plexiglas shield that are placed over the infant in the incubator.
- Plastic wraps should not be used for prolonged periods. Since they may faster an environment that promote bacterial growth when placed in direct contact, i.e. the skin.

Fluid Requirement for Low Birth Weight Babies

Refer Chapter 19: Care of Child with Phototherapy, Page no. 135 and 136.

General Guidelines for Fluid Therapy

Refer Chapter 19: Care of Child with Phototherapy, Page no. 136.

Nurses Responsibilities

- The incubator should be prewarmed to 34°–36.1°C for infants less than 1500 g and 33.9°–35°C for infants more than 1,500 g.
- After the infant is placed, the incubator is set for maintenance of skin temperature between 36.0°–36.5°C.
- The infant need not be fully clothed, a diaper is only put.
- Ensure that servo probe is in place a properly secured to prevent hyperthermia. Reposition the probe when infant is turned; never place a probe under the infant.
- The weaning of infant from incubator should be gradual process.
- The unit should be thoroughly disinfected everyday.
- Record temperature and humidity of the incubator and the responses of infant.

- Do not open the incubator during the routine care. Abrupt change in the temperature can cause untoward metabolic responses in the newborn that may cause apnea.
- Humidity chamber should be drained and replenished daily.

> **POINTS TO NOTE**
>
> - It is important that the incubator should not interfere with observation of the neonate and quality of care.
> - Sensory stimuli like light and pain should be kept to the minimal.
> - When neonate develops fever, the incubator modes have to be changed in normal modes.
> - When the neonate is nursed in prone position, skin sensor is placed over the flank and it should not touch the bed.
> - The neonate in the incubator should not be bathed.

PRACTICE QUESTIONS

1. What is NTE?
2. What are the nurse's responsibilities for the child on an incubator?

MULTIPLE CHOICE QUESTIONS

1. Which of the following is a mechanism of heat transfer?
   a. Convection
   b. Consumption
   c. Confusion
   d. Convergence
2. An incubator is most likely to be used for which of the following?
   a. Neonate less than 5.25 kg and/or gestational age of less than 30 weeks
   b. Neonate less than 1.75 kg and/or gestational age of less than 30 weeks
   c. Neonate less than 1.5 kg and/or gestational age of less than 30 weeks
   d. Neonate less than 15 kg and/or gestational age of less than 30 weeks
3. How long should the baby's temperature be monitored once it has been weaned to an open cot or bassinette?
   a. Every 4 hours
   b. Every hour
   c. Every 30 minutes then hourly
   d. Every 15 minutes then hourly

ANSWER KEY

1. a   2. c   3. d

CHAPTER 21

Care of the Child in Radiant Warmer

PRACTICE COMPETENCIES
On completion of the chapter, the students will be able to:
- Provide quality nursing care to the patients on radiant warmer
  - Prepare the warmer before the baby arrives
- Record the baby's temperature on a regular basis, preferably every two hours

ABSTRACT
Radiant warmer is a body warming device to provide heat to the body. This device helps to maintain the body temperature of the baby and limit the metabolism rate. Heat has a tendency to flow in the heat gradient direction that is from high temperature to low temperature. The heat loss in some new born babies is rapid; hence body warmers provide an artificial support to keep the body temperature constant. In certain areas with very cold climate, babies are kept on radiant warmer for couple of hours immediately after birth to ensure the baby is stabilized after birth.

Keywords: Radiant warmer, incubator, servo probe, phototherapy, servo control system.

Purpose
To maintain body temperature of the newborn.

Equipment
The parts of the radiant warmer are:
1. **Hood:** Hood contains the radiant heat panel. The radiant heat panel will automatically turn on and off to maintain the infants temperature as desired by temperature control.
2. **Panels:** There are four panels, two side panels, head and foot panel.
3. **Bassinet procedure table:** The bassinet may be placed in varying levels of Fowler's or Trendlenberg position by squeezing the handle under the tabletop.
4. **Storage area:** Linen and equipment necessary for the individual care of infant may be stored.
5. **Control panel:**
   a. On and off switch
   b. Power light for power on indication.
   c. Set temperature—to maintain desired skin temperature.
   d. Skin sensor probe

e. Heater output—provides information regarding the amount of heat generated by the incubator/warmer to keep the infant normothermic.
f. Visible/audible alarm speaker—red light flashes/emits audible alarm when temperature measured by thermistor is ± 1°C.

Nurses Responsibilities

- Monitor the infants temperature frequently
- Ensure the servo probe is in place and properly secured to prevent hypo or hyperthermia
- The weaning for infant should be provided normally
- The unit should be thoroughly disinfected.

Fluid Requirement for Low Birth Weight Babies

Refer Chapter 19: Care of Child with Phototherapy, Page no. 135 and 136.

General Guidelines for Fluid Therapy

Note:
1. On the first day the fluid requirements range from 60 to 100 mL/kg. (The difference between the three categories being 20 mL/kg each).
2. The daily increment in all groups is around 15 mL per kg till day 7.
3. Extra 20 to 30 mL/kg fluid should be added for infants nursed under a radiant warmer. For those receiving phototherapy add extra 10 to 15 mL/kg fluid.
4. These are general guidelines; fluid therapy of every baby should be individualized.

Radiant Warmers

- Radiant warmers are designed to provide a warm climate for infants, i.e. humidity.
- Radiant warmers utilize infrared energy from electrically heated elements that are suspended above the child.
- They are often free standing or incorporated into a unit where they are suspended over a base on that lies on insulated mattress.
- Low walls surround the mattress to provide a safe environment for the infant rolling or sliding off the mattress and serve as a barrier against drafts.
- Set the temperature point usually 36.4°C (97.5°F).
- Baby should be unclothed allow only a diaper and dry well before placing in the open unit under the radiant warmer.
- All radiant warmers should have a servo control system, since, it is relatively easy to under heat or over heat the infant that a high energy warming.
- Servo control probe tape or place over the abdomen between the umbilicus and xiphoid process.
- The probe should be covered with aluminum foil and tape it properly.
- The position of the probe is very important.
- Should not place the skin probe over the rib cage, where the subcutaneous tissue is thin because this misplaced and dislodged probes can lead to overheating or under heating.
- A loose probe can lead to overheating of the infant to cause first degree buns.

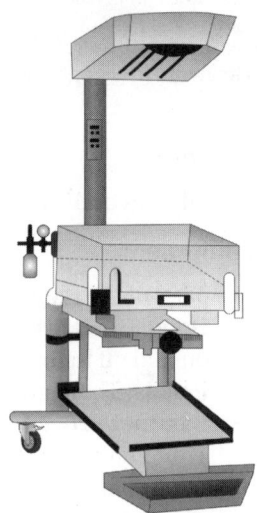

Fig. 21.1: Radiant warmer.

- Monitor the temperature frequently for every one hour and compare that the auxiliary temperature of the body in order to know whether it is that in its normal limits or not.
- If the auxiliary temperature gain 37°C (98.6°F) dress the baby and move him or her from the radiant warmer to an open crib.
- After bringing to the open crib baby should be dress up immediately and cover with the blankets.
- Again recheck the temperature frequently. If there is any variation in newborn's temperature, again you should keep the body in the incubator.

POINTS TO NOTE

Application of skin probe
1. Do's
   - Prepare the skin using an alcohol/spirit swab to ensure good adhesion to the skin.
   - Apply probe over the right hypochondrium area in the supine position.
   - Apply probe to the flank in the prone position.
   - Check sensor probe regularly so as to ensure that it is in place.
   - Ensure that skin probe is free of contact with bed.
   - Cover probe with a reflective cover pad, if available (foil covered foam adhesive pad).
2. Don't
   - Do not apply to bruised skin.
   - Do not apply clear plastic dressings over probe.
   - Do not use fingernails to remove skin surface probes.
   - Do not reuse disposable probes.

PRACTICE QUESTION

1. Nursing care of child with radiant warmer.

MULTIPLE CHOICE QUESTIONS

1. A nurse in delivery room is assisting with the delivery of a new born baby. After the delivery the nurse prepares to prevent heat loss in the new born resulting from evaporation by:
   a. Warming the crib
   b. Turning on overhead radiant warmer
   c. Closing the doors to the room
   d. Drying the infant in a warm blanket
2. An infant is born at 27 weeks' gestation following a pregnancy complicated by preterm labor that progressed despite administration of a tocolytic agent.
   Of the following the most appropriate INITIAL management is to:
   a. Measure transcutaneous oxygen saturation
   b. Perform endotracheal intubation
   c. Place an umbilical arterial catheter
   d. Place the infant in an open bed warmer

ANSWER KEY

1. d   2. d

CHAPTER 22

Ostomy Care

PRACTICE COMPETENCIES

On completion of the chapter, the students will be able to:
- Perform postoperative management of an infant
- Monitor fluid and electrolyte balance
- Carry out enteral feeding.
  - Postoperative complications will relate to wound healing ability, length and type of gut retained, further deterioration of surviving gut, stricture formation and risk of sepsis, as well as individual neonatal characteristics.

ABSTRACT

Caring for children with ostomies comprehensively requires that the healthcare professional understand issues related to normal growth and development as well as more specific medical information about disease processes and ostomy care. Parents should have a working knowledge of routine ostomy care and need guidelines to assist them in recognizing ostomy complications. Complications range from mild to severe. Many patients will experience at least one ostomy related complication during the time they have their diversion. Active support of the child and the parent is essential toward facilitating acceptance and integration of ostomy care in pediatric ostomy clients. This chapter contains colostomy care and irrigation, urostomy care, gastrostomy care.

Keywords: Gastrostomy care, urostomy care, colostomy irrigation, pouches, stoma covers, colostomy care, peritonitis.

COLOSTOMY CARE AND IRRIGATION

Definition

A colostomy is a surgically created of a new opening in the abdominal wall into the colon through which digested food passes.

The opening is called stoma from the Greek word meaning "mouth".

The stool passes through the stoma into a pouch attached to the stoma on the outside of the abdomen.

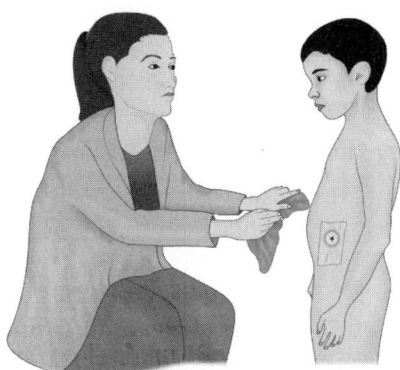

Fig. 22.1: Colostomy in children.

The pouch stoma and skin surrounding the stoma requires care and maintenance by the patient or caregiver.

Purpose
- To provide outlet for intestinal waste.
- To permit escape of feces and flatus when there is an obstruction of the large bowel or a known lesion that will eventually cause obstruction.
- To permit healing of the bowel distal to the colostomy opening since it diverts the fecal contents from the affected area.
- To provide a permanent means of bowel evacuation when the return or anus are non-functional as a result of disease, birth defect or a traumatic condition.

Indications
- Necrotizing enterocolitis
- Imperforate anus
- Intestinal atresia
- Hirschsprung disease
- Intestinal malrotation.

Older Children
- Chronic ulcerative colitis
- Extensive trauma from an automobile accidents
- Peritonitis following abdominal surgery.

Types of Colostomies
- Temporarily and permanent colostomy
- Double barreled and end colostomy
- Wet colostomy and dry colostomy.

Temporary Colostomy

It is normally made for diversion of fecal material. It may be needed to allow the colon to rest and heal for a period of time.
- It may be in place for weeks, months or year.

- ❖ The temporary colostomy will eventually be closed and bowel movements will return to normal.

Permanent Colostomy

It is usually needed when a part of the colon must be removed or cannot be used again.

Precautions: The nurse attending to a colostomy care should wash his or her hands before and after the procedure as well as wear gloves while performing care.

Wet Colostomy

A wet colostomy is used to distinguish of openings. Dry colostomy refers to an opening of the left side of the colon where the fecal content is usually soft and formed. Wet colostomy refers to an opening on the right side of the colon, where the fecal content is liquid.

In addition, the wet colostomy is used for those through which both urine and feces are excreted because of the transplantation of ureters into the colon. This colostomy is never irrigated.

Double Barrel Colostomy

In double barrel colostomy, there are two openings, the proximal and distal segments of the colon. The proximal is functioning and a distal is irrigated to clean.

Types of Pouches used for Colostomies

- ❖ A pouch is worn over a colostomy to collect the stool passed through the stoma.
- ❖ There are a variety sizes and styles of colostomy pouches.
- ❖ Pouches are light weight and odor, proof pouches have a special covering that prevents the pouch from sticking to the body.
- ❖ Some pouches also have charcoal filters while release gas slowly and help to decease gas odor.

Types of Colostomy Pouches

Open-ended Pouch

- ❖ This type of pouch allows you to open the bottom of the pouch to drain the output.
- ❖ The open end is usually closed with a clamp. The open ended open pouch is usually used by people with ascending or transverse colostomies.
- ❖ The output from these colostomies are looser and unpredictable (does not drain at regular time).

Closed-ended Pouch

- ❖ This type of pouch is removed and throw away when the pouch is filled.
- ❖ Closed ended pouches are usually used by people with descending or sigmoid colostomies.
- ❖ The output from these types of colostomies is firm and does not need to be drained.

One piece

A one piece pouch contains the pouch and adhesive skin barrier together as one unit.

- ❖ The adhesive skin barriers is the part of the pouch system that is placed around the stoma and attached to skin.
- ❖ When the pouch is removed and replaced with a new one the new pouch must be attached to the skin.

Two piece
The two piece pouch has two parts an adhesive frange and pouch.
- ❖ The adhesive frange stays in place while the pouch is removed and new pouch is attached to the frange.
- ❖ The pouch does not need to be reattached to the skin each time.
- ❖ The two piece system can be helpful for patient with sensitive skin.

Precut or Cut to Fit Pouches
- ❖ Some pouches have precut holes, so you do not have to cut the opening yourself.
- ❖ Other pouches can be out to fit the size and shape of your stoma.
- ❖ Cut to fit pouches are especially useful right after your surgery because your stroma decrease in size.

Stoma Covers and Caps
- ❖ Stoma caps or covers can be placed on the stoma when the stoma is not active (draining).
- ❖ People with descending or sigmoid colostomies who irrigate may use stoma covers or caps.
- ❖ The cover or cap is attached to the skin in the same way as a pouch.

Preparation
The nurse should instruct the caregivers about the procedure before it is performed.
- ❖ Many parents feel anxious and nervous when first dealing with an ostomy.
- ❖ Encourage the parents or caregivers to ask questions and explain all steps as they are performed.

Change of Pouch
The way in which the caregiver should change the client colostomy pouch depends on the type of pouch use.

Equipment
A tray consists of:
- ❖ A bowl of warm water
- ❖ Dry and wet cotton swabs/soft clean cloth pieces
- ❖ Siloderm ointment/coconut oil/vaseline.

Procedure
If the child wearing an open-ended pouch. The caregiver must empty the contents from pouch into the toilet.
- ❖ Gently remove the pouch by pushing the skin down and away from the adhesive skin barrier with one hand with the other hand, pull the pouch up and away from the stoma.
- ❖ Clean the skin around the stoma with warm water and also use soap.
- ❖ Pat the skin by using soft clean cloth pieces and create a dry surface.
- ❖ Center the pouch over the stoma and press it firmly into place on clean dry skin.
- ❖ Place the old pouch in another plastic bag to be thrown away if the pouch is disposable.

Nursing Management
- ❖ Prepare the child and family about the procedure

- ❖ Adequate explanation given about the indication of stoma, use of colostomy bag
- ❖ Ostomy care can be given into two ways:
    1. Without ostomy bag and
    2. With ostomy bag.
- ❖ During first one or two days following surgery stoma should be exposed to air and checked for bleeding
- ❖ After the child has a liquid stool, clean with soap and water and the skin protected with aluminum paste or zinc oxide as prescribed by the doctor.
- ❖ A dressing made of square of gauze or tissue paper with a hole cut in the middle to fit around the stoma over the protective substance.
- ❖ The purpose of dressing is to absorb fluid
- ❖ It must be replaced after each liquid stool
- ❖ For infants a small ostomy bag or a urine collection bag may be used to collect
- ❖ Larger size bags are available for children and adolescents
- ❖ The skin barrier (stoma adhesive) or other peristomal covering is available which is made of gelatin, pectin and other substance.
- ❖ It is available in powder, paste form to protect the skin
- ❖ The soaps containing perfume, creams should not be used on the skin because they interfere with adhesion of the bag
- ❖ If a sigmoid colostomy has been done on an infant, stools are usually formed, so it is not necessary to use collecting device. Vaseline may be put on the skin around the stoma and a diaper can be applied.

Colostomy Irrigation

Preliminary Assessment

- ❖ Check the name, bed number and other identification of the patient
- ❖ Check the diagnosis and the purpose of irrigation
- ❖ Check the type of colostomy done. Make sure of the proximal and distal loop of the colon
- ❖ Check the patient's ability for self care.
- ❖ Check the doctor's orders for specific instructions and the precautions, if any regarding the colostomy irrigations movement of the patient, etc.
- ❖ Check the understanding of the patient to follow instructions
- ❖ Check the articles available in the patients units.

Equipment

1. Irrigating can with tubing clamp and catheter
2. IV stand
3. A jug with solution at the temperature of 100° to 105°F or 37.8° to 40.6°C.
4. Water soluble jelly
5. Clean cotton swabs
6. Kidney tray and paper bag
7. Dressings, protective ointments, etc.
8. Mackintosh
9. Clean linen as necessary
10. Bucket with disinfecting solution.

Preparation of the Patient and the Environment

1. Explain the procedure to the child attenders and if child is older means tell him how he can cooperate.
2. Make the child sit on a chair in the bathroom. A rubber sheet placed on the lap of the patient can be used as a through leading into the toilet to receive the return flow.
3. Provide privacy.
4. A bath blanket may be kept around the shoulder to prevent chills.
5. Ask the attenders to observe every step. So that they can learn the care of the colostomy. It is desirable to have a family members be present to learn the procedure.
6. Arrange articles conveniently for the nurse and the patient.

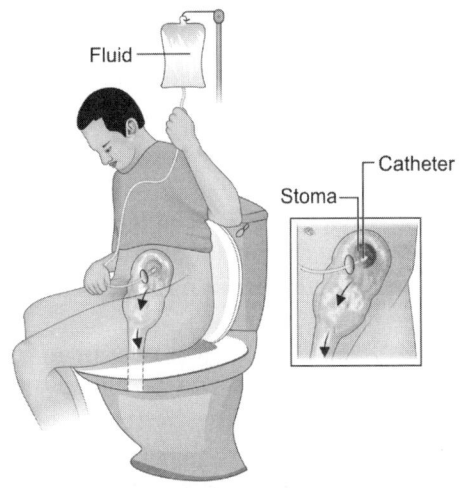

Fig. 22.2: Colostomy irrigation.

Postoperative Care

1. Observation of a stoma and surrounding tissue is important.
2. A stoma is deep pink in color and moist with mucus. The stoma is soft.
3. Irrigation should be done only in preparation for diagnostic tests or surgery and occasionally for the treatment of constipation.
4. Observation of drainage for amount and characteristics is important to provide fluid replacement and prevent dehydration.
5. An abdominal distension may indicate an obstruction and should be reported.
6. Ostomy bag to be checked every 2 hours for leakage and to be changed as soon as leakage is suspected.
7. Teach the parents about the important of emptying the bag when it is ¼ or ½ full and about the treatment of skin breakdown.

Procedure

1. Wash hands.
2. Fill the irrigating can with the solution and hang it at a required height.
3. Expel the air from the tubing and clamp it remove the forth if any, from the solution.
4. Untie the colostomy bag and remove the dressings (not of the incision) if any and discard them into the kidney tray.
5. Clean the skin around the stoma with clean cotton swabs or rag pieces or wash the area with soap and water.
6. Introduce the catheter through the lead and the tip of the catheter is lubricated with water soluble jelly. Lubricants are used sparingly.
7. Pour some solution over stoma.
8. Introduce catheter into the stoma about 4 inches. Do not use any force.
9. Allow the solution to run in slowly involving about 20 minutes.
10. Clamp the tube before the entry of the entire fluid.

11. Remove the catheter from stoma disconnect it from the tubing and place it in the kidney tray.
12. Wait for the return flow divert the attention of patient by providing him play/reading material. The patient may be asked to move from side to side and forward.

After Care of the Patient and the Articles

1. When return flow is complete, remove the mackintosh, clean the skin around the colostomy opening and dry the skin thoroughly.
2. Apply a clean dressing or a clean colostomy bag over the stoma to receive any drainage that may leak out.
3. After making sure that the patient is thoroughly clean, help him to wear his clean dresses.
4. Help the patient to get into his bed. Change the dressing of incision using aseptic technique, make him comfortable. Tidy up the unit.
5. Take all articles to the utility room. Clean all equipment immediately. Rinse them first in cold water then with warm soapy water. Dry and store them in a convenient place for the next use.
6. Patients are instructed for the care and cleaning of the colostomy bags to prolong its life and keep it free or odors. Cleaning with soap or detergent with water and exposing it to fresh air is sufficient. However, it may still be necessary to deodorize the bag with liquid deodorizers available in the market.
7. Chart the procedure in the patient's record with date and time. Specify the amount and the kind of solution, the participation of the patient in the procedure abnormalities, if any noted during the procedure, etc. Record the condition of the skin around the stoma. Record immediately any redness/excoriation of the skin noted and the immediate steps taken to prevent further damage.

■ UROSTOMY CARE

Definition

A urostomy is the removal of the bladder and creation of the surgical opening or stoma to allow urine to drain. Urostomy is the stoma for the urinary system. It is made in where long-time urine through the bladder and urethra is not possible. For example, extensive surgery or obstruction.

Indications

- ❖ Bladder cancer
- ❖ Correct a birth defect
- ❖ A chronic bladder infection.

Purposes

- ❖ Rather than controlled urination a urostomy clients urine will flow naturally out of the body and into collection pouches.
- ❖ Pouching system collect the urine for urostomy clients and come in one or 2 piece bags depending on a patient's needs.
- ❖ Proper care of the pouch requires regular drainage and changing.
- ❖ Drain the pouch when it is between 1/3 and 1/2 full. This will be about every 2-4 hours or more often who drinks a lot of fluids.

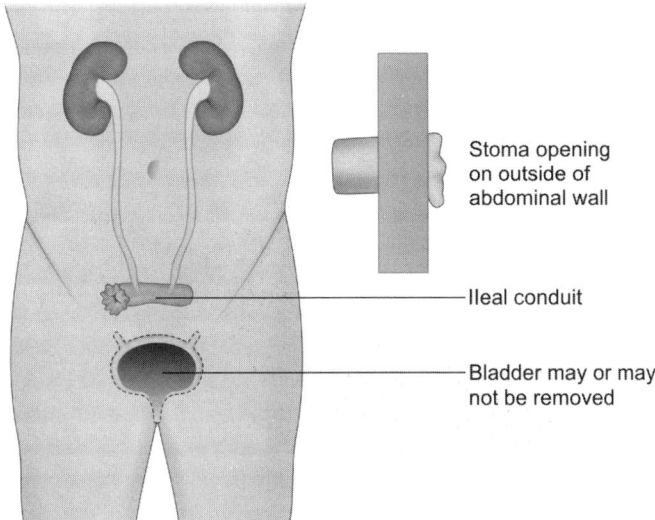

Fig. 22.3: Urostomy.

- To drain open the pouch's valve and empty the urine directly into the toilet.
- Change the pouch every 3–7 days or immediately if there is leakage.
- Remove the old pouch apply the new pouch putting the sticky side to the skin and pressing down to seal all edges.

Equipment

A tray should contain:
- Clean cloth
- Soap
- Skin wipers or powder.

Stoma care
- The stoma needs regular cleaning to prevent irritation caused by regular contact with urine which has a high bacterial count.
- Wipe with a wet cloth while changing the bag will usually be enough.
- Soap is safe, but make sure to rinse well afterward.
- Use skin wipes or powder to protect the skin around the stoma, further and under the pouch barrier.
- Dry the stoma area well before applying pouches.
- Spots of blood around the stoma are not uncommon due to its delicate blood vessels.
- Any bleeding well usually stop quickly.

GASTROSTOMY CARE

A gastrostomy is an opening into the stomach through the abdominal wall into which a self-retaining or jacquet catheter is inserted up to centimeters and is firmly secured in place with adhesive tape.

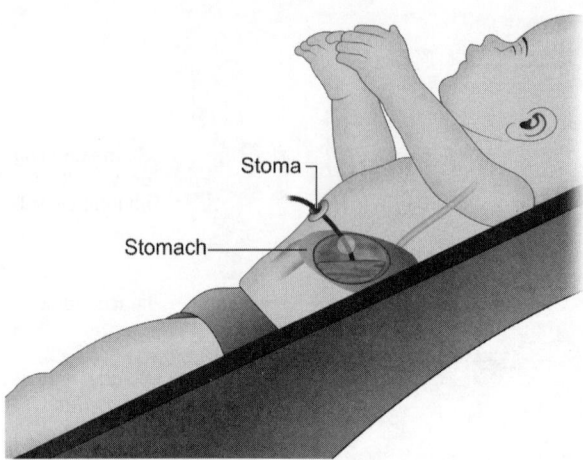

Fig. 22.4: Gastrostomy.

Purposes
- To meet the nutritional needs
- To minimize the infections.

Indications
- Increased metabolic needs and inability to take adequate oral diet—trauma, burns, cancer and sepsis.
- Coma or mechanical ventilation
- Head/neck surgery
- Malabsorption
- Obstruction of esophagus or oropharynx
- Severe anorexia nervosa
- Dysphagia.

Sites of Tube Insertion

Short-term nutritional support
1. (NG) Feeding tubes are passed through the nose or mouth (orogastric) into the stomach and secure in place.
2. Tube placement must be verified before use by X-ray, aspiration of contents for pH, bilirubin concentration auscultation of air injected through tube. The best method is X-ray.
3. If there is a question about tube placement in the respiratory tract, the tube should be removed.
4. Nasoduodenal or nasojejunal tube passed through the nose into duodenum or jejunum and secured in place. X-ray is usually needed to verify correct tube placement.

Long-term nutritional support
1. **Gastrostomy:** Insertion of a tube either surgically or percutaneous endoscopic procedure in the stomach.
2. **Gastrostomy button:** Small device inserted through the gastrostomy stoma to allow for long-term feeding with minimal effect on body image.

3. **Jejunostomy:** Insertion of tube directly into the jejunum either surgically or by a percutaneous endoscopy procedure jejunostomy feedings are generally by continuous infusion using a feeding pump.

Types of Tubes
1. Large bore NG polyurethane tube size 12 to 18 F is very short.
2. Small bore NG tube made of polyurethane, silicone or polyvinyl chloride with a tungsten – weighed tip or non-weighted tip size 6 to 12 F and 30 to 36 inches (76 to 91.5 cm) long.
3. Nasointestinal tube made of silicone, polyurethane or polyvinyl chloride with tungsten – weighted tip size 6 to 12 F and 40 to 60 inches.
4. Gastrostomy tube—catheter made of silicone, polyurethane, polyvinyl chloride or latex; a balloon on the distal end to stabilize tube may be used and ranges from 5 to 30 mL capacity.
5. Gastrostomy button—silicone, ranging from 18 to 28 F and 1 inch (2.5 cm) long, useful for person wanting minimal alteration in body image.
6. Jejunostomy tube—size ranging from 5 to 14 F with or without a balloon (a balloon may obstruct lumen of jejunum). A plain red rubber catheter is occasionally used as a short-term jejunostomy tube and some. Gastrostomy tubes may be used for jejunostomy.

Equipment
- Tube feeding formula
- Graduated containers
- 30–60 mL catheter tipped syringe
- Water
- Stethoscope
- pH strip
- Gavage feeding bag.

Procedure
Preparatory phase
1. Remove formula from refrigerator and allow to come to room temperature
2. Explain procedure
3. Wash hands
4. Protect patient from spillage
5. Shake formula container
6. Elevated head of bed 30°–45°
7. Using the catheter tipped syringe, inject 20–30 cc of air while listening with a stethoscope positioned at the epigastric area (for nasogastric tubes). For nasointestinal tubes 20 cc of air may be injected, but auscultation site may be displaced laterally and inferiorly
8. If NG tube used, aspirate. Stomach contents to cheek gastric residual.

Performance phase
1. For intermittent tube feeding, attach barrel and catheter tipped syringe to be pinch off feeding tube.
2. Fill catheter tipped syringe with formula and allow fluid to flow in by gravity.
3. Pour additional formula into barrel of syringe when it is three quarters empty.

Chapter 22: Ostomy Care

4. After administering the prescribed amount of formula flush tubing with at least 30 cc of water.
5. If using a gavage bag for intermittent feeding, fill bag with prescribed amount of feeding, tubing of air, attach distal end to feeding tube and regulate to run over at least 10-20 minutes.
6. For continuous tube feeding fill bag with 4 hours of tube feeding, flush tubing, attach to volume control infuser according to manufacturer's instructions, attach distal end to feeding tube, and start flush with 30-60 mL of water every 4 hours after first cheeking residual.
7. After intermittent feeding is completed cover end of feeding tube with plug or clamp.

Follow up phase
1. Rinse equipment with warm water, dry and replace every 24 hours or per facility policy.
2. Maintain head of bed elevation for 30-60 minutes after feeding is completed. If continuous feeding, maintain head elevation continuously.
3. Document type and amount of feeding amount of water given and patient tolerance of procedure.
4. Monitor breath sounds, bowel sounds, gastric distention, diarrhea or constipation, intake and output, daily weight and serum chemistry results.

Gastrostomy or Jejunostomy Care

Performance phase
1. Special care ostomy tube insertion site should include:
   a. Cleaning around tube with prescribed cleansing solution every shift and as needed
   b. Applying sterile 4 × 4 gauze pad and taping in place
   c. Applying skin barrier as peristomal skin become excoriated
   d. Tapping of tube to skin or skin barrier with hypoallergenic tape.

Community and Home Care Considerations

Teach patient and family
1. Technique for administration of tube feeding outlined the procedure guidelines
2. Sign and symptoms of potential complications
3. Need to assess tube placement and residual before each feeding
4. Principles of medical asepsis, including careful hand washing, refrigeration of formula, cleaning of equipment with soap and water and through drying between feedings.
5. When the gastrostomy or jejunostomy tube insertion site well healed, surrounding skin can be cleaned with soap and water.
6. Gauze dressing can be applied as needed
7. Leakage around tube or signs of peristomal skin irritation should be reported.

■ URETEROSTOMY AND ENTEROSTOMY CARE

Introduction

A ureterostomy is a surgery to create a urinary diversion (a change in the path by which urine leaves the body). In a ureterostomy, the urine bypasses the bladder and exits the body through a stoma—a surgically created opening—and collects into a pouch worn outside the body.

The procedure is performed to divert the flow of urine away from the bladder when the bladder is not functioning or has been removed. Indications include bladder cancer, spinal cord injury, malfunction of the bladder, and birth defects such as spina bifida.

Definition
Ureterostomy is the creation of a stoma (a new, artificial outlet) for a ureter or kidney.

Types
There are four common types of ureterostomies:
1. *Single ureterostomy*: This procedure brings only one ureter to the surface of the abdomen.
2. *Bilateral ureterostomy*: This procedure brings the two ureters to the surface of the abdomen, one on each side.
3. *Double-barrel ureterostomy*: In this approach, both ureters are brought to the same side of the abdominal surface.
4. *Transuretero-ureterostomy (TUU)*: This procedure brings both ureters to the same side of the abdomen, through the same stoma.

Indications
There are several reasons to recommend a ureterostomy, it includes:
- Have a birth defect, such as spina bifida
- Have had your bladder removed (possibly because of cancer)
- Have a bladder that no longer works properly
- Have a spinal cord injury.

Purpose
The purposes of this procedure are to promote cleanliness and to protect peristomal skin from irritation, breakdown, and infection.

Equipment and Supplies
The following equipment and supplies will be necessary when performing this procedure:
1. Soap and water;
2. Wash basin;
3. Barrier paste;
4. Skin sealant;
5. Gauze pads;
6. Pouch;
7. Bedside urinary drainage bag, and
8. Personal protective equipment (e.g., gowns, gloves, mask, etc., as needed).

Procedure

Steps in procedure	Rationale
1. Place the clean equipment on the bedside stand or overbed table. Arrange the supplies so they can be easily reached	The arrangement of the equipment make it easy to perform the procedure
2. Wash and dry your hands thoroughly	To prevent cross infections
3. Fill the wash basin one-half (1/2) full of warm water. Place the wash basin on the bedside stand within easy reach	To clean the drain bag

Contd...

Contd...

Steps in procedure	Rationale
4. If the child physical or medical condition permits, assist the child into the semi-Fowler's position. Refer to the child's plan of care and/or request information from the nurse supervisor regarding safe positioning for the child	To position the child in comfortable position
5. Put on disposable gloves	To prevent cross infections
6. Remove soiled appliance being careful not to cause unnecessary trauma to peristomal skin. Immediately place a gauze pad over the stomal opening. If stents are present, do not pull. Place gauze pads underneath tips	Placing the gauze pad prevents the pulling of stent over the stomal site
7. Assess the condition of the skin around the stoma	To identify any sort of infection at stomal site
8. Gentle cleanse the surrounding skin with warm water and soap using a washcloth or gauze pad. Pat skin dry with a clean towel	To reduce the skin irritation
9. Apply barrier paste as necessary. Apply skin sealant to skin surrounding stoma. Let dry 1-2 minutes. Insert the new appliance, being sure that it securely adheres to the skin to prevent leakage (*Note*: If stents are present, attach the new appliance to the stents)	The appliances are inserted to prevent leakage from the drain bag
10. Open the drain spout and attach to bedside urinary bag	To drain out urine in to the urinary bag
11. Pour the wash water down the commode. Flush the commode	To flush the commode with the water
12. Discard all disposable items into designated containers	To maintain the standard safety precautions
13. Discard soiled linen into designated container	To clean the soiled linen
14. Clean wash basin and return to designated storage area	To sterilize the used equipment
15. Remove gloves and discard in designated container. Wash and dry your hands thoroughly	To prevent the cross infections
16. Clean the bedside stand and/or overbed table. Return the overbed table to its proper position	To sterilize the stand and the overbed table
17. Wash and dry your hands thoroughly	To prevent cross infections

Documentation

The following information should be recorded in the resident's medical record:
- ❖ The date and time the procedure was performed.
- ❖ The name and title of the individual(s) who performed the procedure.
- ❖ The condition of the skin surrounding the stoma.
- ❖ The type of appliance utilized.
- ❖ All assessment data obtained during the procedure.
- ❖ How the resident tolerated the procedure.
- ❖ If the resident refused the procedure, the reason(s) why and the intervention taken.

Chapter 22: Ostomy Care

ENTEROSTOMY CARE

Definition

This is surgery of the abdominal wall and intestines. An opening is made into the intestines to drain the contents out or put in a feeding tube.

❖ An enterostomy or ostomy (colostomy, ileostomy) is a surgically created opening of the bowel (intestine) to the outside which allows the body to empty stool (poop) and gas. The

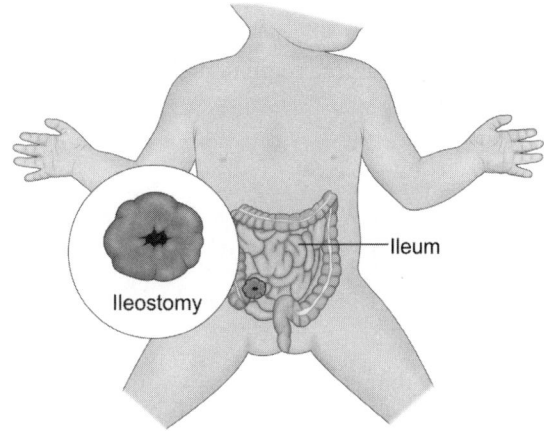

Fig. 22.5: Ileostomy.

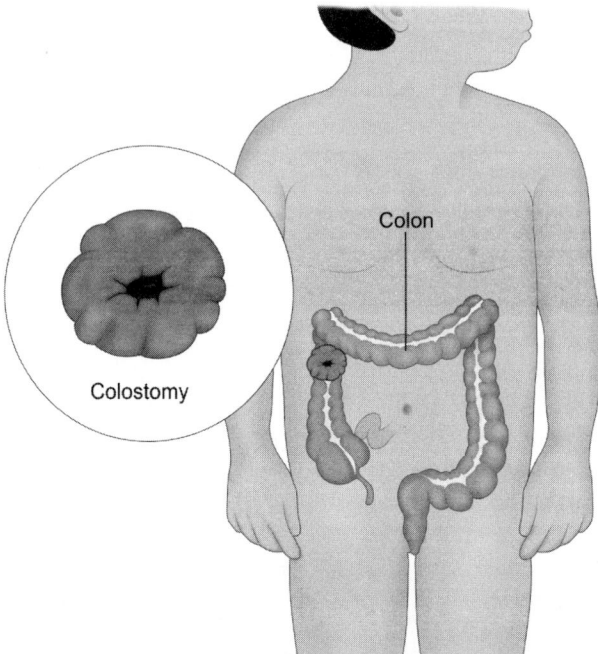

Fig. 22.6: Colostomy.

end of the intestine, which is brought to the surface of the skin on the abdomen, is called the stoma.
- An enterostomy can be temporary or permanent.

Objectives

- To empty and cleanses the colon and rectum.
- To stimulate peristalsis and help develop regular bowel movement.
- To relieve flatulence.

Indications

- Accomplished after surgery to promote regulated evacuation.
- To regulate bowel movement.
- To help avoid constipation.

Equipment

- Enema can and tubing.
- Three emesis basins
- Bath blanket
- Warm water in a basin
- Bath towel
- Bedpans or pail for collecting the return flow
- Irrigating solution
- Newspaper
- Also: Soap, extra rubber sheet, small colon tube, plastic apron, colostomy dressing tray, wash cloth.

Procedure

Nursing interventions	Rationale
Explain the procedure to the patient	To gain the cooperation of the patient
Wash hands	To avoid contamination
Bring equipment to the bedside and provide privacy	To save time and promote the dignity of the patient
Assist the patient to turn on his left side or appropriate side	To allow the nurse to do the procedure without difficulty
Place the emesis basin and newspaper at the foot of the bed	To ensure that the waste are properly disposed
Expose the abdomen, drape the patient with a bath blanker if necessary	Draping is also part in the provision of the patient's privacy
Remove soiled dressings and place them on the emesis basin and newspaper at the foot of the bed	To avoid contamination and control odor
Place the basin for return flow immediately under the colostomy opening. The patient can hold this in place if he is able	Basin must be ready to avoid spillage
Open the clamp on the tubing and allow a small amount of solution to flow into the basin	To release air bubbles in the set-up so that air is not introduced into the colon which would cause crampy pain

Contd...

Contd...

Nursing interventions	Rationale
Lubricate the tip of the colon tube	To facilitate the easy insertion of the tube
Insert the colon tube 6-8 inches into the colostomy opening	To avoid irrigating the intestinal mucosa
Hold the enema can approximately 12 inches above the bed and allow the solution to flow in slowly	To avoid painful cramp usually caused by too rapid flow
When the basin is almost full, quickly remove it and place the second basin in position	To avoid spillage
Empty the first basin immediately	So that it will be ready for use if needed again
After the irrigation is finished, wash the area with soap and water and apply a clean dressing to the area	Cleanliness and dryness will provide the patient with comfort
Return the equipment to the utility room, clean and return to the proper place	This will control odor and prolong life of the equipment

DOCUMENTATION

- Time irrigation administered.
- Kind and amount of solution used for the irrigation.
- Dressing applied.
- Condition of the area.
- Results obtained; amount, color, and consistency of the returns.
- Patient's reaction to procedure.

Possible Complications

Problems from the procedure are rare, but all procedures have some risk. It includes:
- Bleeding
- Blood clots
- Infection
- Skin irritation around the stoma from leaking digestive fluids
- Diarrhea
- Intestinal obstruction
- Hernia the at surgical site
- Blockage or leakage of the tube, requiring replacement
- Adverse reaction to the anesthesia

Post-procedure Care

At the hospital:
- You may need antibiotics. You may also need medications for nausea and pain.
- If you had an enterostomy to help fecal matter exit the bowels, you may have a pouch on the outside of your body. Waste material will be collected in it. You will receive instructions about diet and activity. During the first few days after surgery, you may be restricted from eating.
- The staff will monitor your fluid intake and output to help you avoid dehydration.
- You will wear boots or special socks to help prevent blood clots.
- You will be asked to walk often after surgery.

- You may be asked to use an incentive spirometer, to breathe deeply, and to cough frequently. This will improve lung function.
- Your incision will be examined often for signs of infection.

Preventing Infection
- Washing their hands
- Wearing gloves or masks
- Keeping your incisions covered

There are also steps you can take to reduce your chance of infection such as:
- Washing your hands often and reminding your healthcare providers to do the same
- Reminding your healthcare providers to wear gloves or masks
- Not allowing others to touch your incision

At home:
- Practicing good skin care of the area around the stoma. This will help to prevent infection.
- Caring for the stoma site and changing the ostomy bag if you have one.
- Keeping the area dry until you have permission from your doctor to shower or bathe.

POINTS TO NOTE
- Ureterostomy is the creation of a stoma (a new, artificial outlet) for a ureter or kidney.
- The procedure is performed to divert the flow of urine away from the bladder when the bladder is not functioning or has been removed.
- An enterostomy or ostomy (colostomy, ileostomy) is a surgically created opening of the bowel (intestine) to the outside which allows the body to empty stool (poop) and gas.
- The nurse plays a pivotal role in managing a child with ostomy to reduce the risk of sepsis at the stromal site.

MULTIPLE CHOICE QUESTIONS

1. **A surgical opening from the ureters to divert the urine flow is termed as:**
   a. Urostomy
   b. Jejunostomy
   c. Enterostomy
   d. Ureterostomy

2. **Enterostomy is defined as:**
   a. Opening in the colon
   b. Opening in the stomach
   c. Opening in the ileum
   d. Both a and c

3. **The purpose of creating a enterostomy opening in a child includes all, *except*:**
   a. To empty the stools
   b. To provide gastric feeding
   c. To empty the gas
   d. To reduce the abdominal distension

4. **The complications of enterostomy mainly includes:**
   a. Bleeding
   b. Skin allergy
   c. Vomiting
   d. Diarrhea

ANSWER KEY

1. d   2. d   3. b   4. a

CHAPTER 23

Care of Surgical Wounds, Dressing and Suture Removal

PRACTICE COMPETENCIES
On completion of the chapter, the students will be able to:
- Perform wound dressing.
- Carry out suture removal.

ABSTRACT
The covering of the sutured surgical wound with a sterile dressing is usually considered a routine conclusion to an aseptic operation. The wound is usually left dressed for a minimum of 3 to 5 days. The main purpose of dressing is protection of the wound against bacterial contamination that remains a significant source of postoperative morbidity. This chapter contains care of surgical wounds, dressing and suture removal.

Keywords: Surgical wounds, wound dressing, suture removal, pressure dressing, self-adhesive dressing.

DEFINITION

It is a sterile protective surgical covering, applied to a wound/incision with aseptic technique, with or without medication.

PURPOSES OF DRESSINGS

- To promote wound granulation and healing
- To prevent microorganism from entering the wound
- To decrease the presence of purulent wound drainage
- To absorb fluid and apply medication
- To immobilize and support the wound
- To assist in removal of necrotic tissue
- To provide comfort

TYPES OF DRESSINGS USED

Types of Dressing Used Depends on
- The location, size and type of the wound
- Type and amount of exudate

- ❖ Whether the wound is infected
- ❖ Frequency of changing the dressing.

Gauze

These are most commonly used dressing. They do not interact with wound tissues and thus cause little wound irritation. They are available in different textures and in squares of 10 × 10 cm 5 × 5 cm rectangles—10 × 20 cm and in rolls of various lengths, squares.

Types of Dressings

Wet Dressing

These are preferred in treating wounds that require debridement. This moistens the dressing, increasing the gauze's ability to collect exudates and wounds debris.

Non-adherent Dressing

These dressing have a shiny non-adherent surface that does not stick to incision or wound opening but allows drainage to pass through the softened gauze above.

Self-adhesive Dressing

It is ideal for small superficial wound that do not require debridement.

Advantages:
- ❖ It sticks to undamaged skin
- ❖ It allows the wound surface to breathe
- ❖ It promotes epithelial cell growth
- ❖ It can be removed without damaging the underlying tissues
- ❖ It promotes observation of the wound.

Hydrocolloid (HCD) and Hydrogel Dressings

These types of dressings are occlusive with the following advantages:
- ❖ Absorb drainage through the use of exudates absorbers
- ❖ Maintain wound humidity
- ❖ Slowly liquefy necrotic debris
- ❖ Provide protective cushioning.

Pressure Dressing

Pressure dressing helps in promoting hemostasis. It exerts pressure over an actual bleeding site. It also helps in eliminating dead space in underlying tissues and allows the wounds to heal normally. Once pressure dressing is used, the nurse should keep a constant observation for skin color and pulse in distant extremities.

Equipment

A sterile tray containing:
- ❖ Artery forceps—1
- ❖ Dissecting forceps—2
- ❖ Scissors—1 (surgical)
- ❖ Sinus forceps—1 (as necessary)
- ❖ Suturing cutting scissors—1
- ❖ Small bowl—1
- ❖ Gloves, a mask and a gown

- Cotton balls, gauge pieces cotton pads (as necessary)
- Dressing towels
- Towels clips—4.

An unsterile tray containing:
- Cleaning solutions (as necessary)
- Ointments and powders as prescribed
- Bandages, binders, pins, adhesive plaster and scissors
- A large bowl with a disinfectant solution
- A kidney tray and a paper bag
- A Mackintosh and a towel.

Preparatory Phase
- Wash hands thoroughly, put on mask, gown and gloves
- Place dressing, supplies or articles on a clean flat surface (overhead table)
- Place disposable bags nearby to collect soiled dressings
- Determine what type of dressing is necessary
- Open the dressing tray by peeling a part the edges of the package
- Wash hands thoroughly before and after the procedure.

General instructions for wound dressing
- Maintain a strict aseptic technique to prevent cross infection to and from the wound. All materials touching the wound should be sterile
- All articles should be disinfected thoroughly before and after the procedure
- One set of instruments should be used for one dressing
- Use mask, sterile gloves and gown to minimize wound contamination
- Dressing should not be done immediately after sweeping and dusting; wait at least for 15-20 minutes
- Use individually wrapped sterile dressing and equipment for the wound
- Maintain a sterile field around the wound by spreading sterile towels
- Avoid talking, coughing, sneezing once the wound is opened
- If dressing is adherent to the wound due to secretions or blood, wet it with sterile saline before it is removed
- Observe the discharge from the wound accurately for color, odor, amount and consistency
- Shortening and removal of the drainage tube is done only after doctor's order
- Avoid meal timings for doing dressing. It should be done either half an hour before or after the meal.

Preparation of the patient and environment
- Identify the patient and position him comfortably
- Explain the procedure and provide privacy
- Drape the patient
- Offer a bed pan or urinal prior to dressing
- Close the doors and windows. Put off the fan to prevent draughts
- Keep one assistant for dressing of the large wounds
- Protect the bed with a mackintosh and a treatment towel
- Expose the part as necessary
- Untie the bandage or adhesive and remove only after hand washing
- Turn the patients head to one side to prevent anxiety.

Steps of Procedure

1. Screen and drape the patient
2. Wash hands
3. Collect required articles to the bed side
4. Loosen all adhesive tapes of the old dressing but do not remove the dressing
5. Wash hands
6. Put on mask, gown and gloves as necessary
7. Open the sterile tray
8. Pick up the dissecting forceps and remove the sorted dressing
9. Fold the soiled dressing inwards and place it in the paper bag or covered bin. Discard the dissecting forceps in the bowl of antiseptic lotion
10. Clean the wound from center to periphery
11. Use one gauze for one stroke from up to downwards
12. After thorough cleaning of the wound dry it with a dry gauzy piece
13. Apply medication if ordered
14. Cover the wound with a sterile gauze piece and then with cotton pads
15. Reinforce the dressing on the dependent part where the drainage may be collected
16. Discard artery forceps and dissecting forceps in the bowl of antiseptic lotion
17. Remove gloves and secure the dressing with bandage for adhesive tapes
18. Make the child comfortable and remove all articles from bedside.

Removal of Sutures

- To remove the interrupted sutures or drainage tube there should be doctors instructions
- It is always done after the wound is thoroughly cleaned.

Extra sterile articles needed are:

- Suture cutting scissors—1
- Toothed dissecting forceps—1
- Grasp the knot of the suture with the toothed forceps and pull it gently to expose the portion of the stitch under the skin.
- Cut the suture with the suture cutting scissors between the knot and the skin.
- Pull the thread out as one piece.
- The suture which is already above the skin should not be drawn under the skin
- Every suture should be examined for its completion
- Total number of sutures removed should be counted.

After care of the patient and articles

- Remove the Mackintosh and treatment towel
- Take all articles to the treatment room
- Discard the soiled dressing in the covered container and send it for incineration
- Remove the instruments and other articles from the disinfectant solution and clean them thoroughly
- Dry them and reset the tray and send it for autoclaving
- Replace all articles at the proper place
- Help the patient to dress up and make him comfortable
- Replace the bed linen
- Wash hands

❖ Record the procedure in nurses record, condition of the wound, type and amount of discharge, condition of the suture, etc. If any abnormality is found, report to the surgeon. Keep the unit tidy and clean.

POINTS TO NOTE

- Keep the wound covered with a clean dressing until there is no fluid draining from it.
- Wait about 2–4 days after surgery before showering.
- Avoid soaking in the bathtub or swimming until the next doctor visit.
- Try to keep pets away from the wound.
- Avoid picking or scratching scabs. A scab may itch as the skin underneath heals, but picking or scratching can rip the new skin underneath. The wound will take longer to heal and the scar it leaves may be worse.
- Offer your child healthy foods—especially lots of vitamin-rich fruits and vegetables and lean proteins—while the wound heals. He or she should drink plenty of water and eat whole grains and high fiber diet to avoid constipation.

PRACTICE QUESTIONS

1. List down the purpose of dressings.
2. What are the points need to remember while doing dressing?

MULTIPLE CHOICE QUESTIONS

1. Keloid scars is made up of:
   a. Dense collagen
   b. Loose fibrous tissue
   c. Granulomatous tissue
   d. Loose areolar tissue
2. Following are required for wound healing, *except*:
   a. Zinc
   b. Vitamin C
   c. Calcium
   d. Copper
3. The vitamin which has inhibitory effect on wound healing is:
   a. Vitamin A
   b. Vitamin E
   c. Vitamin C
   d. Vitamin B complex

ANSWER KEY

1. a   2. d   3. b

CHAPTER 24

Catheterization in Children

PRACTICE COMPETENCY

On completion of the chapter, the students will be able to:
○ Perform insertion of an indwelling urethral catheter using aseptic technique

ABSTRACT

Bladder catheterization dates back to 300 BC. There are reports of catheters being made from dried reeds, palm leaves, animal skins and cheese glue. This was followed by the development of metal catheters using gold, tin, lead and silver. More malleable materials become available in 1844 following protection of the vulcanization of rubber. In 1934, Foley designed the inflation balloon to retain the catheter in the bladder. Urinary catheterization is the insertion of a tube in to the bladder, using aseptic technique, for the purpose of evacuating or instilling fluid. Catheterization has physical, mental and social implications beyond the drainage of urine. The promotion of best nursing practice in catheter care is integral to enhancing good patient care. This chapter contains nursing care plan for pediatric catheterization, female urinary catheterization and male urinary catheterization for children.

Keywords: Urinary catheterization, male urethral catheterization, female urethral catheterization, catheter care, removing catheter.

■ INTRODUCTION

A urethral catheter is a hollow tube inserted through the urethra into the bladder for the purpose of urine drainage, instillation of medical treatments or urine output monitoring. Insertion of an indwelling urethral catheter is an invasive procedure that should only be carried out when necessary for individual patient care by a qualified competent healthcare professional using an aseptic none touch technique (ANTT).

Aims of Urethral Catheterization

❖ To promote the child's dignity and comfort
❖ To recognize and minimize risks of secondary complications
❖ Ensure the child has age appropriate explanation of procedure using play therapy and distraction tools where appropriate

- ❖ Ensure parents/carers have adequate explanation of procedure
- ❖ To ensure that a quality service is offered to all patients
- ❖ To ensure that current research based practices are implemented.

Indications for Urethral Catheterization

- ❖ To drain the bladder prior to or following abdominal/pelvic/rectal surgery
- ❖ Prior to investigations
- ❖ To relieve retention of urine
- ❖ To measure accurate urine output
- ❖ To relieve urinary incontinence when no other means is practical.

Factors to Consider Prior to Catheterization

- ❖ Is there an alternative less invasive method of management
- ❖ History of hematuria and or discharge
- ❖ History of urethral obstruction or previous difficult catheterization
- ❖ History of fused or labial adhesions
- ❖ History of recent surgery to the lower urinary tract
- ❖ Patients with congenital abnormalities
- ❖ Trauma to the pelvis or abdomen
- ❖ Inflammation of the genitourinary tract; cystitis, urethritis, vaginal pain
- ❖ Immunocompromised patients
- ❖ Spinal cord injured patients due to risk of autonomic dysreflexia.

If the child has any of the above concerns advice should be sought from the responsible pediatrician.

Documentation

Following catheterization a record must be made in the patient record.

Related to
- ❖ Reason(s) for catheterization
- ❖ Type of catheter used, the size (Ch/Fr), length, material, balloon size, batch number and manufacturer

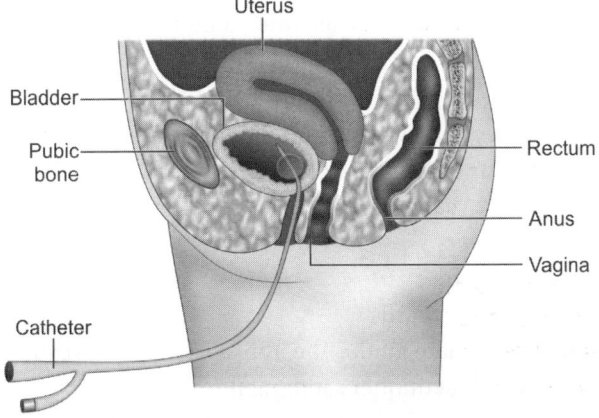

Fig. 24.1: Female child urethral catheterization.

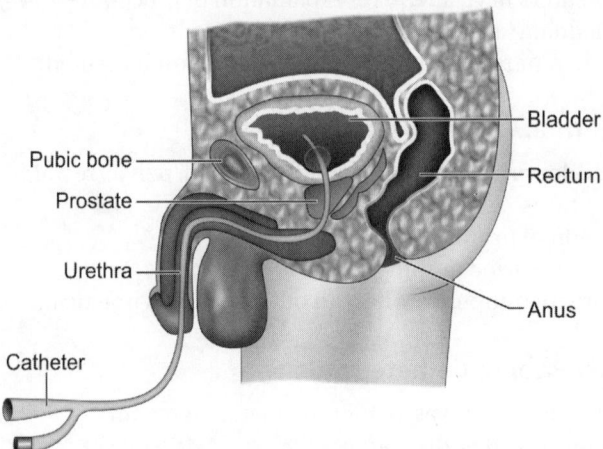

Fig. 24.2: Male child urethral catheterization.

- Cleansing solution and lubricant/anesthetic agent used
- Any problem encountered during procedure
- Volume of urine drained
- Date for reassessment
- Signature of the practitioner who carried out the catheterization.
    Note: Ch = Charriere
    Fr = French
    1 mm = 3 Fr

Catheter Selection

Catheters should be used in line with the manufacturer recommendations in order to avoid product liability (medicines and healthcare products regulatory agency). Selection of catheter depends upon the individual patient's needs, latex allergy, anticipated duration of catheterization and need for bladder washout.

Duration of Catheter

- Short-term (up to 28 days) PTFE bonded latex
- Long-term (up to 12 weeks) silicone elastomer coated.

Catheter Size

Do not use feeding tubes they can become knotted in the bladder and unable to be removed Choose the smallest to provide adequate drainage.

　　　Size 6 Ch...............up to 2 years
　　　Size 8 Ch...............2–10 years
　　　Size 10 Ch............10–14 years
　　　Size 12 Ch............14 years upwards

These sizes are an approximate guide. The appropriate size of catheter should be chosen according to the experienced practitioner's judgment.

Length of Catheter

Pediatric catheters are available up to size 12 Ch and are standard length. For older children using a size 12 Ch then select male or female:
- Pediatric approximately 30 cm
- Female approximately 26 cm
- Male approximately 43 cm

Balloon Size

Instruction on the catheter packaging should be followed
- Routine 5 mL in pediatric catheters
- Adult 10 mL.

PROCEDURE FOR PEDIATRIC URINARY CATHETERIZATION GENERAL GUIDELINES

- Insertion of an indwelling urethral catheter should be carried out by a qualified competent health professional.
- Discuss the proposed procedure with the child and parents/guardians (carer), document consent in medical notes. Check for allergies including latex and any known reactions to anesthetic gels.
- Cultural and religious beliefs need to be considered before performing the catheterization.
- Where a child of any age refuses urethral catheterization the procedure should be delayed if possible.
- Enlist assistance from the hospital play specialist to support the child throughout the procedure.
- Prepare a quiet room, which allows sufficient space for the play specialist and carer to accompany the child.
- Collect catheter dressing pack, normal saline (warmed)—for cleaning, plastic apron, collecting bowl, drainage bag and holder or straps tape, lubricating anesthetic gel
- Select a urethral catheter of the appropriate type and size and water for the balloon.
- Prepare the clinical area (where possible using the treatment room) with the appropriate equipment using an aseptic technique.
- The child should have the procedure explained with age appropriate play preparation, using dolls, catheter tubes, and equipment to demonstrate the process.
- Reassure the child and carer throughout the procedure, stopping any time the child asks for a rest.
- Put on plastic apron disinfect and wash hands with antimicrobial solution, apply sterile gloves and plastic apron.
- Draw up sterile, water into a syringe for the catheter balloon. Some catheters come with a prefilled syringe.
- Check anesthetic gel and volume.
- Position child appropriately—Ideally babies and children are catheterized on the bed with their hips flat on the bed, but alternatively—female toddlers can be held on carer's knee with their legs in the frog position. The child faces forward, leans back upon parent with buttocks almost at the parent's knee.

Female Urethral Catheterization

- Clean the urethral meatus before insertion of the catheter. Use only soap and water or normal saline, using a single downward stroke, using the dominant hand then discard the swab into a yellow clinical waste bag.
- Hold labia firmly open with the other hand and identify the urethral meatus.
- If Nurse feels it is appropriate instil anesthetic gel to the area around and just inside the urethral meatus. (0–2 years: 1–2 mL, 2–5 years: 2–4 mL, 5–10 years: 4–6 mL,10 + years: 6 mL)
- Wait for 3–5 minutes and lubricate catheter with anesthetic gel
- Hold the catheter 8–10 cm from the tip, ensuring the other end is over the collecting bowl and gently insert it into the urethra until urine flows.

Male Urethral Catheterization

- All boys are encouraged to lie on their back on the bed, remove their underwear and sit on the disposable under pad.
- With the non-dominant hand gently retract the foreskin using sterile gauze until the urethral meatus is visible. With the dominant hand clean the glans with a sterile swab and 0.9% normal saline, Instil anesthetic gel into the urethra (0–2 years: 1–2 mL, 2–5 years: 2–4 mL, 5–10 years: 4–6 mL,10 + years: 6 mL) and squeeze the penis gently, wait for 3–5 minutes and lubricate catheter with anesthetic gel.
- Hold the penis upright and firmly at the base. Hold the catheter 15–20 cm from the tip and gently insert it into the urethra. Continue insertion very slowly until resistance is felt, when the catheter reaches the bladder neck. Gently rotate the catheter slightly between the fingers and thumb until the sphincter relaxes and allows the catheter to enter the bladder, resulting in a flow of urine.

In Both Female and Male

- Advance the catheter a further 4 cm. Inflate the balloon with sterile water.
- Connect indwelling urethral catheter to a sterile closed urinary drainage system.
- Position urine drainage bag below the level of the bladder or on a stand that prevents contact with the floor.
- Attach the catheter with tape to the child's groin, avoiding tension to the bladder neck. Ensure movement of the child's leg is not restricted.
- Remove and discard gloves and wash hands with antimicrobial solution.
- Ensure that the child is comfortable.
- Dispose of all equipment according to clinical waste procedures.
- Disinfect and wash hands with antimicrobial solution.
- Document catheter insertion: Reason for catheterization, Parental consent, Catheter type, size (Ch), length, balloon size, material and batch number of the catheter used, cleansing solution used, lubricating agent used, record any problems negotiated during the procedure, volume of urine drained, date and time of catheterization, planned date for re-assessment.

Catheter Care/Urinary Drainage Equipment

- To care for an indwelling catheter, cleanse the urethral area and the catheter itself with soap and water every day. Also thoroughly cleanse the area after all bowel movements.
- Drainage system should always be based on an individual assessment of need.

- Empty the drainage bag often enough to maintain urinary flow and prevent reflux. Use a clean separate container for each patient and avoid contact between tap and the container.
- Change drainage bags when they become discolored, have sediment, offensive smell or are damaged. All bags must be changed following manufacturers recommendations.

When Removing the Catheter

- The qualified practitioner should reassess the need for the catheter on a daily basis. The catheter should be removed as soon as the patient's condition allows
- Explain the procedure to the child/carer. Inform them of post catheter symptoms, i.e. urgency, frequency and discomfort, which are often caused by irritation of the urethra by the catheter. Symptoms should resolve over the following 24–48 hours. If not further investigations may be needed.
- Attach an empty syringe to the balloon port on the catheter, and allow it to fill with the water from the balloon. Do not pull the water out.
- Gently check the catheter is free to be removed, and then proceed to remove the catheter slowly from the bladder and urethra and discard.
- Ensure adequate oral intake and document
- Monitor urine output after removal. The first void should occur within 6–7 hours of removal and document.

> **POINTS TO NOTE**
> - When inserting urinary catheters, be aware of and respect cultural beliefs related to privacy, family involvement, and the request for a same-gender nurse.
> - Inserting a urinary catheter requires visualization and manipulation of anatomical areas that are considered private by most patients.
> - These procedures can cause emotional distress, especially if the patient has experienced any history of abuse or trauma.

PRACTICE QUESTIONS

1. What are the points to consider prior to catheterization?
2. How do you remove the catheter?

MULTIPLE CHOICE QUESTIONS

1. **Acute hemorrhagic cystitis is most commonly caused by:**
   a. *Escherichia coli*
   b. Adenovirus
   c. *Klebsiella*
   d. *Proteus*
2. **You have a child complaining as follows after catheter removal. Which statement suggestive of UTI in child?**
   a. "I pee a lot"
   b. "It burns when I pee"
   c. "I go hours without the urge to pee"
   d. "My pee smells sweet"

3. The primary reason for taping an indwelling catheter laterally to the thigh of a male client is to:
   a. Eliminate pressure at the penoscrotal angle
   b. Prevent the catheter from kinking in the urethra
   c. Prevent accidental catheter removal
   d. Allow the client to turn without kinking the catheter

ANSWER KEY

1. a   2. b   3. a

CHAPTER 25

Insertion of Suppositories

PRACTICE COMPETENCIES
On completion of the chapter, the students will be able to:
- Carry out insertion of suppository in children.
- Promote optimum comfort for the child in children after the insertion of suppository.

ABSTRACT
Suppositories are generally indicated for use in infants and young children. Common medications administered via this route are analgesics, sedatives and anti-emetics. Nursing priorities include individual child assessment, medication knowledge, safe medication practices and the promotion of optimum comfort for the child.

Keywords: Suppositories, child, procedure.

INTRODUCTION
Suppositories are cone shaped or in a semi-solid form, which is intended to body orifices (rectum, vagina, urethra). They melt, soften or dissolve in the body orifices and exert local or systemic effect.

DEFINITION
A suppository is another way to give medication. When your child has a suppository, the medication is put into their rectum. A suppository comes in a solid form that when put in the rectum slowly melts.

A suppository is a plug of medicine designed to melt at body temperature within the rectum (back passage, or bottom).

IDEAL SUPPOSITORY MEASURES
- Melts at body temperature or dissolve in the body fluids
- Non-toxic and non-irritant
- Compatible with any medication
- Releases any medication readily
- Easily moulded and removed from the mould
- Stable to heating above the melting point

- Easy to handle
- Stable on storage.

EQUIPMENT

- Non-sterile gloves
- Water soluble lubricant
- Wash cloth
- Medication/suppository.

INDICATIONS

- Child with frequent vomiting or in NPO
- Child with high grade fever
- Respiratory distress
- Decreased level of consciousness in case of any gastric irritation.

CONTRAINDICATIONS

- Known sensitivity to medication
- Rectal bleeding
- Rectal prolapse
- Increased intracranial pressure
- Coagulopathy
- Neutropenia
- Acute abdominal surgical incisions
- Acute ulcerative colitis recent rectal surgery.

PRE-PROCEDURE GUIDELINES

- Explain the procedure to the patient family members
- Provide privacy to the child
- Perform hand hygiene
- Wear disposable gloves
- Place hygienic sheet or wash cloth under buttock and position the patient in left lateral position
- Cover with a sheet or a blanket and expose only when required.

Table. 25.1: Procedure for insertion of suppositories.

Steps in procedure	Rationale
1. Verify the medication order by the physician thoroughly. Check for allergy to the drug and if present notify to the physician **Alert**: Rectal medication administration is contraindicated in children who are immunosuppressed or thrombocytopenic because of the risk of infection or bleeding	Verifies correct drug dose, route, time and patient. Allergic reactions to patient may be life-threatening

Contd...

Contd...

Steps in procedure	Rationale
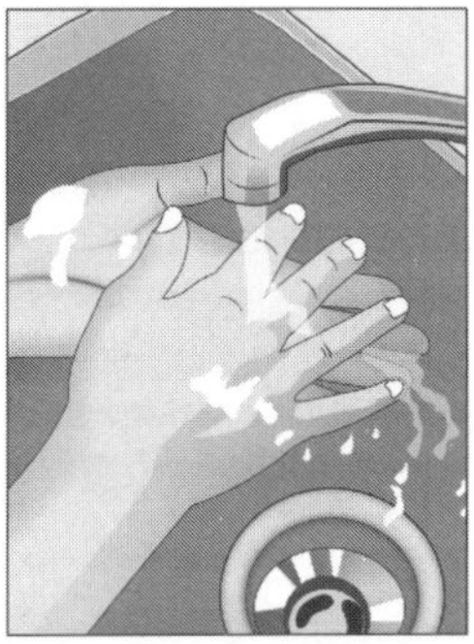 2. Perform hand hygiene	Reduces the transmission of microorganisms

Fig. 25.1: Hand hygiene.

Steps in procedure	Rationale
3. Obtain the medication and read the label to verify with the order, check for the expiry date; if expired do not administer the drug	To decrease chance of medication error, patient route, dose, frequency and time to be administered must be verified each time a medication is administered
4. Check medication form dispensed to ensure that it is appropriate for the child	Suppositories are the most frequent form of rectal administration, although occasionally medication may be administered in an enema form. Child are very susceptible to fluid or electrolyte imbalance
5. Prepare medication for the administration. Avoid cutting if possible. If the suppository must be cut to obtain the ordered dose, then it must be cut length wise	Cutting a suppository length wise helps absorption at the required rate. The drug may not be dispersed with in the suppository
6. Wear the disposable gloves	Protects the administrator from the fecal materials, thus reducing the transmission of microorganisms
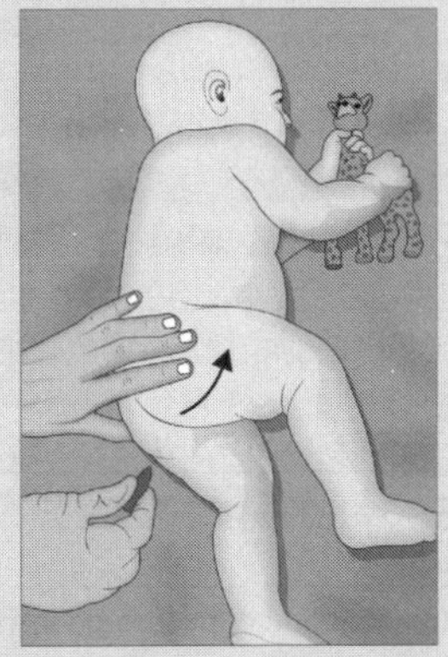 7. Position the child in left lateral position with the right leg flexed or in the knee chest position	Either of these positions exposes the anus and helps to relax the external sphincter for ease of insertion

Fig. 25.2: Left lateral position with right leg flexed.

Contd...

Contd...

Steps in procedure	Rationale
8. Remove the suppository packaging and lubricate the suppository with a water soluble lubricating jelly **Fig. 25.3:** Removing the suppository form packing.	Reduces friction against mucosal surfaces
9. Insert suppository using index or little finger gently not more than 1 cm into the rectum, placing the medication against the rectal wall	The suppository must be passed the internal sphincter to prevent expulsion
10. Hold the child's buttocks together until the child relaxes or loses the urge to push. If the child has a stool with in 30 min, examine the stool for the presence of suppository **Fig. 25.4:** Holding the child's buttocks.	Prevents expulsion of medication
11. Remove the gloves. Dispose the gloves in appropriate bin	To maintain the standard precautions
12. Perform hand hygiene and document the procedure	Reduces the transmission of microorganisms and documentation aids in improving the communication of patient information

COMPLICATIONS

❖ Perforation or injury to the rectum

- ❖ Sepsis
- ❖ Bleeding
- ❖ Adverse reactions to the medication.

> **POINTS TO NOTE**
> - A suppository is a plug of medicine designed to melt at body temperature within the rectum (back passage, or bottom).
> - Insert suppository using index or little finger gently not more than 1 cm into the rectum, placing the medication against the rectal wall.
> - Rectal medication administration is contraindicated in children who are immunosuppressed or thrombocytopenic because of the risk of infection or bleeding.
> - The suppository must be passed the internal sphincter to prevent expulsion.

MULTIPLE CHOICE QUESTIONS

1. **The main purpose of providing the suppository is:**
   a. To provide rectal medication
   b. To reduce inflammation
   c. To promote comfort
   d. To improve circulation
2. **Suppository means:**
   a. Tablet given orally
   b. Intravenous medication
   c. Intramuscular injection
   d. Rectal medication
3. **Possible complication of using rectal suppository:**
   a. Vomitings
   b. Skin inflammation
   c. Fever
   d. Bleeding
4. **Position used to place a suppository to a child:**
   a. Supine position
   b. Lithotomy position
   c. Left lateral position
   d. Prone position

ANSWER KEY

1. a   2. d   3. d   4. c

CHAPTER 26

Oxygen Administration in Children

PRACTICE COMPETENCIES

On completion of the chapter, the students will be able to:
- Maintain targeted SpO_2 levels in children through the provision of supplemental oxygen in a safe and effective way which is tolerated by infants and children
- Monitor SpO_2/SaO_2
- Select the appropriate flow rate and delivery device.
- Ensure adequate clearance of secretions and limit the adverse events of hypothermia and insensible water loss by use of optimal humidification (dependent on mode of oxygen delivery).
- Maintain efficient and economical use of oxygen.

ABSTRACT

Rapid and effective oxygen delivery is an essential component of the care of critically ill or injured children. A variety of systems are available to deliver oxygen to children who are breathing spontaneously. Factors that influence the appropriate choice for any given situation include the dose of oxygen required and how well the child accepts the device. This chapter contains various methods of oxygen administration to children such as face mask, nasal canula, oxygen tent, hood, incubator, and 'T' piece circuit.

Keywords: Oxygen administration in children, face mask, venture mask, nasal pongs, oxygen tent, oxygen hood, incubator "T" piece circuit.

INTRODUCTION

Oxygen is essential for human survival.

Inspired air contains 21% of oxygen.

It is carried in the body largely in combination with hemoglobin and a small quantity is transported in physical solution in plasma.

Each molecules of hemoglobin can bind up to four molecule of oxygen and each gram of hemoglobin can carry approximately 1.34 mL of oxygen.

In persons with normal lungs breathing room air, the dissolved portion of oxygen in plasma is only 2% of total.

If some person is exposed to 100% oxygen, the amount of dissolved oxygen may approach to 10% of whole.

OXYGEN THERAPY

Oxygen may be classified as an element, a gas, and a drug.

Oxygen therapy is the administration of oxygen at concentrations greater than that in room air to treat or prevent hypoxemia (not enough oxygen in the blood).

The WHO recommends that oxygen should be administered to a child with:
Central cyanosis/inability to drink
Grunting in infant < 2 months of age
Tachypnea, restlessness, chest in drawing

Oxygen saturation (arterial blood)
Newborn 40–90%
Thereafter 95–99%

Additional Benefits of Oxygen Therapy
- Increased clarity
- Relieves nausea
- Can prevent heart failure in people with severe lung disease
- Allows the bodies organs to carry out normal functions.

Long-term Benefits of Oxygen Therapy
- Prolongs life by reducing heart strain
- Decreases shortness of breath
- Oxygen retards the aging of human cells
- Oxygen helps relieve headaches
- Oxygen alleviates tiredness
- Oxygen boosts the immune system
- Oxygen supports breathing of air in cases of asthma and allergies
- Oxygen helps in cases of depression
- Oxygen improves physical performance by up to 25%.

Levels in the blood decrease, and the patient may need supplemental oxygen.
- Oxygen therapy is a key treatment in respiratory care.
- To increase oxygen saturation in tissues where the saturation levels are too low.

INDICATIONS
- Hypoxia—the blood oxygen levels < 92%
- Hypercapnia—increased carbon dioxide levels
  Oxygen therapy is used to decrease work to breathing by increasing alveolar oxygen tension.

Indications for Oxygen Therapy
Any individual with one or more of the following:
- Peri and postcardiac or respiratory arrest blood oxygen levels (oxygen saturation levels of < 92%)
- Acute and chronic hypoxemia (PaO_2 < 65 mm Hg, SaO_2 < 92%)
  Signs and symptoms of shock
  Low cardiac output and metabolic acidosis (HCO_3 < 18 mmol/L)
  Chronic type two respiratory failure (hypoxia and hypercapnia)

Despite a lack of supportive data, oxygen is also administered in the following conditions:
Dyspnea without hypoxemia
    Postoperatively, dependent on instruction from surgical team
    Treatment of pneumothorax
    Chronic lung disease
    Congenital heart disease with pulmonary hypertension
    Pulmonary hypertension secondary to respiratory disease
    Interstitial lung disease
    Obliterative bronchiolitis
    Cystic fibrosis and other causes of severe bronchiectasis
    Obstructive sleep apnea and other sleep related disorders
    Palliative care for symptom relief.

Types of Oxygen Therapy

High Concentration Oxygen Therapy

Up to 60% results in the reduced risk of hypoventilation and retention of carbon dioxide. High concentration oxygen therapy can have detrimental effects on the respiratory system, particularly after prolonged usage and can lead to respiratory distress due to absorption atelectasis (collapse of alveolus due to blockage). In the premature infant retrolental fibroplasias can be a side effect due to vasoconstriction and could lead to permanent blindness.

Low Concentration Oxygen Therapy (Controlled Oxygen Therapy)

Used to correct hypoxemia by using an accurate amount of oxygen without depleting existing maintenance of carbon dioxide and respiratory acidosis. Blood gases should be used to measure the precise concentration of oxygen.

Long-term Oxygen Therapy (LTOT)

The provision of continuous oxygen therapy for patients with chronic hypoxemia, requirements vary between 24 hour dependency and dependency during periods of sleep. Principally aims to improve symptoms and prevent harm from chronic hypoxemia. Any child likely to require LTOT for longer than 3 weeks should be considered for domiciliary oxygen.

METHODS OF OXYGEN THERAPY

The selection of an appropriate oxygen delivery system must take into account, clinical condition, the patient's size, needs and therapeutic goals:
    High concentration oxygen is usually delivered via incubator or humidified head box for concentrations below 50%, oxygen can be delivered via nasal cannula.
  A. Face mask
  B. Nasal cannula
  C. Oxygen tent
  D. Hood
  E. Incubator
  F. T-piece circuit
  G. Transtracheal oxygen delivery

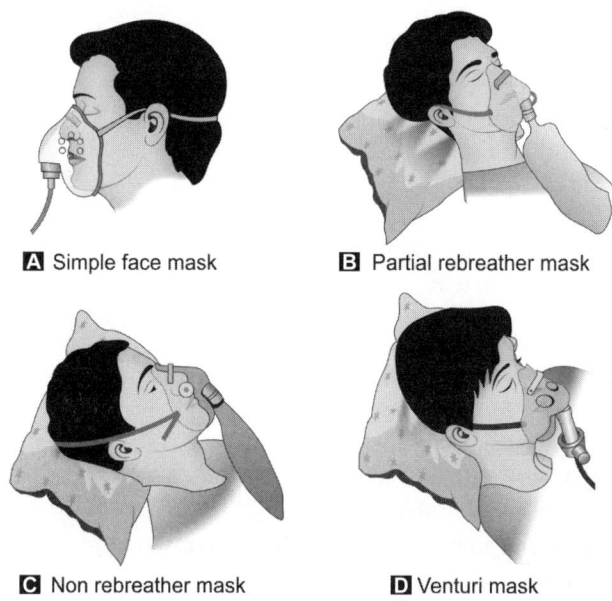

Figs. 26.1A to D: Types of oxygen masks.

A. Face Mask

- ❖ It cover the client's nose and mouth may be used for oxygen inhalation.
- ❖ Exhalation ports on the sides of the mask allow exhaled carbon dioxide to escape.

Types of Face Masks

Simple face mask: Delivers oxygen concentrations from 40 to 60% at liter flows of 5 to 8 liters per minute, respectively.

Partial rebreather mask: Delivers oxygen concentration of 60 to 90% at liter flows of 6 to 10 liters per minute, respectively.

Non-rebreather mask: Delivers the highest oxygen concentration possible 90 to 100%, by means other than intubation or mechanical ventilation, at liter flows of 10 to 15 liters per minute.

Venturi mask: Delivers oxygen concentration varying from 24 to 40% or 50% at liter flows of 4 to 10 liters per minute.

These are designed to deliver a fixed percentage of O_2 (24%, 28%, 35%, 40%, 50%).
- ❖ Operate according to the Venturi principle.
- ❖ O_2 flowing through a narrow orifice contain room air at up to 150 L/min via vents in the mask connector.
- ❖ The gas flow and the Venturi valve determine the O_2 concentration.
- ❖ Humidification is not necessary due to the large amounts of room air entered.
- ❖ These masks are particularly useful for chronic airflow limitation (CAL) patients, whose stimulus to breathe is controlled by a degree of hypoxia (hypoxic drive) because the mask delivers high volume of oxygen.

Equipment: Disposable face mask, oxygen source.

Procedure

1. **Prepare patient**
   - Utilize standard infection control precautions
   - Position, reassure, inform consent
   - Appropriate to condition
2. **Prepare equipment**
   - Remove mask from package
   - Secure mask tubing to oxygen source
   - Turn on oxygen and set to a minimum of 8 L/min
   - Extend elastic strap
   - Ensure malleable nose adjustment opened out.
3. **Application of mask**
   - Hold mask with one hand and stretch elastic strap
   - Place elastic strap over patient's head and above ears
   - Gently place mask over patient's face, fitting nose
   - Adjustment to afford comfortable fit.
4. **Adjust elastic strap to support mask in position but not too tight.**
   - Secure oxygen tubing. To prevent dislodgement.
5. **Ensure oxygen flow rate is appropriate to patient's condition.**

B. Nasal Cannula

- Also called nasal prongs.
- Is the most common inexpensive device used to administer oxygen.
- It is easy to apply and does not interfere with the client's ability to eat or talk.
- It delivers a relatively low concentration of oxygen which is 24 to 45% at flow rates of 2 to 6 liters per minute.

Equipment

- Oxygen cylinder with regulator fitments
- Opening key
- Humidifier
- Nasal tubes
- Rubber tubing
- Adhesive tape
- Cylinder step
- Oxygen mask, if available.

Procedure

- Explain the procedure and tell them why it is require check the cylinder; open the valve away from patient.
- Fill humidifier half filled with water.
- Attach the tubing of humidifier and oxygen cylinder and outlet of humidifier to the patient.
- Unscrew regulator and allow release of oxygen from cylinder which can be observed from bubbling of water in humidifying bottle.

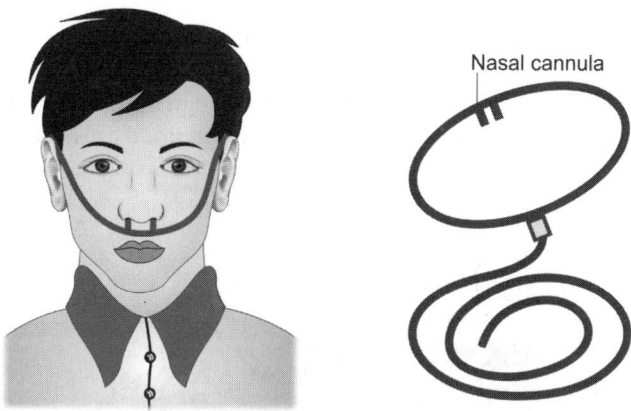

Fig. 26.2: Infant with nasal cannula.

C. Oxygen Tent

An oxygen tent consists of a canopy over the patient's bed that may cover the patientfully or partially and it is connected to a supply of oxygen.

The canopies are transparent and enables the nurse to observe the patient. The lower part of the canopy is tucked under bed to prevent the escape of oxygen. There are advantages and disadvantages of tent.

Advantages

- Oxygen tent provides an environment for the patient with controlled oxygen concentration, temperature regulation and humidity control.
- It allows freedom for free movement in bed.

Disadvantages

- It requires high volume of oxygen (10 to 12 L/min)
- Loss of desired concentration each time tent is opened.
- There is an increased chances of fire.
- It requires much time and effort to clean and maintain the tent.

The infant incubator like an oxygen tent designed to maintain a constant temperature in the environment of the infant.

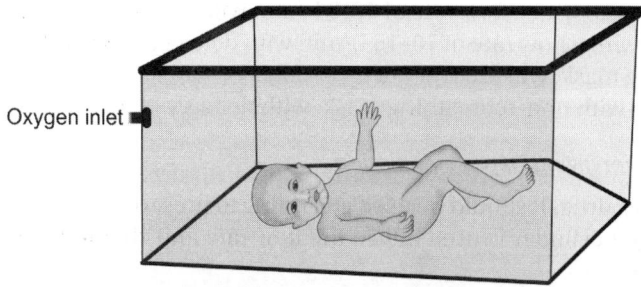

Fig. 26.3: Infant in oxygen tent.

D. Hood

Oxygen hoods are clear, plastic cylinders that encompass the infant's head. Oxygen concentrations of 80 to 90% can be achieved with oxygen flow rates of ≥10 to 15 L/mt. Oxygen enters the hood through a gas inlet. Exhaled gas exists through the opening at the neck. The hood is usually well tolerated by newborns. Infants in an oxygen hood are accessible for monitoring and other care.

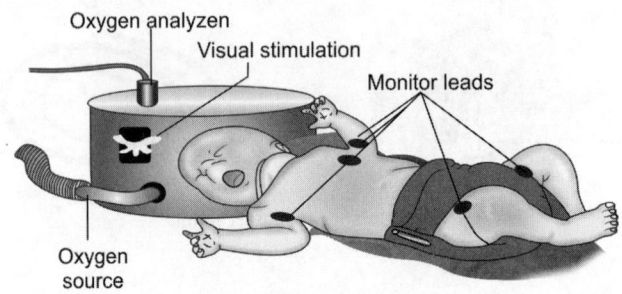

Fig. 26.4: Infant in oxygen hood.

E. Incubator

If a neonate is placed in an incubator and requires oxygen it can be provided with oxygen through a part for passing the air.

- The humidified oxygen is administered in to the incubator.
- The incubator is used to provide a controlled environment for the neonate.
- Adjust the oxygen flow to achieve the desired concentration.

F. T-Piece Circuit

- Deliver fixed percentage of oxygen (according to gas flow rates) via an endotracheal or tracheostomy tube.
- Deliver variable percentage of oxygen via CIG, Hudson or tracheostomy mask.

G. Transtracheal Oxygen Delivery

The percentages of oxygen delivered through various methods are:

- Nasal cannula: with a flow rate of 1–6 L/min with maximum delivery 45%.
- Nasal catheter: with a flow rate of 1–6 L/min with maximum delivery 45%
- Face mask: with a flow rate of 5–10 L/min with delivery of 35–60%
- Venture type mask: with a flow rate of 5–10 L/min with delivery of 25–60%
- Oxygen hood: with a flow rate of 10–15 L/min with delivery of 80–90%
- On-rebreathing mask: with delivery of up to 90%.
- Anesthesia bag with non-rebreathing mask: with delivery of up to 95%.

General Instructions for giving Oxygen Inhalation

- Oxygen acts as a drug. It should be used according to prescription.
- When an oxygen cylinder is used adjust the flow rate and should be used with regulator and humidifier.
- Every part of the apparatus should be clean to prevent infection.
- Use disposable nasal catheters.

- Change the nasal catheters at least every 8 hours.
- Lubricate the nasal catheter sparingly while the oxygen is flowing.
- During the administration of oxygen the valve controlling the rate of flow should not be handled.
- Oxygen administration must never be stopped until the factors that caused hypoxia is reversed.
- When the oxygen therapy is discontinued it should be done carefully and gradually.
- For all patients receiving oxygen inhalation the temperature should be taken rectally.
- Pay attention constantly while flowing the oxygen.
- Prevent the deprivation of oxygen resulting from the depletion of oxygen from this cylinder keep ready another cylinder.
- For fear of retrolental fibroplasia the premature babies are given oxygen inhalation for a short period.
- When oxygen is administered through nasal catheter it should not be passed beyond the uvula.

Nurses Responsibility in Administration of Oxygen

- Check the name, bed number and other identifications
- Check the diagnosis and need for oxygen therapy
- Check the doctors orders for initiation of therapy
- Assess the child for signs of clinical anoxia
- Assess the patients vital signs
- Check the results of arterial blood gas analysis
- Note any signs of pulmonary dysfunction
- Inspect anterior nares for irritation
- Inspect the skin and nose and surrounding areas for any skin lesions
- Check the patients mental status and ability to follow instructions
- Check the articles available in the unit.

After Care of the Patient

- Stay with child until she is recovered
- Keep the child warm and comfort
- Evaluate the child's progress by child's monitoring of vital signs
- Watch the child for any detorioratory symptoms after removal of oxygen
- Record the procedure date and time
- Request for an arterial blood gas analysis at specified intervals to treat hypoxia
- Clean the all articles and take it and replace it in utility room
- Clean the nasal catheter with cold water then warm water.

Complications

1. **Retrolental fibroplasia:** A high concentration of oxygen for prolonged period can damage the immature retinal blood vessels in premature infants.
2. **Carbon monoxide narcosis:**
   - Pulmonary congestion
   - Bronchiolar edema
   - Broncopulmonary necrotizing bronchiolitis
   - Oxygen toxicity
   - Pulmonary diseases and seizure disorders.

Chapter 26: Oxygen Administration in Children

> ### POINTS TO NOTE
>
> **Oxygen safety:** Oxygen is not a flammable gas but it does support combustion (rapid burning). Due to this the following rules should be followed:
> - Do not smoke in the vicinity of oxygen equipment.
> - Do not use aerosol sprays in the same room as the oxygen equipment.
> - Turn off oxygen immediately when not in use.
> - Oxygen is heavier than air and will pool in fabric making the material more flammable. Therefore, never leave the nasal prongs or mask under or on bed coverings or cushions whilst the oxygen is being supplied.
> - Oxygen cylinders should be secured safely to avoid injury.
> - Do not store oxygen cylinders in hot places.
> - Keep the oxygen equipment out of reach of children.
> - Do not use any petroleum products or petroleum by products, e.g., petroleum jelly/vaseline whilst using oxygen.

PRACTICE QUESTIONS

1. What are the benefits of oxygen therapy?
2. What are the indications for oxygen therapy?
3. What are the complications of oxygen therapy?

MULTIPLE CHOICE QUESTIONS

1. Which of the following statements regarding emergency oxygen therapy is true?
    a. Oxygen should be used as a treatment for breathlessness
    b. Oxygen therapy should always be prescribed
    c. Nonrebreathe oxygen mask is the delivery device of choice in critical illness
    d. Nasal cannula is the oxygen delivery device of choice in critical illness
2. Which of the following is not a feature of life-threatening asthma?
    a. Hypoxia
    b. Hypocapnia
    c. Silent chest
    d. Cyanosis
3. Which oxygen delivery system is for high flow oxygen?
    a. Nasal cannula
    b. Venturi mask
    c. Partial nonrebreather
    d. Simple mask
4. Which oxygen delivery system would you use for the lowest flow of oxygen?
    a. Simple face mask
    b. Nasal cannula
    c. Nonrebreather
    d. Partial nonrebreather

ANSWER KEY

1. c   2. b   3. b   4. b

CHAPTER 27

Cardiopulmonary Resuscitation

PRACTICE COMPETENCIES
On completion of the chapter, the students will be able to:
- Recognize a deteriorating infant and prevent cardiac arrest.
- Perform immediate basic life support maneuvers and act as an active member of the resuscitating team.
- Provide family care during cardiopulmonary resuscitation.

ABSTRACT
Pediatric resuscitation offers a challenge to the pediatric critical care nurse. Participating in resuscitation attempts requires specialized knowledge and skills. For best survival and quality of life, pediatric basic life support should be part of a community effort that includes prevention, early cardiopulmonary resuscitation, prompt access to the emergency response system, and rapid pediatric life support. This chapter contains objectives, purposes, indication, preparation for resuscitation, equipment required; initial steps of resuscitation, techniques of chest compression are included.

Keywords: Cardiopulmonary resuscitation, TABC of resuscitation, positive pressure ventilation, chest compression with two finger, and thumb technique.

■ INTRODUCTION

As you know the birth propels the newborn from a cocoon of warm weightless fluid environment to that of cold, dry and highly stressful environment by cutting the umbilical cord. It is the first few minutes of a newborn life that can be critical. This is the time when newborn is making an abrupt transition from the mother's uterus to the extrauterine life. The major problem that can arise during this time is birth asphyxia. The way in which an asphyxiated neonate is managed in the first few minutes of life can have consequences over an entire life time directly affecting quality of the life.

Every neonate has right to have resuscitation performed at a high level of competence. This means that the proper equipment must be immediately available in the delivery room. Remember, majority of the newborns cry spontaneously and require no treatment at all not even suction. Occasionally newborn that does not cry spontaneously and do not establish effective cardiopulmonary circulation, need resuscitation, based on newborn condition.

■ OBJECTIVES

After completing this practical, you the student should be able to:
- Identify the signs that indicate the need for resuscitation

- Assemble the appropriate equipment needed for resuscitation, and
- Resuscitate the newborn successfully.

PURPOSES

The main purpose of resuscitation is to initiate respiration in a newborn, who is asphyxiated or spontaneous breathing has not been initiated.

INDICATIONS

Antepartum Factors

- Maternal diabetes
- Pregnancy induced hypertension
- Previous Rh sensitization
- Bleeding in second or third trimester
- Post-term gestation
- Maternal age less than 16 years or more
- Multiple pregnancies
- Severe anemia
- Chronic hypertension
- Previous still birth
- Maternal infection
- Maternal drug abuse.

Intrapartum Factors

- Abnormal presentation
- Premature labor
- Foul smelling amniotic fluid
- Precipitate labor
- Prolapsed cord
- Abruptio placenta
- Meconium stained amniotic fluid.

PREPARATION FOR RESUSCITATION

Two trained personnel capable of working together to perform all aspects of resuscitation; it may be nurse and pediatrician or two skilled nurses.
- Source of heat either radiant warmer or 200 watt bulb.
- Adequate lighting and place to work.

EQUIPMENT REQUIRED

- Minimum two clean dry and warm sheets for each newborn
- Ambu bag and mask
- Infant laryngoscope
- Endotracheal tube of three different sizes
- Sterile suction catheter 12–14
- Oral mucous suction

- Oxygen source
- Emergency drugs (epinephrine, naloxone hydrochloride, normal saline)
- Ventilator
- Leucoplast
- Scissor
- Appropriate sized gloves.

THE TABC OF RESUSCITATION

The steps in resuscitation follows the well known TABC's of cardiopulmonary resuscitation:
T : Temperature maintenance
A : Ensuring/establishing an open airway
B : Initiating breathing
C : Maintaining circulation.

Now how you can maintain this:
T : Temperature maintenance is ensured by placing the newborn under preheated radiant warmer or 200 watt bulb.
A : The patency and adequacy of airways is established by proper positioning of the newborn, i.e. slight extension of neck by placing a roll or towel under the shoulder. Suction the mouth, nose and in some instances the trachea. If necessary insert an endotracheal tube to ensure an open airway.
B : Breathing can be initiated by using tactile stimulation or positive pressure ventilation can be used if necessary using bag and mask ventilation.
C : Circulation can be maintained by giving chest compression and medication.

SIGNS TO EVALUATE FOR RESUSCITATION

As soon as the newborn is delivered, you have to evaluate the newborn's condition, so that you can decide and take the necessary action. It is continuous process of assessment, action, evaluation, decision and further action.

Initial assessment performed within a few seconds after birth, determines whether some degree of resuscitation is required for the newborn. The five questions to be answered are:
1. Is the amniotic fluid of meconium?
2. Is the newborn breathing or crying?
3. Is there a good muscle tone?
4. Is the color pink?
5. Was the newborn at term?

INITIAL STEPS OF RESUSCITATION

- Provision of warmth
- Positioning
- Clearing the airway
- Tactile stimulation
- Administration of oxygen.

Provision of Warmth

- Ensure that radiant warmer is in working condition and preheated, and kept ready for use.
- Check and keep warm linen ready to receive the newborn, and for drying the newborn. Keep one sheet for drying the newborn and wrap the newborn in other sheet after removing wet sheet.
- As soon as the newborn is delivered, receive in dry and warm linen.
- Place the newborn under preheated radiant warmer or 200 watt bulb which ever is available.

Position

Position the newborn's neck slightly extended by placing a rolled towel under the newborn's shoulder to raise it about 2–2.5 cm above the mattress. Care should be taken to prevent hyperextension or underextension of the neck, because this may block the airway and decrease the air entry.

Clearance of the Airway

The appropriate method of clearing the airway depends on the presence or absence of meconium and the newborn's level of activity.

If no Meconium

Suction the secretions from the airway by wiping the nose and mouth, i.e. with the clean gauze piece or with suction catheter 12 or 14 French. If secretions are copious:
- Turn the head to one side.
- Suction the mouth, oropharynx and then the nose.
  If nose is suctioned first, the newborn may take the breath and secretions from the mouth can easily aspirate.
- Avoid vigorous suctioning and stimulation of the posterior pharyngeal wall as this may lead to vagal stimulation and cause bradycardia or apnea.
- Suction pressure should not exceed 80–100 mm Hg.

If Meconium is Present

- Suction the mouth, nose and posterior pharynx after the delivery of head, and the delivery of shoulders.
- Position the patient for successful CPR. The victim should be supine on firm, flat surface. Stabilize the neck.
- Open airway.
  a. **Head tilt–chin lift:** The rescuer should place the hand on the victim's forehead and tilt the head back gently into a sniffing (or) neutral position in an infant and slightly further back in a child. The child's chin is lifted upward. Care must be taken not to close the mouth.
  b. **Jaw thrust:** The rescuer should place two (or) three fingers under each side of the lower jaw at its angles and lift the jaw upwards.

Tactile Stimulation

- If the newborn fails to establish spontaneous and effective respiration even after drying, positioning and suctioning stimulate breathing by tactile stimulation.

❖ Safe and appropriate method of providing tactile stimulation is slapping/flicking the sole of the feet or gently rubbing the back of the newborn. If after one (or) two flicks newborn cries it indicates establishment of breathing. If no response occurs, discontinue and immediately start with bag and mask ventilation.

Administration of Oxygen

A newborn who has central cyanosis should initially receive high concentration of oxygen. To give free flow oxygen regulates the rate of flow at 6 L/min either by oxygen mask or oxygen tubing. Kept half inch from the newborns face. Slowly the newborn start turning pink. Once the newborn becomes pink the oxygen should be gradually withdrawn, the newborn can remain pink while breathing room air.

❖ Initial steps of the resuscitation should not take more than 30 seconds.
❖ After initial steps of resuscitation, check respiration heart rate and color.
❖ Count the heart rate for 6 seconds multiply by 10 to get heart rate per minute.
❖ If newborn is spontaneously breathing, i.e. heart rate >100 per min, i.e. no central cyanosis, further resuscitation is not required.
❖ If newborn is apneic after 30 seconds of initial steps, heart rate is below 100/min or cyanosis is present despite 100% free flow oxygen. This indicates need for assisted ventilation by bag and mask.

■ POSITIVE PRESSURE VENTILATION BAG AND MASK

Indications

Apnea after 30 seconds of initial steps of resuscitation heart rate below 100/min persistent central cyanosis despite 100% free flow oxygen.

■ TECHNIQUE OF POSITIVE PRESSURE VENTILATION

Ensure that mask of the right size is available. Use cushioned round mask or anatomical mask should cover the mouth. Nose and tip of the chin but not the eyes.

Self-inflating bag does not require a compressed gas source to fill, it is designed to inflate automatically as you release your grip on the bag.

Stand at the head end or on the side of the newborn observe that the bag does not block your view of the neonate chest. Allow you to observe the rise and fall of the chest during the resuscitation.

The mask should be applied, i.e. slight pressure to avoid the leakage. Hold the mask using thumb, index, and the middle finger of the left hand while supporting the chin, i.e. ring and the little finger. Ensure air tight seal is achieved. Compress the bag using finger tip. Avoid compressing the bag using your palm of the hand.

Compress the bag to cause visible expansion of the chest. The best guide to adequate pressure during bag and mask ventilation is an easy rise and fall of the chest, i.e. each breath.

The rate of positive pressure ventilation should be 40–60/min and while compressing the bag say squeeze and while releasing the pressure count two three. This sequence will give a rate of 40–60 breaths/min.

Observe that the rise and fall of the chest is noticeable as it indicates the mask is sealed and the lungs are getting inflated.

If there is no improvement in color, heart rate or breathing, it is possible that the chest is not expanding adequately. It can be due to following reasons:
- In adequate seal that there is air leak from the mask. The mask may not be of the right size or not properly applied.
- Blocked airway due to wrong position or accumulation of secretion.
- Inadequate pressure.

The corrective action for inadequate or no chest raise during bag and mask ventilation are as follows:
- Reapply mask using slight downward pressure
- Reposition the head
- Check for secretion, suction mouth and nose
- Ventilation with mouth slight downward pressure
- Reposition the head
- Check for secretion, suction mouth and nose
- Ventilate, i.e. mouth slightly open
- Increase pressure of ventilation
- Recheck or replace the resuscitation bag.

Check for improvement, i.e. is indicated by:
- Increased heart rate
- Spontaneous breathing
- Improvement in color

After 30 minutes of positive pressure ventilation assess the heart rate, color and breathing. If color is improving, and also spontaneous is seen with heart rate more than 100 beats/min, then stop positive pressure ventilation but continue free flow oxygen.

If heart rate is between 60–100/min, continue positive pressure ventilation.

If heart rate is below 60/min continue positive pressure ventilation and start chest compression.

Bag and mask ventilation causes abdominal distention as air not only enters the lungs but also escapes into stomach via esophagus. Distended abdomen presses from the diaphragm and comprise ventilation. Thereafter, if ventilation continues for more than two minutes, an orogastric tube (6 feeding tube size 6–8 French) should be inserted and left to decompress the stomach.

CHEST COMPRESSION

The decision to initiate chest compression is based on neonate heart rate. Chest compression is indicated when heart rate is below 60 beats/min after 30 seconds of positive pressure ventilation, i.e. 100% oxygen.

TECHNIQUE OF CHEST COMPRESSION

Ensure that the neonate's back is firmly supported, so that heart can be compressed between the sternum and spine. Two trained personnel are needed, i.e. one for chest compression and another for positive pressure ventilation.

There are two ways of chest compression.

Two finger method: The tip of the middle and the index finger should be used for compression. Other hand can be placed under the back of the neonate to provide support.

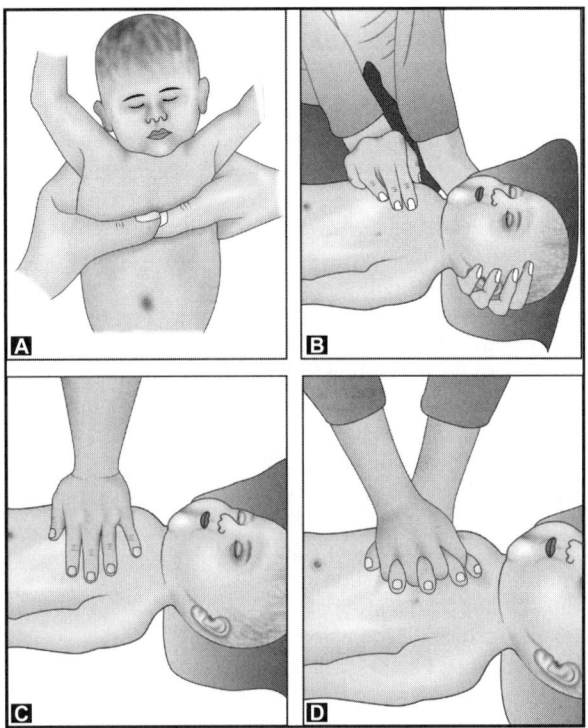

Figs. 27.1A to D: Chest compressions: (A) Premature infant (thumb method); (B) Infant (finger method); (C) Young child; (D) Older child/adolescent.

Thumb technique: Thumbs of both hands are placed either side by side or one over the other, i.e. fingers encircling the ribcage.

Site: Lower one third of the sternum, i.e. the area just below the inter nipple line and above the xiphisternum.

Rate of compression: The sternum be compressed at the rate of 120 beats/min and the ventilation is given at the rate of 40–60 breaths/min. Rate of cardiac massage should be coordinated with ventilator support, i.e. three chest compression and one breath.

One and two and three squeeze should be the squeeze followed for chest compression and positive pressure ventilation.

Compress the chest to a depth of one third of the anterior. Posterior diameter of the chest.

After 30 seconds of chest compression and ventilation, evaluate heart rate and make your decision based on the heart rate:

If heart rate is below 60/min, continue chest compression and ventilation.

If heart rate is above 60/min, discontinue chest compression whereas ventilation should be continued till the heart rate is above 100/min and neonate is breathing spontaneously.

If the technique of chest compression is incorrect it can cause trauma to the heart, or liver.

Excessive pressure over the ribs and xiphoid can lead to broken ribs, laceration of liver and pneumothorax.

POINTS TO NOTE

Precautions during resuscitation:
- Never delay in evaluating the baby's condition at birth, assess for respiration, heart rate and color immediately.
- Remember, first few breaths require two to three times pressure than succeeding breath to remove fetal lung fluid.
- Anticipating the need for resuscitation and adequate preparation are vital for further action.
- Maintain asepsis and universal precautions.
- Every action should be based on evaluation and decision.
- Follow the principle of successful resuscitation.
- Never allow the baby to be hypothermic.
- Do not keep the baby in head down position for long time.
- Avoid vigorous and continuous suctioning.
- Refrain from harmful practices during tactile stimulation.
- Never use full palmer grasp for giving bag and mask ventilation.
- Don't blow your lungs into baby's mouth.
- Call for assistant whenever you need or in difficulty.
- Be consistent in compressing the chest for rate and depth.
- Stop the unsuccessful attempts of intubation immediately
- Stablize the baby with PPV and then reattempt.
- Don't leave an open endotracheal tube in place.
- Never give sodium-bicarbonate till the ventilation is established. It must also be followed by ventilation.
- Epinephrine and volume expanders should be given before Sodi-bicarb injection.
- Remember, the treatment of metabolic acidosis.
- Evaluate respiration, heart rate and color and take decision before initiation of any further action.
- Keep record of all findings and actions.

PRACTICE QUESTIONS

1. How will you evaluate resuscitation procedure?
2. What is the technique of chest compression for a neonate?

MULTIPLE CHOICE QUESTIONS

1. **What is the first action on commencing resuscitation of a newborn baby?**
   a. Follow ABC approach
   b. Dry and cover baby
   c. Commence chest compressions
   d. Insert a Guedel airway
2. **During resuscitation in an infant, ratio of chest compression and ventilation breath should be:**
   a. 1:1
   b. 1:3
   c. 5:1
   d. 4:1
3. **How many liters of oxygen should be administered via a bag valve mask for young child?**
   a. 5 liters
   b. 10 liters
   c. 15 liters
   d. 20 liters

ANSWER KEY

1. b   2. c   3. c

CHAPTER 28

Endotracheal Intubation

PRACTICE COMPETENCIES
On completion of the chapter, the students will be able to:
○ Assist the doctor in the procedure by preparing the patient and keeping articles ready for use.

ABSTRACT
Endotracheal intubation usually requires two qualified healthcare professionals, one to insert endotracheal tube in to the trachea and another person to assist. This procedure outlines the responsibilities of the assistant who will prepare and monitor the patient, assemble the equipment required, act as an extra set of hands (especially when vocal cords are being visualized and immediately following tube placement), and ensure patient safety. A third healthcare professional may be needed for medication administration or other tasks as directed. This chapter contains indications, technique of endotracheal intubation, procedure of endotracheal intubation, and medications.

Keywords: Endotracheal intubation, size of endotracheal tubes, orotracheal intubation.

INDICATIONS
- To suction trachea in presence of meconium when the newborn is not vigorous.
- Suspected congenital diaphragmatic hernia requiring ventilation.
- Non-response to bag and mask ventilation
- Prolonged positive pressure ventilation is required
- To administer epinephrine if required to stimulate the heart.

TECHNIQUE OF INTUBATION
Selected the correct size of endotracheal tube and ensure availability of straight blade laryngoscope of size zero for preterm and one for term neonate. The appropriate diameter of the endotracheal tube on the basis of weight of neonate is given below.

Selecting the size of endotracheal tube
- Neonate with birth weight of less than 1000 g requires 2.5 mm internal diameter of ET
- Neonate with birth weight of 1000 to 2000 g requires 3 mm internal diameter of ET
- Neonate with birth weight of 2000 to 3000 g requires 3.5 mm internal diameter of ET
- Neonate with birth weight of more than 3000 g requires 4 mm internal diameter of ET.

With the help of laryngoscope, introduce the endotracheal tube to a level, so that the vocal cord guide is placed at the level of vocal cord.

Confirm the tube placement by ventilating the neonate, with correctly placed tube air entry is heard on both sides of the chest and air is not heard entering the stomach. After confirmation of correct placement of tube, endotracheal tube length outside should be around 4 centimeters.

■ PROCEDURE OF ENDOTRACHEAL INTUBATION

In most situations, orotracheal intubation is done which is easier, but it can get dislodged readily, nasotracheal intubation is more difficult and cumbersome, but is useful when prolonged ventilation is required. The shortening of the tube reduces dead space and prevents kinking. The endotracheal tube connector should be fitted on the cut end of the tube. The suction source should be readily available to provide 100 cm H_2O negative pressure.

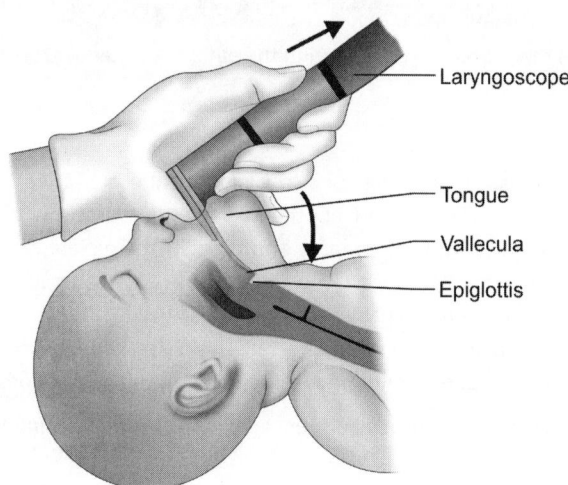

Fig. 28.1: Insertion of laryngoscope.

■ OROTRACHEAL INTUBATION

- ❖ Place the infant supine, i.e. slightly extended by placing a roll of towel under the shoulders.
- ❖ Stand beyond the head end of the baby, i.e. is placed near the edge of the table.
- ❖ Before intubation, improve the oxygenation and condition of the baby by administration of 100% O_2 through bag and mask ventilation for 3–4 min.
- ❖ Turn on the laryngoscope light and hold the laryngoscope in your left hand, i.e. the blade pointing away from you.
- ❖ Stabilize the infants head, i.e. your right hand.
- ❖ The laryngoscope blade is advanced beyond the base of the tongue till it rests in the vellecula (area between the base of the tongue and the epiglottis).
- ❖ At this point, the entire blade is lifted by pulling it forward in the direction of the handle and not by tilting the handle backward.
- ❖ By lifting the epiglottis, i.e. the tip of the blade and by applying gentle pressure over the avoided area (by the little and ring finger of the hand holding the laryngoscope or by an assistant) the glottis opening, i.e. all its landmarks is exposed to the view.

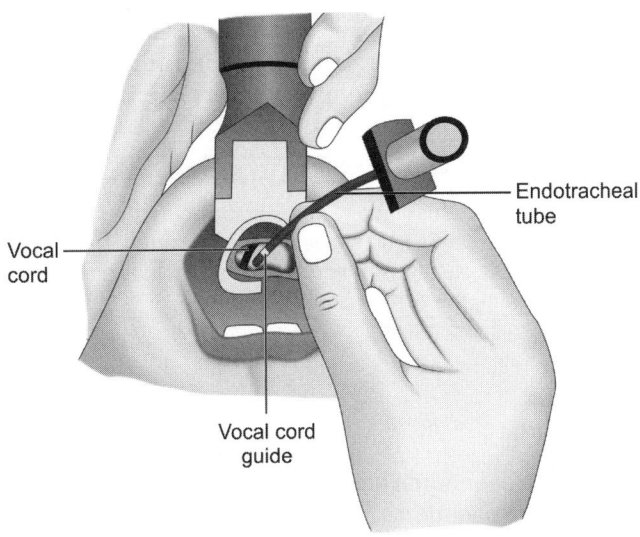

Fig. 28.2: Insertion of endotracheal tube.

- ❖ The secretions, if any, should be sucked before the endotracheal tube is inserted.
- ❖ Hold the endotracheal tube in your right hand and introduce it in to the right side of the infant's mouth.
- ❖ Keep the glottis in view and insert the tube until the vocal cord guide is at the level of the vocal cords.
- ❖ Hold the tube firmly at the lips, i.e. fingers of yours right hand while keeping the baby's head stabilized.
- ❖ Gently remove the laryngoscope, i.e. displaying the tube.
- ❖ Note the centimeter mark on the tube at the level of the lips as future guide, so that it is readily identified when the tube slips out.
- ❖ Connect the endotracheal tube to a bag and ventilate the infant.
- ❖ There should be a slight rise of the chest, i.e. each ventilation, i.e. equal breath sounds on both sides of the chest (at the level of the nipples) and without any air entering the stomach or abdominal distension.
- ❖ If the breath sounds are unilateral or unequal on two sides, the tube should be withdrawn by 1 cm and its placement is rechecked.
- ❖ It is not unusual for the undetached tube to enter the esophagus when no breath sounds are heard in the chest and air is heard entering the stomach and causing abdominal distension.
- ❖ The procedure should be repeated again to insert the tube into the trachea.

▮ MEDICATIONS

The role of drug is very limited in neonatal resuscitation. In few neonate who fail to improve, i.e. ventilation and chest compression the medication becomes necessary. Adrenaline, nalaxone and volume expanders should be available in the labor room. Dexamethasone, atropine, calcium, dextrose, etc. are not indicated for resuscitation in the labor room.

Adrenaline is indicated when the heart rate is below 60 per minute, despite chest compression and positive pressure ventilation for 30 seconds. It is given through intratracheal or intravenous route but never through cardiac route. Administer 0.1–0.2 mL/kg of 1:10000 dissolution.

Nalaxone hydrochloride is indicated in neonate, i.e. poor respiratory effort but good heart rate (>100/min) and who is pink, and there is history of narcotic administration (morphine or pethedine) to the mother, i.e. in past four hours of delivery administer 0.1 mL/kg.

> **POINTS TO NOTE**
>
> ➤ **Analgesia/sedation:** Some infants may require a presuction bolus of analgesia or sedation where the need is anticipated; however urgent suction should not be deferred. The need for this intervention is based on clinical assessment. Nursing comfort measures, such as positioning and containment, should also be utilized following the suction procedure.
> ➤ Parents can help to support, contain and comfort the neonate while the nurse is carrying out the procedure.

PRACTICE QUESTIONS

1. What are the indications for endotracheal intubation?
2. How do you select the size of endotracheal tube for neonates?

MULTIPLE CHOICE QUESTIONS

1. Which of the following are potential complications associated with intubation?
   a. Hypotension
   b. Raised intracranial pressure
   c. Aspiration
   d. All of the above
2. What procedure should be performed after intubation to confirm the position of the endotracheal tube?
   a. Gastric pH measurement
   b. Respiratory rate measurement
   c. Arterial blood gas analysis
   d. Chest X-ray
3. Which of the following are indications for emergency intubation?
   a. Respiratory failure and cool peripheries
   b. Respiratory failure and oliguria
   c. Respiratory failure and severe illness of any cause
   d. Respiratory failure and low intracranial pressure.

ANSWER KEY

1. d   2. d   3. c

CHAPTER 29

Endotracheal Tube Suctioning

PRACTICE COMPETENCIES

On completion of the chapter, the students will be able to:
- Perform endotracheal tube (ETT) suction to clear secretions using aspetic technique
- Maintain airway patency
- Optimize oxygenation and ventilation in a ventilated patient.
- Maximize the amount of secretions removed with minimal adverse effects associated with the procedure.

ABSTRACT

Endotracheal tube (ETT) suction is necessary to clear secretions and to maintain airway patency, and to therefore optimize oxygenation and ventilation in a ventilated patient. ETT suction is a common procedure carried out on intubated infants. Effective suctioning is an essential aspect of airway management in the intubated critically ill child. There are many associated risks and complications. The recommendations prior to suctioning include comprehensive patient assessment and patient preparation. The recommendations during suctioning include appropriate catheter selection, depth of insertion, suction pressure, duration of procedure and number of suction passes. Prevention of infection and maintenance of asepsis, i.e., hand washing, wearing gloves, aprons and goggles are also essential.

Keywords: Suctioning, procedure, nurses responsibilities, infant/child.

■ INTRODUCTION

Effective suctioning is an essential aspect of airway management in the intubated critically ill child. They are unable to maintain a patent airway as glottic closure is compromised, preventing cough reflex, increasing secretions and also compromising their ability to clear endotracheal secretions.

■ DEFINITION

Suctioning is described as the mechanical aspiration of pulmonary secretions from a patient with an artificial airway in position.

■ INDICATIONS FOR SUCTIONING

The decision to suction should be based on individual patient assessment and the following clinical signs that may indicate the need for suctioning. Suctioning should be done as rarely as possible and as frequently as needed.

- Visible or audible secretions—rattling or bubbling sounds, audible with or without a stethoscope
- Decreased oxygen saturation levels
- Bradycardia/tachycardia
- Increased pCO_2
- Deteriorating blood gas values
- Changes in respiratory rate and pattern with increase respiratory distress
- Change of color (cyanosis, pallor, mottled)
- Suspected endotracheal tube obstruction
- Ventilator alarms, i.e., increased proximal airway pressure/decreased tidal volume
- Decreased breath sounds/absent chest movement
- Increased airway pressure when ventilated (decreased tidal volumes)
- Decreased chest excursion/asymmetry
- Patient agitation.

ESSENTIAL EQUIPMENT

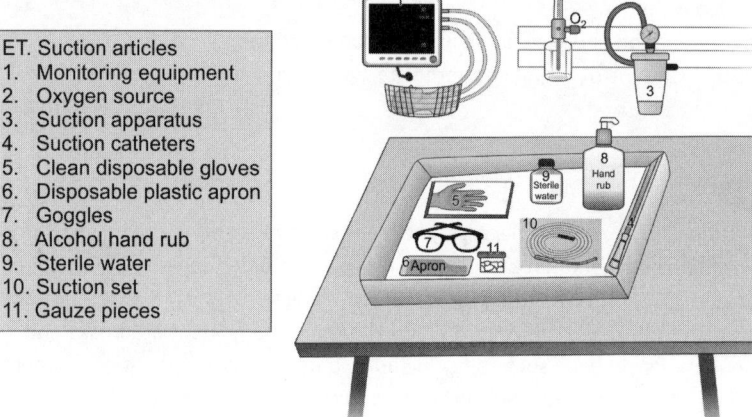

ET. Suction articles
1. Monitoring equipment
2. Oxygen source
3. Suction apparatus
4. Suction catheters
5. Clean disposable gloves
6. Disposable plastic apron
7. Goggles
8. Alcohol hand rub
9. Sterile water
10. Suction set
11. Gauze pieces

Fig. 29.1: Endotracheal tube suction articles.

- Oxygen source/oxygen mixer for preterm/neonates
- Monitoring equipment—oxygen saturation, heart rate and blood pressure
- Suction apparatus
- Appropriately sized suction catheters
- Selection of clean disposable gloves
- Disposable plastic apron
- Goggles
- Alcohol hand rub
- Sterile water for irrigation

Precautions with Endotracheal Suctioning

- Raised intracranial pressure (ICP)
- Pulmonary hypertension
- Pulmonary edema
- Pulmonary hemorrhage

These conditions may be exacerbated by suctioning and extra-precautions taken.

Potential Complications of Suctioning

Respiratory
- ❖ Hypoxia
- ❖ Bronchospasm
- ❖ Tracheobronchial mucosal trauma resulting in potential pulmonary hemorrhage
- ❖ Contamination of airway leading to nosocomial infection
- ❖ Unplanned extubation
- ❖ Atelectasis (loss of ciliary function/glottis closure)
- ❖ Right upper lobe collapse (excessive suction pressures)
- ❖ Pneumothorax

Cardiovascular
- ❖ Vagal response bradycardia
- ❖ Hemodynamic instability
- ❖ Pulmonary vasoconstriction.

Neurological
- ❖ Changes in cerebral blood flow velocity/raised intracranial pressure
- ❖ Decreased oxygen availability in cerebral blood flow increases risk of intraventricular hemorrhage (IVH) and hypoxic ischemic encephalopathy infection
- ❖ Nosocomial infections

Pain
- ❖ Behavioral pain response in infants

Table 29.1: Endotracheal intubation.

Action	Rationale
Preprocedure	
Comprehensive respiratory assessment	To assess the need for suctioning
Explain procedure to patient/parents.	To minimize anxiety and stress
Preparation of patient—physical, psychological and pharmacological, i.e., sedation	To reduce risk of complications
Ensure all necessary equipment is available - see list above	To ensure effectiveness of procedure and minimize risk of complications
Ensure the correct suction pressure is set Neonate 50–80 mm Hg Pediatric 80–100 mm Hg Older child 100–120 mm Hg	High negative suction pressures and deep suctioning may cause right upper lobe collapse in children. Also high pressures may damage respiratory mucosa and cause destruction of epithelial cilia of the airway
Calculate appropriate sized suction catheter, double the size of the endotracheal tube (ET) | ETT size (mm) | Suction catheter size | |---|---| | 2.5 | 5 fg | | 3.0 | 6 fg | | 3.5 | 7 fg | | 4.0-4.5 | 8 fg |	To ensure effectiveness of procedure and minimize risk of complications. To guarantee maximum of 50% of internal diameter which creates less negative pressure and prevents hypoxia and right upper lobe collapse/atelectasis. It also limits the risk of mucosal trauma. Too big a suction catheter has been demonstrated to reduce the tidal volume to <10%.
• Decontaminate hands prior to procedure • Put on apron and goggles	Maintenance of asepsis and prevention of cross infection. Protection of practitioner
Oxygen saturations, chest expansion and underlying disease should be used to determine the need for pre-oxygenation and/or hyperinflation.	

Chapter 29: Endotracheal Tube Suctioning

Action	Rationale
Standard suction support hyperoxygenation is 30% above patients' baseline oxygen requirements using Servo I ventilation **Note:** Preterm infants ensure maximum of 10-20% pre oxygenation	Suction support does not provide hyperinflation
Also reduce hyper oxygenation in the cardiac patient with unbalanced circulation, i.e., hypoplastic left heart syndrome	To prevent hyperoxemia and oxygen freeradical damage which may increase the risk of retinopathy of prematurity (ROP), periventricular leukomalacia (PVL) and chronic lung disease
	To prevent systemic steal or over perfusion of circulation to the lungs in infants with hypoplastic left heart syndrome (HLHS).
Hyperventilate (up to five breaths) using are breathing circuit as clinical indicated **Note:** This is NOT a routine practice	To prevent hypoxemia. It also increases the residual capacity of the lungs and reduces the risk of atelectasis and shunting
Apply non-sterile glove to the dominate hand.	To maintain non-touch technique
Determine insertion approximately 0.5–1 cm beyond the length of the endotracheal tube (*shallow suctioning*)	Shallow suction is recommended in the literature. Superior benefit of deep suctioning over shallow suctioning has not been demonstrated and more adverse events may be associated with it. Deep suctioning stimulates vagal nerve predisposing infant to bradycardia and hypotension. It prolongs coughing, increasing intrathoracic pressure and decreasing venous return. Also increased risk of mucosal and cilia trauma, inflammation and infection. Desaturation may also occur
Check against a predetermined length, i.e., paper tape measure posted at bedside	
Remove the catheter from its sheath using dominate hand.	

Table 29.2: Endotracheal suctioning procedure.

Action	Rationale
Suctioning procedure	
Two practitioner technique is recommended on infant/child who is acutely ill/unstable and high-risk of not tolerating the procedure, without profound decrease in heart rate, blood pressure and oxygen saturation	
Monitoring Monitor vital signs, i.e., heart rate and oxygen saturations.	To have a baseline set of observations and allow monitoring throughout the procedure
Disconnect patient from ventilator and introduce suction catheter gently to required depth	To prevent mucosal damage
Withdraw the suction catheter gently applying continuous suction pressure by placing the thumb over the suction control port, maximum 5-10 seconds. Observe the secretions for color, consistency and amount **Note:** Do NOT rotate the suction catheter	To ensure patency of endotracheal tube and prevent hypoxia. Take into consideration the patient's own respiratory/ventilation rate and clinical state. Suction catheters have multiple - eyes (holes) in their diameters and therefore the rotating method is not necessary
Recovery period should be given when more than one catheter pass is needed and no more than three passes during any one suctioning session	To allow oxygen levels to return to baseline and minimize mucosal damage

Action	Rationale
Suction catheter passes should be kept to a minimum and should not exceed 3 passes	The literature lacks consensus on the number of passes a single catheter can be used for, ranging from a single pass to multiple passes. Research studies have shown no increase in nosocomial infection after using a single catheter for up to 24 hours
A new sterile catheter is used for each suctioning session unless contaminated	A new suction catheter must be used for oral nasal and endotracheal insertion
Oropharyngeal/nasopharyngeal suctioning Oropharyngeal suctioning should be carried out first.	To reduce the amount of negative pressure in the lung and to reduce the level of hypoxia
Attach manual rebreathing circuit to patient and provide manual ventilation following suctioning as clinically indicated, observing airway pressures on manometer dial for infants.	Reoxygenating to reverse hypoxia or hypercarbia that may have developed. To reduce the risk of barotrauma.
Note: Routine Instillation of normal saline 0.9% prior to suctioning is NOT recommended.	*The literature does not support this practice.* Detrimental effects demonstrated in adults and of no theoretical benefit in Pediatrics.
	Sputum and saline do not mix
	• No increase in amount of secretion obtained when saline instilled • It adversely effects tissue and arterial oxygenation • Infants/children have experienced significantly greater desaturation following normal saline 0.9% instillation and may last up to 2 minutes • It dislodges bacterial colonies contributing to lower airway contamination increased incidence of bradycardia and need for increased $FI.O_2$

Action	Rationale
Post procedure Monitor the infant/child's oxygen saturation levels and heart rate for any decrease indicating hypoxemia throughout the procedure.	Early and timely intervention for instability.
Wean oxygen if increased, to baseline	To reduce risk of complications
Dispose of the suction catheter in the clinical waste bin and rinse tubing by dipping it in a small container of sterile water, dispose gloves in the clinical waste bin adhering to universal health and safety precautions. NB: Discard container with sterile water after each suctioning episode.	To prevent cross infection.
Evaluate effectiveness by conducting a comprehensive post suctioning respiratory assessment, including breath sounds.	To ensure effectiveness of the procedure.
Wash hands after procedure.	Maintenance of asepsis.
Document procedure and findings—color, consistency and amount of secretions.	Document effectiveness of procedure. Continuation of nursing care and maintains accountability through accurate recording of nursing intervention.
Allow patient 20-30 mins before taking a blood gas. Allow patient 20-30 mins before taking a blood gas.	To ensure an accurate sample

NURSES RESPONSIBILITIES

- Observe for the signs and symptoms of need to perform ET tube care—solid or loose tape: pressure sores on nose, lips or corner of mouth, and excess nasal or oral secretions.
- Observe for factors that increases the risk of complications from ET tube—type and size of tube, movement of tube up and down trachea (in and out) duration of tube placement, cuff over inflation or under inflation, presence of facial trauma, malnutrition and neck or thoracic radiation.
- Assess child knowledge of procedure.
- Obtain other nurses assistance in the procedure.
- Explain the procedure and client's participation including importance of the following—not biting or moving ET tube with tongue, trying not to cough when tape is off ET tube, keeping hands down and not pulling on tubing, removal of tape from face can be uncomfortable.
- Assist client to assume position comfortable for both nurse and client (usually supine or semi-Fowlers)
- Wash hands and administer endotracheal, nasopharyngeal and oropharyngeal suction.

POINTS TO NOTE

- Suctioning is described as the mechanical aspiration of pulmonary secretions from a patient with an artificial airway in position.
- Withdraw the suction catheter gently applying continuous suction pressure by placing the thumb over the suction control port, maximum 5–10 seconds.
- Insert approximately 0.5–1 cm beyond the length of the endotracheal tube
- High negative suction pressures and deep suctioning may cause right upper lobe collapse in children. Also high pressures may damage respiratory mucosa and cause destruction of epithelial cilia of the airway.
- Monitor the infant/child's oxygen saturation levels and heart rate for any decrease indicating hypoxemia throughout the procedure.

Analgesia/Sedation
- Some infants may require a presuction bolus of analgesia or sedation where the need is anticipated; however urgent suction should not be deferred. The need for this intervention is based on clinical assessment. Nursing comfort measures, such as positioning and containment, should also be utilized following the suction procedure.
- Parents can help to support, contain and comfort the neonate while the nurse is carrying out the procedure.

MULTIPLE CHOICE QUESTIONS

1. ET suctioning is performed to:
   a. Reduce inflammation
   b. Improve circulation
   c. Reduce heart rate
   d. Reduce secretions that blocks airway
2. Maximum time to place the suction catheter in ET tube:
   a. 5 minutes
   b. 10 seconds
   c. 4 minutes
   d. 30 seconds

3. **Pressure used for suctioning neonates:**
   a. 50–80 mm Hg
   b. 20–30 mm Hg
   c. 40–80 mm Hg
   d. 10–20 mm Hg
4. **Possible complication of performing suctioning frequently:**
   a. Blockage of airway
   b. Bleeding
   c. Elevated saturation
   d. Reduce temperature
5. **Airway patency in intubated child is maintained by:**
   a. Humidification
   b. Chest physiotherapy
   c. Intubation
   d. Endotracheal suctioning
6. **Endotracheal suctioning is a:**
   a. Invasive procedure
   b. Emergency procedure
   c. Noninvasive procedure
   d. Unsterile procedure
7. **Endotracheal suctioning is usually performed, *except*:**
   a. Intensive care unit
   b. Emergency department
   c. Outpatient department
   d. Operation theater
8. **Reason why ET suctioning will be done before feeding in children is to:**
   a. Favor intestinal absorption
   b. Prevent aspiration
   c. Prevent asphyxia
   d. Avoid crying
9. **Commonly the need of ET tube suctioning in children is assessed by:**
   a. Auscultation and inspection
   b. Inspection and palpation
   c. Inspection and percussion
   d. Auscultation and percussion
10. **Contraindication for ET tube suctioning is:**
    a. Tonsillitis
    b. Sinusitis
    c. Epiglottitis
    d. Epistaxis
11. **Recommended protective equipment while ET tube suctioning are:**
    a. Gloves, eyewear and hand washing
    b. Mask, footwear and apron
    c. Gloves, mask and hand washing
    d. Gloves, eyewear and mask
12. **The purpose of thumb control valve in ET tube suctioning is:**
    a. For easy holding
    b. Allowing intermittent suction

c. Allowing continuous suction
d. Creating good negative pressure
13. **Humidification recommended before ET tube suctioning is:**
    a. Prevent dehydration
    b. Lubrication during suctioning
    c. Loosening secretion
    d. Decreasing discomfort suctioning
14. **After ET tube suctioning following assessments are mandatory, *except*:**
    a. Central venous pressure
    b. Vitals checking and color
    c. Auscultation of lungs
    d. Viscosity and amount of secretion

ANSWER KEY

1. d	2. b	3. a	4. b	5. d	6. a
7. c	8. b	9. a	10. c	11. d	12. b
13. c	14. a				

CHAPTER 30

Care of Child on Ventilator

PRACTICE COMPETENCIES
On completion of the chapter, the students will be able to:
- Provide effective nursing care to the child on ventilator.
- Monitor vital signs
- Perform suctioning using aseptic technique

ABSTRACT
In modern intensive care management of critical problems, most of the patients need artificial ventilation during the stage of their illness. With the availability of a variety of ventilators and increasing medical expertize, mechanical ventilation has become easier today. Although it is a life saving intervention, mechanical ventilation can also cause serious complications. Ventilator assisted pneumonia was about 41% among device associated infections. With preventive measures, early detection and effective management of these problems can be easily alleviated and survival can be improved. This chapter contains indications, definitions for terminology, types of ventilator support, care of infants on ventilator, complications during ventilator support, and nursing management during extubation.

Keywords: Care of child on ventilator, continuous positive airway pressure, mechanical ventilation, blood gases, endotracheal tube suction, extubation.

INTRODUCTION
- Assisted ventilation is an invasive life support procedure with multiple effects on the cardiopulmonary system.
- Use of any ventilator strategy an understanding of how ventilator changes affect blood gas values and knowledge of the pathophysiology of common neonatal pulmonary disorders.
- A close collaborative approach is needed between physicians, nurses, and the respiratory therapists for successful ventilation.
- Assisted ventilation includes continuous positive airway pressure (CPAP) and intermittent mandatory ventilation (IMV).

INDICATIONS
The main reason is respiratory failure. This occurs commonly in newborns in:
- Hyaline membrane disease

- Pneumonia
- Meconium and other aspiration syndromes
- Perinatal hypoxia
- Shock
- Extreme prematurity.

DEFINITIONS

FiO_2: Fraction inspired oxygen concentration. Air has 21% oxygen. A baby can receive air (21%), 100% oxygen or any concentration, of oxygen in between these two, through a ventilator. This is usually marked on a round dial in ventilators. FiO_2 is percentage of oxygen expressed as a fraction of 1. Thus, 40% oxygen concentration is expressed as a FiO_2 of 1.0. Measuring the FiO_2 gives us an idea of how much oxygen the baby requires to inhale, to maintain normal arterial oxygen saturation.

ABG: Arterial blood gas can be obtained either by the arterial stab method or from an indwelling arterial cannula. Best indicator of pH. PaO_2 and $PaCO_2$

CBG: Capillary blood gas gives a lower pH value and higher $PaCO_2$ value. When compared to ABG

VBG: Venous blood gas, provides information about pH and $PaCO_2$ but not PaO_2

PaO_2: Partial pressure of oxygen

$PaCO_2$: Partial pressure of carbon dioxide

BE: Base excess a minus value indicates the extent of base deficit, A base deficit of more than 3.0 indicates a metabolic acidosis.

Normal blood gas in room air (measured in mm of Hg)
Arterial blood gas
pH : 7.35–7.45
PaO_2 : 53–65
$PaCO_2$: 35–45

Capillary blood gas
pH : 7.30–7.35
PaO_2 : 40–00
$PaCO_2$: 40–45

Venous blood gas
pH : 7.25–7.30
PaO_2 : 30–45
$PaCO_2$: 45–50

O_2 Sat: Oxygen saturation expressed as a percentage. It can range from zero to 100. This is measured by doing a blood gas analysis or by using a pulse oximeter

Do not confuse with FiO_2 and PaO_2.

$TcPO_2$: Transcutaneous oxygen is measured by using an instrument which directly measures the PaO_2 when the electrode is attached to the skin

$TcPCO_2$: Transcutaneous carbon dioxide. It is similar to $TcPO_2$ but measures the $PaCO_2$

IMV: Intermittent mandatory ventilation. It needs an endotracheal tube insertion with pressure and rate settings in a ventilator

CPAP: Continuous positive airway pressure. This form of ventilation which can be done by using nasal prongs, nasopharyngeal or endotracheal tube.

TYPES OF VENTILATORY SUPPORT

Continuous positive airway pressure (CPAP): This can be provided by all neonatal ventilators and some homemade devices. CPAP can be given by nasal prongs, nasopharyngeal prongs and through the endotracheal tube. This method of ventilation causes less barotrauma than intermittent mandatory ventilation. Only nasal and nasopharyngeal CPAP is discussed here.

Indications
- Treatment of early or mild respiratory distress syndrome (RDS)
- Moderately frequent apneic spells
- After recent extubation
- For weaning chronic ventilator dependent Infants
- CPAP is rarely of benefit in pneumonia, meconium aspiration, chronic lung disease or severe apnea.

Technique
- Nasal prongs, single or double nasopharyngeal prongs and endotracheal tubes are used to administer CPAP.
- The single nasopharyngeal prong is a 3.0 or 3.5 mm endotracheal tube. This is cut to reach up to the nasopharynx. The advantages of this method are that the other nostril is free for a nasogastric tube and the mouth is left open as a safety "blow-off valve. However, frequent suctioning is needed as it blocks easily.
- In this device, gas flows through the circuit at 5–8 liters per minute. The amount of CPAP is adjusted by tightening the gate clip and by varying the distance below the water surface of the tube in the water bottle.

Complications
- Nasal trauma can lead to nostril stenosis
- Feeding problems occur because gas distends the stomach. Insert an open nasogastric tube to decompress the abdomen
- non-cooperation is common, especially from big babies
- CPAP should be undertaken with caution in units with no facility for recognition of deterioration and institution of IMV.

Mechanical Ventilation

Also called intermittent mandatory ventilation (IMV). The type of ventilators used most frequently in the newborn nursery are pressure limited, time cycled and with continuous flow.

Principle

A continuous flow of filtered, heated and humidified air-oxygen mixture is circulated from the infant's airway. The maximum pressure called peak inspiratory pressure (PIP) and minimum pressure called peak end expiratory pressure (PEEP) are selected. The rate, duration of inspiration (inspiratory time or I time) and ratio of inspiratory and expiratory times (I: E ratio) are also set.

Indications

- Any situation when infant is unable to ventilate on his own
- Prolonged apnea
- PaO_2 of less than 50 mm Hg in a FiO_2 of more than 0.8 and/or $PaCO_2$ of more than 60 mm Hg with acidemia (pH less than 7.2).

Advantages

- The continuous flow of gas allows infant to have spontaneous respirations between ventilator breaths
- Good control is maintained over ventilator pressures
- The system is relatively simple.

Disadvantages

- Spontaneous breathing by infants may interfere with adequate ventilation
- Needs endotracheal intubation
- Invasive and causes barotraumas.

■ CARE OF INFANTS ON VENTILATOR

- **General principles**
  - Infants requiring assisted ventilation must never be left unattended
  - The cardio respiratory monitor should be in continuous operation whilst the infant is being ventilated and all alarms must be operational. This, of course, does not replace good clinical observation
  - Observations are to be recorded hourly and whenever, there are changes in settings.
- **Objectives of good ventilator care**
  - Maintaining a patent airway
  - Adequate ventilation with required oxygen concentration
  - Adequate suctioning of secretions from tracheobronchial tree to prevent obstruction
  - Maintaining fluid and electrolyte balance
  - Preventing hypothermia
  - Preventing infection.
- **Equipment**
  - Open cot with radiant warmer ventilator
  - Ventilator circuit and humidifier
  - Cardio respiratory monitor
  - Equipment for intubation
  - Transcutaneous oxygen monitor or pulse oximeter
  - Emergency pneumothorax pack
  - Suction equipment.

Management

- Confirm the ventilatory settings with the doctor
- Observe ventilatory settings and oxygen concentration hourly and record in a flow chart
- Secure the endotracheal tube (ETT) adequately, avoiding traction on tube
- Avoid kinks in circuit tubing

- Remove water condensation in circuit frequently
- Monitor the temperature of inspired gases
- Top up humidification chamber frequently
- Maintain strict fluid balance chart
- Use the transcutaneous oxygen or pulse oximeter continuously, if available
- Keep alarms on in the ventilator at all times
- Perform frequent blood gas estimations. Stable babies need at least once in four to six hourly estimations.

Blood gases are mandatory twenty minutes after any change in ventilator settings
- Change infant's position every four hours
- Perform oral and nasal toilet every four hours
- Weigh infants daily using a sling scale
- Change circuits, humidification chambers and filters every 48 hours, if possible
- Send weekly endotracheal aspirates for bacteriological culture and sensitivity, as per unit protocol.

VENTILATOR SIGHS

- A sigh is an additional ventilator breath introduced manually to increase tidal volume. It is used to prevent atelectasis (collapse) of the lung
- Sighing is to be performed on any infant receiving IMV when the ventilator rate is more than 10 breaths per minute
- Sighs can be performed for two breaths every half hour. To perform a sigh, increase the set peak inspiratory pressure (PIP) by 5 and hold at that pressure for two breaths.

Read just PIP to the previous set level
Caution should be exercised in sighing infants receiving 35–40 cm of PIP. Check with doctor before sighing in such cases.

ENDOTRACHEAL TUBE SUCTION

General Principles

- An endotracheal tube in situ is a foreign body which will stimulate the production of mucoid material and block the narrow orifice of the ETT
- Hence, careful suctioning of the ETT is necessary to prevent obstruction

Signs of Excessive Secretions and Blocked ETT

- Cyanosis, restlessness, retractions, tachypnea, nasal flaring, diminished breath sounds and hypotonia
- Cyanosis and bradycardia that do not respond to stimulation, increased FiO_2 and rate
- Rales and rhonchi on auscultation
- Audible crackles without stethoscope.

Equipment

- Self-inflating bag (Ambu or Laerdal) connected to oxygen
- Sterile towel
- Sterile gloves
- Suction catheters

5 G for ETT < 3.5 mm
6 G for ETT > 3.5 mm
- One 2 mL syringe
- One 21 gauge needle
- One 2 mL ampule N saline
- 100 mL water for irrigation.

Technique

- Two staff nurses or one nurse and one doctor perform this procedure
- Infants on rates below 20 must have I:E ratio altered to 1:1 and rates increased to twenty
- All infants must have oxygen increased to 100% for 5 seconds immediately prior to suction and following completion of procedure
- Routine hand wash is performed
- Equipment is assembled on a sterile towel
- Suction is turned on with pressure not exceeding 60–80 mm Hg
- Both lung fields are auscultated
- Required length of catheter is measured for insertion into ETT and marked with a tincture benzoin swab
- 0.2 mL normal saline is instilled into the ETT and several breaths are allowed on ventilator
- The suction catheter is moistened with sterile water and without contaminating inserted into the ETT without force or suction
- Suction is applied while catheter is gently rotated and withdrawn. The whole suctioning procedure must not last more than 10 seconds.
- The infant's condition is continuously observed by assistant and pulse oximeter/TCM monitor throughout the procedure. If there is hypoxia the procedure is abandoned and baby reconnected to the ventilator.

Ventilator settings are adjusted to previous settings
- Suctioning procedure is repeated only, if necessary
- Oropharynx is now gently suctioned
- Suction tube is discarded.

Precautions

- Suctioning of the airway can cause irritation and excessive production of secretions
- Excessive suctioning can cause hypoxia.

COMPLICATIONS DURING VENTILATION

- Blocked or kinked endotracheal tube
- Displaced endotracheal tube
- Ventilator malfunction
- Overheating of inspired gases
- Leak in circuit
- Condensation in tubing resulting in aspiration
- Air leak syndromes, e.g., pneumothorax
- Infections
- Oxygen toxicity
- Bronchopulmonary dysplasia.

BRADYCARDIA DURING VENTILATION

- Observe the monitor alarm and confirm the situation clinically
- Check that the ventilator circuit is correctly assembled and the ventilator is functioning
- Position the infant flat and check the position of the endotracheal tube by auscultation
- Transilluminate the chest if there is suspicion of a pneumothorax
- If there is no improvement, increase ventilation parameters in this order
  - Rate by 10 breaths per minute
  - PIP by 2 cm water
  - FiO_2 as required
- Call for assistance
- Prepare for extubation and re-intubation, if no improvement
- Maintain thermoneutral environment
- Prepare, administer and record resuscitative drugs, if necessary
- Ensure the event is well documented

EXTUBATION

The procedure is performed by the doctor. The resuscitation is readily available for emergency reintubation, if required.

- **Equipment**
  - Head box of appropriate size or prongs for CPAP, whichever is required
  - Humidifier-base and tubing
  - Oxygen tubing and connector
  - Oxygen analyzer
  - Sterile container and scalped blade
  - Self-inflating bag and mask
  - Size 10 G suction catheter
  - Resuscitation trolley.
- **Procedure**
  - Empty stomach prior to extubation
  - Ensure a good intravenous line is in situ
  - Aspirate contents of the stomach
  - Attach self-inflating bag to 2 L/min oxygen flow. Connect to blender, if available
  - Suction endotracheal tube immediately prior to extubation and send aspirate for culture
  - Loosen strapping from the infants face
  - Suction the oropharynx
  - Doctor withdraws the ETT
  - Place head box or nasal prongs as ordered.

Nursing management of an extubated patient

- Position infant head down for six hours
- Perform hourly chest physiotherapy and gentle oropharyngeal suction, for six hours
- Continue chest physiotherapy at frequent intervals thereafter for the next 24 hours
- Commence feeding six hours later, if ordered. Do not nurse baby head down once feeding commences
- Perform ABG half an hour after extubation. Unless otherwise indicated
- Give all infants, who have been ventilated for more than 24 hours, humidified gases for at least another 24 hours.
- Do a chest X-ray 6 hours after extubation.

POINTS TO NOTE

- Review communications from the professional healthcare team.
- Check ventilator settings.
- Suction the patient as needed.
- Evaluate sedation and pain needs.
- Use techniques to avoid infection.
- Check and recheck the patency of the airway.
- Monitor vital signs for hemodynamic instability.

PRACTICE QUESTIONS

1. What are the indications for ventilator support?
2. What are the normal values of ABG?
3. What are the signs of blocked endotracheal tube?
4. How do you take care of a child after extubation?

MULTIPLE CHOICE QUESTIONS

1. **One of the following modes of ventilation "locks out" the patient's efforts to breathe:**
   A. Controlled mandatory ventilation
   B. Synchronous intermittent mandatory ventilation
   C. Assist control mode
   D. Pressure control mode
2. **One of the following modes of ventilation has the risk of the patient getting respiratory alkalosis:**
   A. Controlled mandatory ventilation
   B. Synchronous intermittent mandatory ventilation
   C. Assist control mode
   D. Pressure control mode
3. **One of the following modes of ventilation reduces the work of breathing by overcoming the resistance created by ventilator tubing:**
   A. Controlled mandatory ventilation
   B. Synchronous intermittent mandatory ventilation
   C. Assist control mode
   D. Pressure support mode
4. **Ventilators have two major functions:**
   a. Volume, SIMV
   b. Volume, pressure
   c. Pressure, PSV-Pro
   d. Barotraumas alert: volume alert
5. **What is the normal range of $PaCO_2$?**
   a. 30–40 mm Hg
   b. 22–26 mm Hg
   c. 35–45 mm Hg
   d. 33–43 mm Hg

6. An unconscious baby is receiving mechanical ventilation Which nursing diagnosis takes priority:
   a. Self–care deficit related to unconsciousness
   b. Risk for impaired skin integrity related to immobility
   c. Ineffective airway clearance related to the inability to expectorate
   d. Imbalanced nutrition: less than body requirements related to inability to swallow

ANSWER KEY

1. a   2. c   3. d   4. b   5. c   6. c

CHAPTER 31

Intravenous Therapy

PRACTICE COMPETENCIES

On completion of the chapter, the students will be able to:
- Perform insertion, monitoring and maintenance of intravenous access in children.
- Improve cannulation skills.

ABSTRACT

Intravenous therapy is a complex nursing treatment that most children in an acute care setting have at one time or another during their hospital stay. The importance of correctly identifying veins, catheter selection, dressings, and potential complications are all issues that nurses face on a daily basis. This chapter contains indications, common IV solutions, additives, procedure and nursing care with IV infusion.

Keywords: Intravenous therapy, additives for IV, skin necrosis, sloughing, tissue infiltration, hypoglycemia, air embolism, cold stress, infusion pump.

INDICATIONS FOR IV THERAPY

- Supply parenteral fluids to:
  - Maintain daily requirements
  - Restore losses
  - Replace ongoing losses
  - Maintain electrolyte balances
  - Correct fluid and electrolyte disturbances.
- Administer blood and its components
- Administer parenteral medication (e.g. antibiotics, chemotherapy, analgesics)
- Administer total parenteral nutrition (TPN)
- Provide intravenous access in case of an emergency
- Provide access for diagnostic purposes (e.g. dye injection prior to a procedure)

COMMON IV SOLUTIONS

- Sodium chloride 0.9% (0.9 NaCl)
- Sodium chloride 0.45% (0.45 NaCl)
- Dextrose 5%/sodium chloride 0.9% (D5W/0.9 NaCl)
- Dextrose 5%/sodium chloride 0.45% (D5W/0.45 NaCl)

- Dextrose 5%/sodium chloride 0.2% (D5W/0.2 NaCl)
- Dextrose 5% in water (D5W)

COMMON IV ADDITIVES

- KCl — Potassium chloride
- Mg^{++} — Magnesium
- Ca^{++} — Calcium
- PO_4 — Phosphate
- $NaHCO_3$ — Sodium bicarbonate

EQUIPMENT

1. Basic dressing pack
2. Cannula, e.g. 22 G or 24 G Jelco
3. 2 mL and 5 mL syringes
4. Extension tube set
5. Skin preparation
    i. Alcoholic chlorhexidine if the infant's weight >1500 g
    ii. Aqueous chlorhexidine if the infant's weight <1500 g
    iii. 2 alcohol swabs
    iv. Use betadine and alcohol or spirit if chlorhexidine solution is not available.
6. Strapping
7. Splint
8. Parenteral administration set
9. Parenteral solution and additives as ordered
10. Hook for pack
11. Infusion pump attached to support
12. Restraint for limb, if necessary
13. Razor, if scalp vein is used
14. Overhead light
15. Warmth.

PREPARATIONS

1. Prepare the above equipment
2. Prepare the IV solution as follows:
    a. Check orders
    b. The staff nurse prepares the solution. Two nursing staff must cross-check/prepare solution
    c. Using aseptic technique, insert additives as ordered in the pack. Mix well. Attach signed additive label to the pack.
    d. Additives must be compatible with each other and with the solution.
    e. No drugs are to be added to the parenteral nutrition bottle. However, medications may be added to the buret by either the medical staff or by the charge nurse.
3. Prepare the skin as follows:
    a. Clean the site with alcohol/spirit
    b. Clean the site again with betadine/chlorhexidine solution
    c. Clean again with alcohol/spirit
    d. The site is now ready for insertion of needle/cannula.

HINTS FOR PROLONGED IV INFUSIONS

1. Prepare all requirements prior to insertion of the cannula. This helps to prevent clot formation and loss of infusion.
2. Connect to the administration set as soon as possible and flush with saline/dextrose until the line can be connected to infusion pump.
3. Strap the cannula securely to prevent its accidental removal. Support the site (especially limb) to prevent the infant dislodging the line.
4. Keep a watch for infiltration of fluid in subcutaneous tissue as well as evidence of infection.

Potential Hazards of Infiltration of Fluid Administration

1. Skin necrosis and sloughing may result from the following:
   a. Tight strapping (ischemia)
   b. Injection of irritant solution, especially, if osmolality exceeds serum osmolality (280 mmol/L), e.g. 10% dextrose (500 mmol/L) or $NaHCO_3$ 8.4% (1680 mmol/L). Solutions should be diluted more than half the serum osmolality value.
   c. Inadvertent intra-arterial infusion
   d. Continued extravascular infusion.
2. Infection.
3. Tissue infiltration resulting in hypoglycemia. Monitor reflotest dextrostrips.
4. Cold stress especially if there is a delay in cannulation.
5. Air embolism.

Nursing Care

1. Maintain the limb in a comfortable and functional position to prevent nerve damage, structural problems, and accidental dislodgement of IV line.
2. If unsure of infusion pump, please refer to equipment manual.
3. Prevent entry of infection into the line.
4. Check for order changes frequently. If ordered, the administration set may need to be reprimed, so that the infant receives altered solution immediately and not hours later (due to "old" fluid in administration set).
5. Hourly observations of the fluid/hour, progressive total and ordered total are a must.
6. Maintain the following:
   a. Type of fluid and rate/hour
   b. Hourly total
   c. Progressive total
   d. Infusion pump setting
   e. Amount of positive or negative balance.
7. Check the infusion site hourly report and record increasing swelling, erythema and leakage around the site or ischemia.
8. If a buret is used, do not fill over 100 mL routinely. Refill when buret has 10 mL left.
9. Expel any air from the infusion line.

Notes

1. Prime giving sets as instructed in "Infusion pump" section.
2. When checking parenteral fluid, note the following:

a. Correct fluid for correct patient
b. Additives
c. Expiry date of solution
d. Date of orders (new orders every 24 hours).
3. Filters are never used for CVC or arterial lines.
4. Parenteral solution packs are emptied and discarded when changed or when the infusion is terminated.

> **POINTS TO NOTE**
> - It is a nurse's responsibility to ensure the safe monitoring and management of child's IV line.
> - Nurses will be checking the IV at least once every hour, including throughout the night.
> - Parents and caregivers can help with IV monitoring by ensuring their child does not pull the line, watching for pain or numbness, keeping the IV site dry, keeping the IV site visible and alerting the nurse when concerns or problems arise.
> - Be aware of the signs of an IV line not working properly and the symptoms your child may experience.

PRACTICE QUESTIONS
1. What are the indications for IV therapy?
2. How do you prepare for IV therapy?
3. What are the common IV solutions used?
4. What are the common IV additives used?

MULTIPLE CHOICE QUESTIONS
1. **What is the first step in the insertion of a peripheral IV line or saline lock?**
    a. Get permission from the patient /family member
    b. Obtain a physician's order
    c. Educate the patient about the need for IV access
    d. Provide privacy
2. **After applying the tourniquet, if the vein feels hard or rope like:**
    a. Use it, it is the best choice for an IV
    b. Stretch it to prevent rolling
    c. Select another site
    d. Have the child relax his/her fist
3. **While in the process of inserting an IV, which of the following is not acceptable?**
    a. Enter the skin at a 30–40° angle
    b. A devise may be reused as long as it is in the same site as the original attempt
    c. Enter the skin directly over the vein
    d. Enter the skin slightly adjacent to the vein and direct the needle into the side of the vein wall.

ANSWER KEY

1. b   2. c   3. b

CHAPTER 32

Blood-Drawing Technique in the Neonate

PRACTICE COMPETENCIES
On completion of the chapter, the students will be able to:
- Perform venipuncture and cannulation for the purpose of blood sampling in neonates.
- Provide comfort to the baby.

ABSTRACT
The choice of site and procedure depends on the volume of blood needed for the procedure and the type of laboratory test to be done. Venipuncture is the method of choice for blood sampling in term neonates, however it requires an experienced and trained phlebotomist and if not available, a physician may need to draw blood sample. Patient immobilization is crucial to the safety of the neonate undergoing phlebotomy, and to the success of the procedure. A helper is essential for properly immobilizing the patient for venipuncture or finger prick. This chapter contains procedure for heel puncture, antecubital venous stick, and arterial puncture.

Keywords: Heel puncture, neonatal osteomyelitis, antecubital venous stick, extravasation, hematoma, arterial puncture, infection, bleeding, scarring.

■ HEEL PUNCTURE

The newborn's calcaneus (heel bone) does not extend medial to a line drawn posteriorly from the middle of the great toe or lateral to a line drawn posteriorly between the 4th and 5th toes, To avoid puncturing the calcaneus, the skin puncture should be performed outside of these two lines.

Purpose
1. Micro volumes of blood are desirable and now possible to avoid causing anemia.
2. Veins should be reserved for parenteral therapy.
3. Frequent sampling of blood may be necessary to monitor acid-base status in sick infants, i.e. with RDS.
4. Venipuncture may be hazardous in such infants, e.g. may cause hypoxemia.
5. If the area is warmed properly, the capillaries can become "arteriolized". The oxygen content measured from arteriolized samples when the levels are in the middle ranges, i.e. approximately 40 to 60 mm Hg.

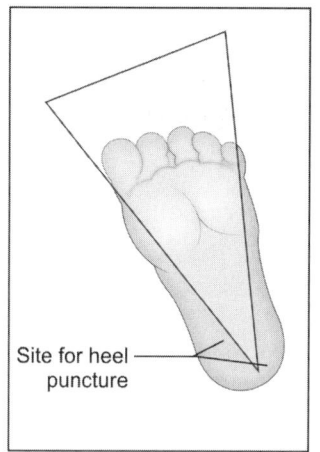
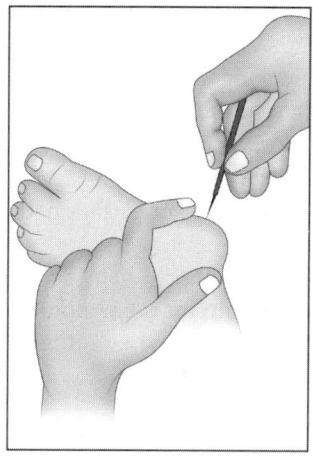

Fig. 32.1: Optimal site for heel puncture of newborn.

Limits

1. Volume of blood required for tests may exceed the volume available from single puncture. Volume available per single-puncture depends on size and health of infant.
2. Blood from skin puncture may be invalid to use:
   a. When exact PaO_2 measurement required
   b. Certain enzymes.

BLOOD-DRAWING TECHNIQUES IN THE NEONATE

Procedure

1. Preparation:
   - Explain the procedure to the mother and obtain verbal consent.
   - Advise the mother she may be present while the procedure is done.
   - Check the identity of the neonate with the laboratory test request form.
   - Perform hand hygiene and done gloves

   Additional information:
   - If a skilled phlebotomist is available venipuncture is the preferred method for obtaining blood in term neonates.
   - It causes less pain to the neonate, takes less time to do and is associated with less maternal anxiety.

2. Choosing a site for the heel prick:
   - Use the most medial or lateral portions of the planter surface of the heel
   - Limit the depth of the puncture wound by using an automated lancet.

   Additional information:
   - Using the lateral or medial edges of plantar area of the foot decreases the risk of damage to the calcaneus.
   - The recommended maximum lancet depth is 2.4 mm when used on the lateral or medial edges of plantar area of the foot.

- Serious complications of the heel prick can include necrotizing chondritis, calcaneal osteomyelitis, and soft tissue damage.
- Only consider using the whole plantar surface of the foot (using automated lancets of 2.2 mm in length or less) for neonates over 33 weeks gestation if they are having multiple / frequent heel pricks.

    Additional information:
    - Do not use the posterior surface of the foot because the calcaneum is more superficial at this area.

3. Preparation of the neonate:

   Methods to reduce pain for the neonate:
   - Skin-to-skin contact with the mother
   - Swaddling/containment
   - Breastfeeding
   - Administration of sucrose/glucose

   Additional information:
   - Skin-to-skin contact for 10–15 minutes prior to heel stab is an effective, easily implemented and safe method to reduce pain in the neonate.
   - Breastfeeding or breast milk should be offered to alleviate procedural pain in neonates.
   - Administration of sucrose/glucose has a similar effect at reducing pain.

   3.1. Position the neonate: Ensure the foot is lower than the body.

   Additional information:
   - Assists with blood flow.

4. Taking the blood sample:
   - Choose a puncture site—do not use a previous puncture site.
   - Clean the heel site (i.e. gauze and water) if the foot appears unclean (e.g. fecal material).
   - Encircle the foot with the palm of the hand and the index finger.
   - Make a quick puncture with the automated lancet device.
   - Wipe off the first drop of blood with a gauze swab
   - Allow enough time for capillary refill of the heel and only gently "pump" the heel, if necessary to continue the blood flow.
   - Apply gentle digital pressure with a gauze swab to puncture site if bleeding continues after procedure.
   - Wipe the heel and apply gauze over the puncture site holding until the bleeding stops.
   - Document as required

   Additional information:
   - Alcohol impregnated wipes should not be used for newborn screening test or glucose reading as the alcohol can effect the test accuracy. It has been associated with chemical burns in premature infants.
   - Automated lancets causes less bruising and facilitate faster healing of the foot.
   - The first drop of blood may be diluted by interstitial fluid.
   - Squeezing the heel causes or increases pain for the neonate can cause hemolysis and soft tissue damage.
   - Avoid the use of adhesive tape or band aids as they cause pain on removal

COMPLICATIONS

1. Neonatal osteomyelitis of the calcaneus (extreme rarity relative to high frequency of use of heel puncture)

2. Macerated heels
3. Infection
4. Inclusion cysts found at follow-up (no disability)
5. Bleeding from site of puncture
6. Abnormal laboratory values.

Prevention of Complications

1. Aseptic technique
2. Proper location and depth of puncture
3. Avoidance of "milking" heel to obtain blood
4. Apply pressure to the site after the procedure until bleeding stops.

Antecubital Venous Stick

When technique to be utilized
1. When amount of blood needed exceeds volume available from single heelstick puncture.
2. When blood culture needed and obtaining blood from UAC is not possible.
3. When coagulation studies are needed and obtaining blood from UAC is not possible.

When technique not to be utilized
1. In infants weighing <1250 g who need their veins saved for central line placement.
2. When contraindicated by condition of the site, i.e., lesions.
3. When contraindicated by physician order for any other reason.

Methods

1. Examine the area for potential venous site. Look for visible antecubital veins.
2. Apply a clean rubber band as tourniquet to distend the vein.
3. Prepare the skin with povidone-iodine and leave on for more than 1 minute.
4. Wipe with isopropanol/water 70%. Wipe dry with sterile gauze.
5. For blood cultures, do not remove povidone-iodine solution.
6. If the position of the needle is directed by the finger, the finger should be cleansed in the same manner. Do not touch the area at all if blood culture to be obtained.
7. No. 25 butterfly needle is inserted into the vein with bevel up and tourniquet removed when blood return is observed.
8. Remove blood to be tested with a syringe.
9. Remove the needle and hold the insertion site with sterile gauze until the bleeding stops.
10. Do not apply band-aid to this area.
11. For obtaining blood culture if insertion attempt need be repeated, use a new sterile butterfly needle each time.

Complications

1. Extravasation of blood
2. Hematoma
3. Infection.

Prevention of Complications

1. If extravasation of blood is seen, i.e. "vein blows", withdraw needle and apply pressure to the area for approximately 5 minutes before re-attempting stick.

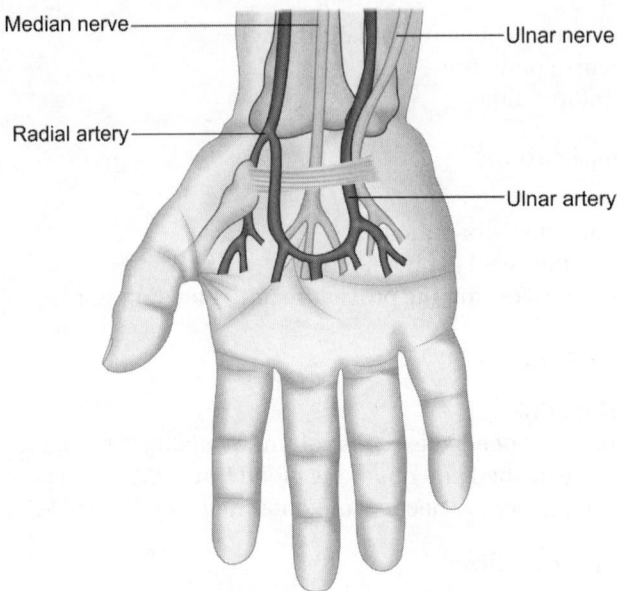

Fig. 32.2: Site for visualization for radial artery.

2. Aseptic technique.
3. No more than three attempts should be made by one person.

ARTERIAL PUNCTURE

Importance: Accurate method of obtaining arterial blood gas (ABG) analysis for assessment of respiratory status.
1. **Radial artery**
   a. Preserves collateral circulation to the hand via the ulnar artery
   b. Avoid area of median nerve (lie midline), ulnar nerve and ulnar artery.
2. **Temporal artery**
   a. Alternative site
   b. Avoids area of peripheral nerves.

Methods

1. *Palpate for pulse:* Assess the strength and position. If attempting a radial artery puncture, palpate for ulnar pulse. Do not proceed to puncture the radial artery if ulnar pulse is not palpable.
2. *Cleanse the area:* With povidone-iodine solution and allow it to dry. Wipe povidone-iodine solution off with an alcohol swab (70% isopropanol) unless blood culture is to be drawn.
3. *Radial artery:* Attempt puncture with bevel of the needle up 45° angle, with the wrist. extended.
4. *Temporal artery:* Needle should be at less than 30° angle with the scalp.
5. *Posterior tibial artery:* Not to be attempted unless attempted radial and temporal arterial punctures have failed. Must have a neonatologist's approval.

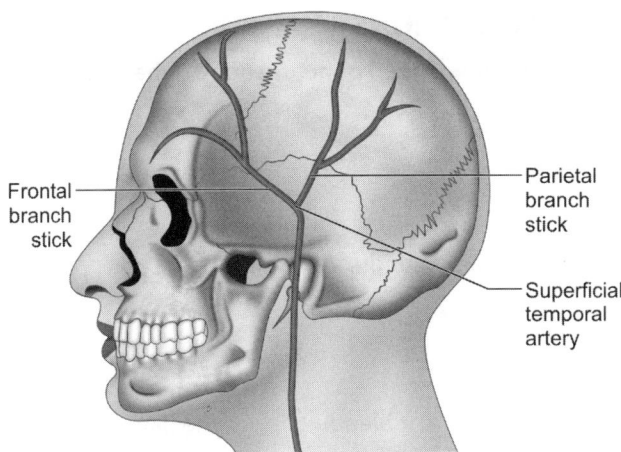

Figs. 32.3: Location of temporal artery (frontal and parietal branch stick).

6. *Continue to palpate pulse*: Insert the needle and guide towards the pulse. If no blood returns, pull back slowly and re-attempt.
7. Attach the syringe (heparinized for ABG) and drawback gently and slowly discarding the initial drop of blood (to clear heparin), then obtain sample.

Follow-up After Puncture

1. Withdraw the needle and apply pressure with a sterile gauze over the puncture site until bleeding stops, approximately 5 minutes.
2. Do not apply band-aid to arterial puncture site.

Complications

1. Scarring
2. Hematoma
3. Infection
4. Bleeding.

Prevention of Complications

1. Apply pressure after puncture
2. Rotate sites to allow healing and to prevent scarring
3. No more than three attempts to be made by one person.

POINTS TO NOTE

➤ Drawing 5 or 10 mL from a newborn can be difficult and potentially harmful.
➤ To get a sample of capillary blood, some practical skills and knowledge how to avoid unnecessary pain, injury and stress in a newborn baby is needed.

PRACTICE QUESTIONS

1. What are the complications of blood drawing in a neonate?
2. How do you obtain blood for ABG in a neonate?

MULTIPLE CHOICE QUESTIONS

1. What is the maximum recommended puncture depth when performing a heel stick on an infant?
   a. 0.5 mm
   b. 1 mm
   c. 3 mm
   d. 2 mm
2. The smallest veins in the human body are known as:
   a. Villi
   b. Bronchioles
   c. Venules
   d. Lymph glands
3. In case of shock in newborn and if bleeding is not the likely cause then do the following, *except:*
   a. Establish IV access
   b. Give IV normal saline or Ringer lactate 10 mL/kg over 10 minutes
   c. Give IV normal saline or Ringer lactate 20 mL/kg over 60 minutes
   d. Give 10% dextrose at maintenance rate
4. A term newborn 2,560 g is admitted at 4 hours with heart rate 200/minute, cold extremities, capillary fill time of 4 seconds. The resident shifts the baby inside the neonatal intensive care unit and starts oxygen and other resuscitative measures. On asking the history from the relatives, the resident realizes that the neonate was born by LSCS done for placenta previa and the mother had come with severe bleeding per vaginum to the hospital and the baby referred after birth to the NICU. Which is the most appropriate NEXT STEP for management?
   a. Give IV normal saline 10 mL/kg over 60 minutes
   b. Give IV normal saline/Ringer lactate 10 mL/kg over 10 minutes
   c. Arrange blood 10 mL/kg and transfuse over 30 minutes
   d. Immediately give 20 mL/kg O negative packed RBC over 30 minutes

ANSWER KEY

1. d   2. c   3. c   4. b

CHAPTER 33

Central Venous Catheters and Long Lines

PRACTICE COMPETENCIES

On completion of the chapter, the students will be able to:
- Perform appropriate selection of catheter, patient preparation and choice of skin antisepsis.
- Provide appropriate care to the lines using aseptic techniques.

ABSTRACT

Central lines are inserted when a child requires frequent and/or long-term venous access, for example, the administration of TPN, cytotoxic drugs or frequent antibiotics. Catheter related blood stream infection remains an important health problem for hospitalized children. Caring for a child with a central venous catheter may be a little scary at first. This chapter contains nursing care of a child with CVC and long lines.

Keywords: Central venous catheters, syringe pump, CVC dressing.

DEFINITIONS

A central venous catheter (CVC) is of the Vygon type or of any other make available locally.

A "long" line is a silastic catheter extending further than a limb or any parenteral catheter inserted in the theater.

A "short" line is confined to a limb and has not been inserted under a general anesthesia.

Long and short lines must be determined by contrast radiographic examination.

Care of Lines

1. Site dressings are to be changed on alternate days.
2. Connection dressings are to be changed once per day.
3. No filters are to be used in the line.
4. For CVC lines, a full sterile technique is to be used including the use of a sterile gown.
5. For long lines, use sterile technique without using a sterile gown.
6. For short lines, use a surgically clean technique as for peripheral infusions.

Changing Connection Dressing

Requirements

1. Sterile gown if CVC line
2. Mask

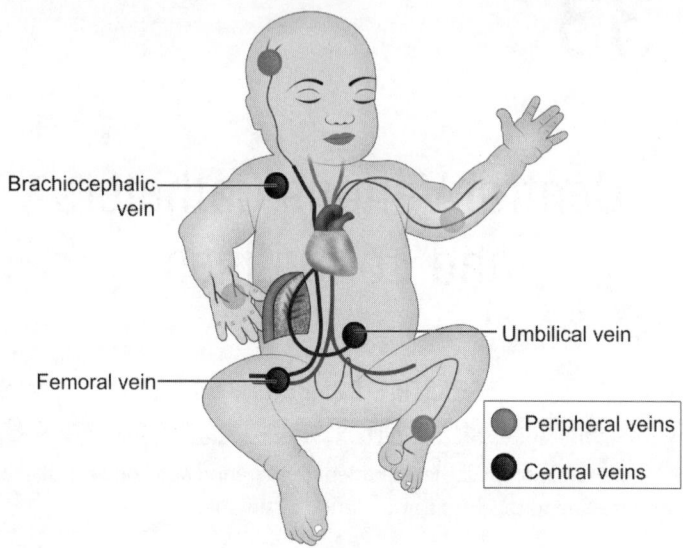

Fig. 33.1: Central venous sites.

3. Sterile, surgical gloves
4. Dressing pack
5. Betadine solution
6. Sterile scissors/scalpel blade
7. Dressing
8. Tape
9. Parenteral fluid
10. Appropriate luer lock (LL) administration set
11. 3-way stopcocks-luer lock
12. Sterile towels—2
13. An operator and an assistant are both required for this procedure.

Procedure

1. Scrub, wear gown, apron and glove.
2. Cut dressing in half using scissors or scalpel.
3. Cut one or two slits in the edge to correspond to tap(s) site.
4. Remove current dressing, and hold the line, so that the connections can easily be swabbed.
5. Swab connections with betadine solution and place swabbed connections on a sterile drape.
6. Apply betadine solution on the dressing, so that it is covered in the solution but does not drip.
7. Attach 3-way stopcock to the new administration set. Close off all clamps and taps.
8. Have an assistant to hold the IV pack, so that it can easily be punctured without being contaminated.
9. Completely prime administration set, so that there is no air-bubble, then wrap end of the line in second sterile drape.
10. Occlude line to the patient (without damaging the connections)-and turn 3-way stopcock to off position.
11. Disconnect the old line.
12. Reconnect the new line including the infusion pump connections.
13. Release tubing, place stopcock in correct position for administration of the parenteral fluid, release clamps and turn the infusion pump on.

14. Redress the site as follows:
    a. Wrap dressing around connections, so that the slits correspond to tape sites. The plastic surface should be in contact with the taps.
    b. Place adequate amount of tape under the dressing. Cut slits to correspond to the tape sites.
    c. Fold over, the edge of both sides of the tape (for easy removal next day).
    d. Place adhesive surfaces of the tape together.
    e. Ensure the line is functioning. Check the tape position and the infusion pump.

PROCEDURE IF INTRALIPID IS USED

Procedures

1. Use syringe pump
2. Prime the line to remove all air from the tube
3. Attach to main 3-way stopcock in the parenteral line
4. Do not completely cover the connection sitewith dressing
5. Turn the 3-way stopcock on to both intralipid and dextrose saline to the patient.

To Administer Medications through These Lines

1. Clean the outer area of the tap with betadine swab.
2. Using sterile gloves, remove cap, place syringe or luer lock extension tube into port and give the medication (when flushing pre and postmedication use a swab and no-touch technique).
3. Clean port with a sterile cotton bud and cap with a new sterile cap.
   Note that no blood sampling or blood transfusion must ever be done via CVC line.

Removal of Lines

1. CVC and long lines are removed only by the medical staff.
2. Short lines may be removed by the nursing staff who have been instructed.

Procedure for Changing CVC Dressing

Requirements

1. Mask
2. Sterile gown
3. Surgical gloves
4. Dressing pack—may need extra gauze
5. Gauze
6. Betadine ointment
7. Sterile scissors/scalpel blade
8. Tape.

Note that extreme care must be taken as most CVC or long lines are not sutured into place. The cotton bud present with CVC lines should not be disturbed.

Procedures

1. Scrub, gown and glove
2. Carefully remove the soiled dressing
3. Slit the gauze/dressing and paint with betadine
4. Swab the site

POINTS TO NOTE

- When a continuous infusion is not in progress it is necessary to instill a heparin lock to maintain CVC patency. The strength of the heparin will depend on various factors such as, catheter type, the time between heparin instillation, and patient characteristics.
- Partial or complete occlusion of a CVC is due to kinking, malposition, medication precipitation or lipid occlusion, should be ruled out as a potential cause of occlusion.
- Removal of a percutaneous CVC should be undertaken by staff, who are knowledgeable and skilled in this procedure.
- All cuffed and surgically placed CVCs, e.g., Hickman lines, Portacaths, must be removed in the operating room.

5. Apply gauze/dressing
6. Cover with tape.

PRACTICE QUESTION

1. How do you change connection dressing of central venous catheter?

MULTIPLE CHOICE QUESTIONS

1. Which of the following is not a complication of CVC insertion?
   a. Pneumothorax
   b. Bloodstream infection
   c. Aspiration pneumonia
   d. Hemothorax
2. When preparing the skin prior to CVC insertion, you should:
   a. Not wear gloves
   b. Wear nonsterile gloves
   c. Wearing sterile gloves
   d. Ask the child to wear mask
3. Chlorhexidine skin preparation should not be used in which patient population?
   a. Cancer patients
   b. Trauma patients
   c. Children less than 2 months of age
   d. Any children

ANSWER KEY

1. c   2. c   3. c

CHAPTER 34

Umbilical Arterial Catheterization

PRACTICE COMPETENCIES
On completion of the chapter, the students will be able to:
- Identify the anatomical structures of the umbilical cord pertinent to umbilical arterial catheterization.
- Describe the preparation, and technique in regards to performing an umbilical arterial catheterization.
- Explain the potential complications of umbilical arterial catheterization.
- Describe interprofessional team strategies for improving care coordination and communication to advance the care of a critically ill newborn and improve outcomes.

ABSTRACT
Umbilical arterial catheterization is a common procedure within the NICU. The umbilical artery can be used for arterial access during the first 5–7 days of life. It is rarely used beyond 7–10 days. Umbilical artery catheterization provides direct access to the arterial blood supply and allows accurate measurement of arterial blood pressure, a source of arterial blood sampling and intravascular access for fluids and medications. This chapter contains the procedure of umbilical arterial catheterization.

Keywords: Thrombosis, embolism, hemorrhage, alcoholic chlorhexidine, acid-base blood gases, umbilical arterial catheterization.

INDICATIONS
It is indicated in serious neonatal illnesses where major acute disturbance in acid-base blood gases, and fluid electrolyte balance are to be expected. It has several uses which are as follows:
1. Acid-base and oxygenation monitoring
2. Arterial blood pressure monitoring
3. Blood sampling for other investigations

Equipment
1. **Arterial tray contains:**
   a. 1 scalpel blade holder
   b. 1 probe
   c. 4 mosquito artery forceps—2 curved, 2 straight
   d. 2 pair dissecting forceps—toothed, non-toothed
   e. 1 iris forceps
   f. 1 pair scissors
   g. 1 needle holder

h. Cotton swabs
i. Gauze, swabs.
2. **Extra equipment for procedure:**
   a. 1 drape (sterile)
   b. 1 scalpel blade
   c. 1 umbilical artery catheter
      3.5 Fr for <1500 g baby
      5 Fr for >1500 g baby
   d. 1 blood pressure monitoring kit
   e. 1 disposable LL 3-way stopcock
   f. 1 × 10 mL syringe
   g. 1 packet 3/0 black silk suture
   h. Skin preparation solution
      - alcoholic chlorhexidine or betadine for infants >1500 g
      - aqueous chlorhexidine or betadine for infants <1500 g for the first week of life
   i. Strapping bridge
   j. Parenteral administrations set infusion pump
   k. Infusion pump
   l. Order parenteral solution
   m. Add 1 unit/mL heparin to parenteral solution
   n. Drug additive label
   o. Other additives as ordered.
3. **Other requirements**
   a. Surgical mask
   b. Sterile gown
   c. Sterile gloves.
4. **General equipment**
   a. Adequate lighting
   b. Radiant warmer
   c. Vital signs monitor/pulse oximeter
   d. Oxygen, air, and suction equipment
   e. Restraint
   f. Ventilation bag and mask.

Techniques

General preparation check and assemble all the necessary items.

Preparation to secure hemostatic: A circumferential suture is placed around base of cord and tied loosely (through Wharton's jelly not through skin). To control bleeding from umbilical vein, apply digital pressure on the supraumbilical area.

Division of cord: Slice the cord across with scalpel, 1 to 1.5 cm from skin margin. Identification of umbilical vessels. When the cut surface is blotted dry the umbilical vessels can be identified easily
   a. The single thin walled oval umbilical vein
   b. Two smaller thick walled round arteries generally constricted so the lumen appears pinpoint.

Preparation of the umbilical catheter: Heparinized solution is drawn into a syringe and flushed through the selected catheter with 3-way LL stopcock attached.

Insertion of arterial catheter: The orifice is opened with fine forceps or probe dilator, and catheter is gently threaded into place. Obstruction may be encountered at either the level of the anterior abdominal wall or the bladder. This can usually be overcome by 30 to 60 seconds of gentle, steady pressure. Avoid excessive pressure or repeated probings. If unsuccessful, call the next senior doctor.

Position of catheter tip: Place in the descending aorta above the origin of the inferior mesenteric and renal arteries between L 3—L 4 (to avoid occlusion or thrombolytic complications affecting them). The correct position is above T 12 on the radiograph.

Ensure patency of catheter: Do not leave the catheter full of blood. Flush with heparinized solution and connect to the infusion pump as soon as possible.

Secure catheter: Tighten purse-string suture around umbilical stump and tie ends to the catheter. Secure the catheter to skin by taping "bridge fashion" as illustrated in Figure.

Radiograph of abdomen: Always check the location of the catheter radiologically after the procedure.

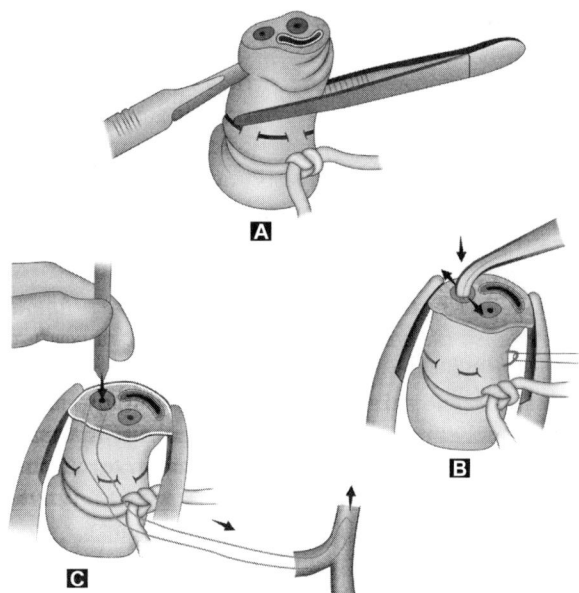

Figs. 34.1A to C: Umbilical arterial catheterization: (A) Cutting the umbilical cord; (B) Preparation of umbilical artery; (C) Stabilization of umbilical catheter.

COMPLICATIONS

1. Hemorrhage due to oozing from the umbilical stump or accidental disconnection of the catheter or any open connections
2. Vasospasm of the femoral artery causing blanching of toes and foot
3. Embolization from an infected blood clot or air in the infusion system
4. *Thrombosis:* This may occlude the following:
    a. Femoral artery—limb ischemia, gangrene

b. Renal artery—hypertension, hematuria, renal failure
   c. Mesenteric artery—gut ischemia, necrotizing enterocolitis.
5. Vascular perforation of the umbilical arteries, hematoma formation and retrograde arterial bleeding
6. Infection—prophylactic antibiotics are not required.

Precautions

1. Note any blanching of limbs, toes or buttocks and report immediately
   a. Massage blanched areas
   b. If one limb is involved, warm the opposite limb to induce reflex vasodilation of affected limb
   c. If physical therapy fails, withdraw the catheter 0.5 to 1 cm and observe
   d. Remove the catheter if ischemia persists
2. Interruption to infusion must be for as short a time as possible
3. Be certain that there are no leaks in the system otherwise. Hemorrhage or clot formation results. Filters are not used for IA lines. All connections must be luer lock.

Removal of Arterial Catheter

The catheter is withdrawn slowly. Press firmly just below the umbilicus for at least 5 minutes and check cautiously. Apply triceps spray and 1 layer of gauze, if there is no further bleeding.

> **POINTS TO NOTE**
>
> Continuation of the umbilical arterial catheter beyond five days is not recommended due to the risk of infection and thrombosis associated with its prolonged use.

■ PRACTICE QUESTIONS

1. What are indications for umbilical arterial catheterization?
2. What are the complications of umbilical arterial catheterization?
3. What are the precautions you take while doing umbilical arterial catheterization?

■ MULTIPLE CHOICE QUESTIONS

1. A healthy 23-year-old pregnant woman gives birth to a male infant vaginally at 29 weeks of gestation due to preterm labor and prolonged premature rupture of membranes. The infant required continuous positive airway pressure support. Umbilical venous and arterial lines were placed, and he was started on antibiotics and total parenteral nutrition. Physical examination is significant for tachypnea, retractions, and bruising over the back and buttocks. At three hours of life, the bedside nurse noted that the left lower extremity is pale and cool. The examination revealed that the femoral pulse on the left is not palpable. Which of the following is the most appropriate next step in the management of the complication being described here?
   a. Application of topical nitroglycerine over the toes of the left foot
   b. Application of warm compress over the right foot
   c. Removal of the umbilical arterial catheter
   d. Initiation of thrombolytics with careful monitoring of coagulation panel

2. A 6-day-old male newborn was admitted to the neonatal intensive care unit (NICU) due to generalized jaundice. His total bilirubin increase rate was 26 micromol/L/hour. He was scheduled for an exchange transfusion. Following an umbilical venous catheter placement, his vital signs are a respiratory rate of 45 breaths per minute, heart rate of 152 beats per minute, blood pressure of 98/60 mm Hg, and temperature of 37.2°C (98.9° F). What is the next step in the management?
   a. Administer a fluid bolus via the umbilical venous catheter
   b. Emergent laparotomy with a transverse incision
   c. Obtain an abdominal ultrasound
   d. Obtain an abdominal X-ray

ANSWER KEY

1. c   2. d

CHAPTER 35

Umbilical Vein Catheterization

PRACTICE COMPETENCIES
On completion of the chapter, the students will be able to:
- Identify the indications and contraindications for umbilical vein catheterization.
- Describe the technique of umbilical vein catheterization.
- Review the appropriate evaluation of the potential complications of umbilical vein catheterization.
- Summarize interprofessional team strategies for improving care coordination and communication to advance umbilical vein catheterization and improve outcomes.

ABSTRACT
Umbilical vein catheterization has been used by neonatal specialists for many years to monitor central pressure, infusion of fluids, and administration of medications during and following neonatal resuscitation. Since, the umbilical vein remains patent for up to one week after birth, it offers an effective route for vascular access in the neonate, and even more so in the premature neonate. The procedure does require specialized equipment, training and confirmation of correct placement by X-ray. This chapter contains procedure of umbilical vein and artery catheterization with rationale.

Keywords: Umbilical vein catheterization, umbilical arterial catheterization.

Choice of catheter: Size of 3.5 Fr or 5.0 Fr is generally recommended for catheterization of the umbilical vein.

Preparation of umbilical catheter: Throughout the procedure of insertion, the catheter is kept filled with fluid and with a syringe attached to the end. If the catheter tip is in the central venous system, there is a large negative pressure generated in it, if the infant takes a deep inspiration as in a sigh or with crying. If the catheter is opened to atmospheric pressure at such a time, this sucks air into the right heart and causes an air embolism.

Location of catheter tip: The best location is beyond the ductus venosus in to inferior vena cava above the diaphragm. Placement of the catheter tip in the portal circulation is undesirable.
a. If wedge shows desirable length of the catheter in a small vein in the liver, it may cause a local area of infarction.
b. Blood flow is slower in the portal system than in the WC so thrombosis or injury from hypertonic infusions are more likely.
c. Portal venous pressure is higher than central venous pressure, its measurement gives no useful information about the cardiovascular state of the infant.

ARTERIAL/VENOUS CATHETER INSERTION: UMBILICAL
(Assisting With)

Policy
- Umbilical catheters will be placed in procedure room whenever possible.
- Infants <29 weeks, admitted from LDR, will have their umbilical catheters placed while inside the food grade polyethylene bag (for thermoregulation). Two X-ray views are required to confirm line placement: AP and lateral.
- For infants <32 weeks and ≤1000 g, follow the skin preparation for immature skin.
- Placement and removal of umbilical catheters is a physician responsibility.

Equipment Required
Gather Equipment
1. Intravenous solutions
    i. For umbilical arterial line
        – 0.45% NaCl with heparin 1 unit/mL
        – for umbilical venous line and depending on the number of lumens available
    ii. Primene C
    iii. D10W with/without heparin 1 unit/mL; plain or with electrolytes
    iv. Other solutions including 0.9% NaCl, nutralipids and medication infusions
2. Umbilical line cart
3. Sterile gown (for physician)
4. Sterile gloves (for physician)
5. Caps (2)
6. Masks (2)
7. Umbilical arterial tray
8. Single lumen umbilical catheter for arterial line (3.5 Fr or 5.0 Fr) and single, double or triple lumen
    – umbilical catheter for venous line (3.5 Fr or 5.0 Fr)
    – 9. 3.0 silk suture

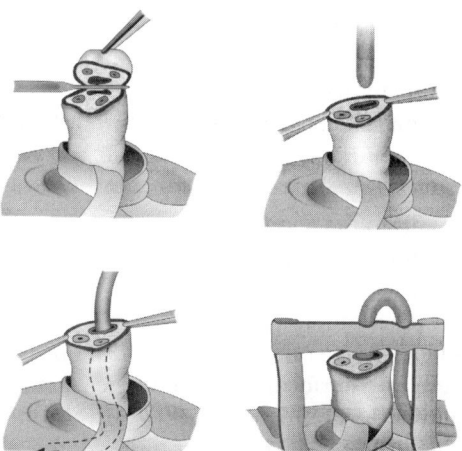

Fig. 35.1: Umbilical venous catheterization.

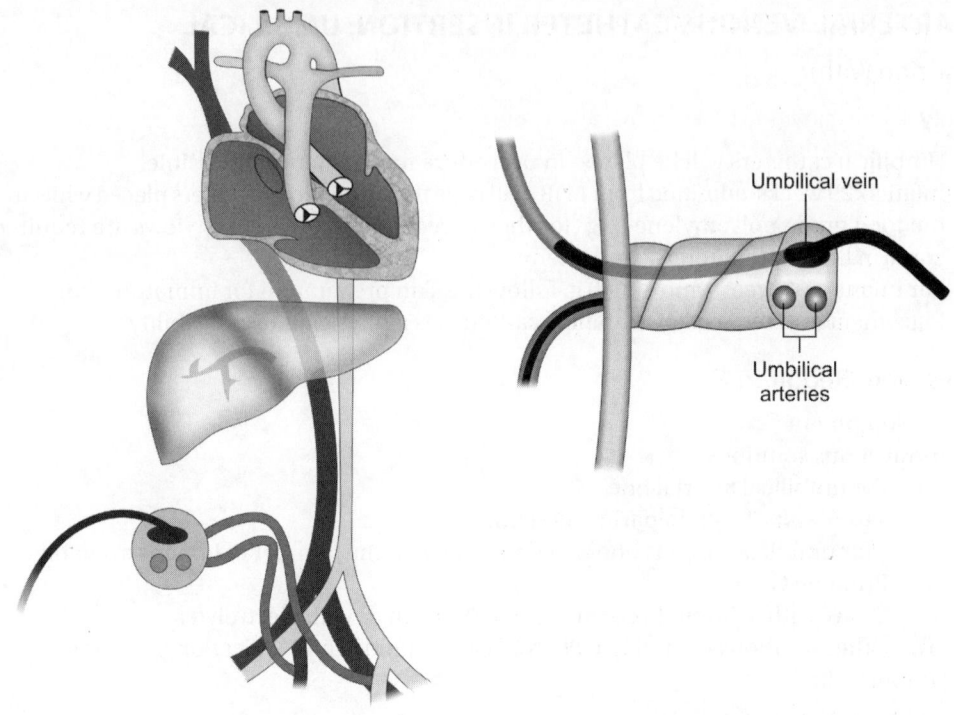

Fig. 35.2: Correct placement of umbilical venous catheter.

10. 10 mL prefilled 0.9% NaCl syringe(s)
11. 3-way stopcock (for arterial line only)
12. Dexidin 2 antiseptic solution (2% chlorhexidine gluconate in 4% isopropyl alcohol solution)
13. Sterile 0.9% NaCl or sterile water (as required)
14. Hydrocolloid duoderm dressing
15. Paper tape
16. 70% isopropyl alcohol and paper towel (for cleaning working surface)
17. Blood collection tubes such as blood culture bottle, gas syringe and EDTA tubes
18. X-ray and blood work requisitions
19. NICU Central Line Insertion Checklist and NICU Central Catheters Registry

Procedure

1. Bring the umbilical line cart to the bedside.
2. Assemble and organize equipment/supplies.
3. Prepare infusions for lines.
4. Restrain infant in supine position.
5. Adjust radiant warmer light to give maximum visualization.
6. Obtain baseline vital signs and perform focused physical assessment.
7. Safely position the infant with careful attention to airway monitoring and maintenance. Ensure head and ETT are visible to the observer under drapes.
8. Follow neonatal intensive care unit (NICU) central line insertion checklist.
9. Clean working surface with 70% alcohol and paper towel.

10. Wash hands for 1 minute.
11. Prepare sterile tray: Open umbilical arterial tray open and add sterile disposable blade to tray add equipment # 8 to # 13 tray.
12. Assist physician to gown, glove and drape.
13. Assist as required to: Measure the depth of catheter insertion(s). Hold umbilical cord with cord clamp attached up and away from abdomen using a Kelly clamp. Ensure physician cleans the umbilical cord and the adjacent skin with antiseptic dexidin 2 solution according to the NICU policy and preparation of skin: antiseptic protocol: Clean/prepare site with dexidin 2 solution for 30 seconds. Allow site to air dry for up to 60 seconds.
14. For infants ≤ 1000 g: Clean/prepare site with dexidin 2 solution for 30 seconds. Rinse cleansed area with sterile 0.9% NaCl or sterile water immediately after antisepsis. Allow site to air dry for up to 60 seconds.
15. Monitor vital signs throughout the procedure.

Once catheters are sutured in place: Umbilical arterial catheter

16. Assistant physician in obtaining blood samples as needed and deposit in appropriate labeled container.
17. Connect infusion directly to umbilical arterial catheter once stopcock is removed.
18. Start infusion at minimum infusion rate required for arterial line infusion.

Umbilical venous catheter:

19. Intermittently flush the catheter using 0.9% NaCl flush to keep the catheter patent or start maintenance infusion(s) at minimal rate prior to X-ray confirmation.
20. Remove sterile drapes. Inspect toes, buttocks, and back for any signs of circulatory compromise.
21. Send X-ray requisition

Once catheter placements are confirmed:

22. Re-set infusion rates per ordered.
23. Calibrate arterial catheter blood pressure transducer and set alarm limits.
24. Secure catheters
25. Loop catheter and tape in a " bridge" fashion
26. Loose the umbilical tape slowly and observe for bleeding.
27. Leave diaper unsecured at sides
28. Discard of equipment and supplies appropriately.

DOCUMENTATION

In NICU Central Catheters Registry

- Time
- Catheter type and size
- Depth of each catheter insertion
- X-ray and final tip location (physician to provide or fill in the information)
- Physician's name.

In Registered Nurses' Notes

- The insertion procedure
- Circulation of buttocks, legs, toes, strength of femoral pulses before and after catheter placement.

Chapter 35: Umbilical Vein Catheterization

In Flow sheet

Blood tests and blood loss.

> **POINTS TO NOTE**
> - The nurse should ensure that all infusions take place in an aseptic manner.
> - The wound site dressings have to be changed regularly.
> - The stump site requires observation for bleeding.
> - If there is any change in the functioning of the line, nursing should report it to the physician.

PRACTICE QUESTIONS

1. What is the policy for assisting umbilical venous catheter insertion?
2. What do you document in NICU chart after umbilical venous catheterization?

MULTIPLE CHOICE QUESTIONS

1. A 7-day-old term male presents to the emergency department with vomiting and severe dehydration. Resuscitation attempts require intravenous (IV) access, and the nursing staff has not been able to obtain a peripheral IV or intraosseous access. After carefully assessing the situation, the provider decides to place an umbilical vein catheter. The umbilical vein is correctly identified, and a preflashed catheter is placed 1–2 cm past the point of blood return. Shortly after placing the line, the nursing staff obtains IV access. The intensive care fellow asks the provider to remove the catheter before the child goes to the intensive care unit. The catheter is removed, and the child suddenly becomes hypotensive and arrests. What step in removal would have helped to prevent this complication?
    a. Flushing the catheter with normal saline while slowly removing it.
    b. Placing the patient in reverse Trendlenberg while removing the catheter
    c. Using umbilical tape to apply pressure on the umbilical stump while removing the catheter
    d. Advancing the catheter 5 cm before removing
2. A full-term 3,800 g neonate requires resuscitation following an uneventful vaginal delivery. Attempts at obtaining peripheral intravenous access have been unsuccessful. The decision is made to insert an umbilical vein catheter. Which of the following addresses the correct diameter of the catheter and length of insertion in the abdominal cavity?
    a. 3.5 French, 11 cm
    b. 5 French, 5 cm
    c. 3.5 French, 5 cm
    d. 5 French, 11 cm

ANSWER KEY

1. c   2. b

CHAPTER 36

Umbilical Cord Blood Collection and Analysis

PRACTICE COMPETENCIES

On completion of the chapter, the students will be able to:

- Understand and perform sample collection of blood from the cord for testing. These tests may measure a variety of substances and check for infections or other disorders:
  - Blood gas analysis: This helps to see if a baby's blood has a healthy level of oxygen and other substances.
  - Bilirubin levels: High bilirubin level indicates sign of liver disease
  - Blood culture: To rule out infection
  - Complete blood count
  - To detect illegal or misused prescription drugs during pregnancy, if found in cord blood healthcare provider can take steps to treat the baby and help avoid complications such as developmental delays.

ABSTRACT

Umbilical cord pH and blood gas values provide valuable information regarding the status of the infant at birth; base excess determination quantifies the magnitude of metabolic acidosis, the putative risk factor for central neurological injury. Asphyxia is a condition of impaired blood gas exchange and if not resolved will lead to progressive hypoxemia and hypercapnia. Asphyxia may occur in a transient fashion with no pathological impact, but significant exposure leads to tissue oxygen depletion, accumulation of fixed acids and eventually metabolic acidosis. An intrapartum event sufficient to cause cerebral palsy may be defined by evidence of metabolic acidosis in the fetal umbilical arterial cord blood obtained at birth with a pH of less than 7, and a base deficit greater than or equal to 12 mmol/L. Analysis of routine paired cord blood samples for all births allows early and appropriate intervention for the neonate when required, and also provides information for medicolegal issues. This chapter contains the procedure of umbilical cord blood collection, and also collection of umbilical samples during infusion.

Keywords: Umbilical cord blood collection, blood gas sampling, intrapartum asphyxia, cord blood pH, hypercapnia.

AT BIRTH

AIM: To collect cord blood samples at birth that will enable the detection of respiratory and metabolic acidosis if present following birth.

BACKGROUND INFORMATION

Umbilical cord pH and blood gas values provide valuable information regarding the status of the infant at birth; base excess determination quantifies the magnitude of metabolic acidosis, the putative risk factor for central neurological injury. Asphyxia is a condition of impaired blood gas exchange and if not resolved will lead to progressive hypoxemia and hypercapnia. Asphyxia may occur in a transient fashion with no pathological impact, but significant exposure leads to tissue oxygen depletion, accumulation of fixed acids and eventually metabolic acidosis. Moderate or severe newborn encephalopathy, respiratory complications, and complex complications increase, when the base deficit is between 12–16 mmol/L.

An intrapartum event sufficient to cause cerebral palsy may be defined by evidence of metabolic acidosis in the fetal umbilical arterial cord blood obtained at birth with a pH of less than 7, and a base deficit greater than or equal to 12 mmol/L.

Analysis of routine paired cord blood samples for all births allows early and appropriate intervention for the neonate when required, and also provides information for medicolegal issues.

Epidemiological studies have shown that about 10% of cases of diagnosed cerebral palsy cases in term infants result from intrapartum asphyxia, and despite the widespread use of electronic fetal monitoring and the increased cesarean section rate. Over the last 30 years the rate of cerebral palsy has not declined in term infants.

Note:
1. Collection of arterial and venous cord blood samples are taken for all births whenever possible.
2. It is preferable to obtain both arterial and venous umbilical cord blood samples for analysis. If only one sample is taken it is preferable that it is the arterial sample.

POST-BIRTH SPECIMEN COLLECTION/EXAMINATION

Equipment Required

- Gloves
- Heparinized syringes × 2
- Needles 21 g × 2
- Face shield
- 5 clamps
- Optional ice and water.

Procedure

1. Immediately after birth while the placenta is still in situ and ideally before the baby's first breath, place four (4) Howard Kelly forceps on the cord to isolate a 20 cm segment in the middle.
   Additional information
   - Delayed umbilical cord clamping may result in significant decreases in arterial blood pH, and increases in arterial blood PCO_2 and base excess.

2. Cut between the two sets of clamps, so that the isolated segment is independent, and both the baby and the placenta still have a clamp in place.
   Additional information
   - Isolating and excising a section of cord allows sampling of cord gases to be delayed until after delivery of the placenta.
3. Continue usual post-birth care of the baby.
4. Collect cord blood (from the placental end of the cord) into a red/pink-topped bottle (EDTA tube).
5. Collect blood for cord blood pH and gas analysis by:
   a. Placing an additional clamp in the middle of the isolated segment of cord to crate two separate sections and
   b. Collecting two samples of blood, one arterial and one venous, from one of the isolated sections.
   Additional information
   - A second segment of cord may be required for repeat sampling.
6. When collecting the blood:
   a. Use heparinized syringes
   b. Take blood from the artery first
   c. Collect a larger quantity of blood from the vein and
   d. Remove all air bubbles from the samples by gently rolling the syringe between the fingers
   Note: Ensure the syringe is upright and the safe cap is in situ prior to doing this.
   Additional information
   - Blood will clot in the syringe unless heparinized and pre-packaged heparinized syringes provide a cost-effective consistent preparation and the correct amount of heparin.
   - The umbilical artery has a smaller lumen, thicker wall, and contains less blood than the umbilical vein. The umbilical vein is more distended and may provide some support for the artery.
   - Arterial blood most accurately reflects the fetal status, while the venous sample reflects the maternal—acid base status and placental function. Aids in subsequent sample identification.
7. Analyze the samples as soon as possible after their collection. if there is likely to be a delay in analyzing the specimens, place the syringes in a "slurry" of crushed ice and water.
   Additional information
   - Arterial and venous blood stored in a doubly clamped segment of cord at room temperature can be measured reliably for up to 60 minutes after birth.
   - Placing the syringes on ice may minimize changes form continued metabolism. Blood sampling for lactate concentration in arterial and venous umbilical cord blood may become unreliable if not analyzed within 20 minutes of birth.
   - Fetal carbon dioxide is removed from the arterial blood in the placenta, therefore the umbilical venous blood should have slightly higher pH and a lower carbon dioxide level than the umbilical arterial blood.
8. Check the results are compatible with one arterial and one venous sample by ensuring that the:
   a. Arterial pH is < the venous pH (by at least a difference of 0.022 units) and
   b. Arterial PCO_2 is > the venous PCO_2 (by at least difference of 5.3 mm Hg).
9. If the sample does not meet the criteria of S. No. 7, repeat the blood collection from the second segment of isolated cord.
10. Record the results.

NORMAL CORD BLOOD GAS AND pH (DURING AND POST-LABOR)

Umbilical Artery

pH	:	7.10–7.38
Base excess	:	–9.0–1.8 mmol/L
PO_2	:	4.1–31.7 mm Hg
PCO_2	:	39.1–73.5 mm Hg

Umbilical Vein

pH	:	7.20–744
Base excess	:	–7.7–1.9 mmol/L
PO_2	:	30.4–57.2 mm Hg
PCO_2	:	14.1–43.3 mm Hg

Normal arterial cord blood lactate = < 6.1 mmol/L.

POINTS TO NOTE

The collection, processing, and banking of cord blood for immediate or future clinical use can be herein have met and passed regulatory scrutiny (including AABB accreditation). Such regulatory compliance comes at a price but is essential in providing the assurance to clients and the transplant physician that each sample is banked under optimal conditions and will continue to be in optimal condition years later, if needed.

PRACTICE QUESTIONS

1. What are the normal values of umbilical artery cord blood gas and pH?
2. What are the normal values of umbilical vein cord blood gas and pH?

MULTIPLE CHOICE QUESTIONS

1. A cord blood gas analysis is being performed during the delivery of a full-term newborn after recurrent variable decelerations were noted on fetal heart rate tracings, as recommended by the American College of Obstetricians and Gynecologists (ACOG) and the American Academy of Pediatrics (AAP). Which of the following sampling methods is the most reliable for the interpretation of cord blood gases?
   a. Sampling of venous cord blood immediately after delivery from a doubly clamped umbilical segment
   b. Sampling of venous cord blood at 30 minutes after delivery from a doubly clamped umbilical segment
   c. Sampling of both arterial and venous cord blood immediately after delivery from a doubly clamped umbilical segment
   d. Sampling of both arterial and venous cord blood at 30 minutes after delivery from an unclamped umbilical segment.
2. The delivery of a full-term newborn was complicated by prolapse of the umbilical cord. The baby was born non-vigorous and required intubation and resuscitation in the delivery room, after which he was immediately admitted to the neonatal intensive care unit for further management. A venous cord blood sample was drawn for analysis immediately after delivery from a doubly clamped segment. The pH was found to be 7.23 with a base deficit of 5.5. Which of the following statements is most accurate regarding the interpretation of this cord blood gas?

a. This cord blood gas is reassuring and rules out any fetal hypoxic injury
b. The arterial cord blood gas pH is expected to be also equal to 7.23
c. This venous cord blood gas cannot be interpreted alone: an arteriovenous pH difference is expected, with the arterial pH being much higher than 7.23
d. This venous cord blood gas cannot be interpreted alone: an arteriovenous pH difference is expected, with the arterial pH being much lower than 7.23

ANSWER KEY

1. c   2. d

CHAPTER 37

Thoracic Drainage for Tension Pneumothorax

PRACTICE COMPETENCIES
On completion of the chapter, the students will be able to:
- Assess the tubing beneath the patient to prevent fluid-filled dependent loops.
- Promote drainage by keeping the chest drainage tube below the level of the patient's chest.

ABSTRACT
Chest drains and chest drainage systems are used frequently in the pediatric intensive care unit. There are many reasons for chest drain insertion, but primarily they are used, whenever there are specific conditions that interfere with the normal mechanism of lung expansion and altered intrathoracic pressures. Pleural chest tubes are inserted to evacuate blood, pus, air and fluid, from the thoracic cavity, to re-establish negative pressure in the intrapleural space and thereby expand the lungs following collapse resulting from surgery or trauma. Mediastinal chest tubes are placed in the mediastinum following open heart surgery, via a medial sternotomy in order to prevent accumulation of blood and clots around the heart, which could cause cardiac tamponade: a life-threatening situation. There are many different types of chest drains available including one-way flutter valve drains such as the Heimlich device or portable drains. However, for the majority of patients in the pediatric intensive care and high dependency units an underwater seal chest drainage system will be used. These systems provide an underwater seal, fluid collection chamber and suction chamber. In pediatric intensive care and high dependency, it is the bed side nurses' role to ensure the patient is cared for safely once chest drains have been inserted. Although insertion of a chest drain may be necessary to help restore adequate oxygenation and promote lung re-expansion in the patient, there are potential risks and complications that the nurse must be aware of. This guideline is intended as a resource for staff involved in caring for children in the pediatric intensive care and high dependency units that require an underwater seal chest drain in situ. This chapter contains procedure for insertion of drainage tube, care during accidental removal of chest drain, care during accidental disconnection/damage to the drainage system, care during chest drain site infection and cell wall injury, care of infection of drain tract, and care during chest drain tube blockage.

Keywords: Thoracic drainage, tension pneumothorax, thoracostomy tube, removal of thoracostomy tube, accidental removal of chest drain, accidental disconnection of chest drain, child with air leak, chest drain tubing blockage.

INDICATIONS

Tension pneumothorax.

Equipment

1. **Emergency relief of pneumothorax**
   a. Aspiration with a needle and syringe usually gives only very brief relief, particularly in infants with severe lung disease who require assisted ventilation
   b. 1 × 23 G butterfly infusion set/Jelco 22 G
   c. 1 × 5 mL ampule of normal saline
   d. 1 × 3-way stopcock
   e. 1 × alcohol swab.
2. **Formal thoracostomy drainage**
   Tray contains:
   a. Scalpel blade holder
   b. 4 mosquito artery forceps—2 curved, 2 straight
   c. 1 pair of dissection forceps
   d. 1 pair of vein scissors
   e. 1 pair suture scissors
   f. 1 small needle holder
   g. 2 towel clips
   h. 2 bowls
   i. Cotton swabs
   j. Gauze swabs.

   Extra equipment
   a. 1 scalpel blade no. 11
   b. 1 packet suture material—3/0 silk with needle
   c. 1 drainage bottle holder
   d. 1 low pressure suction unit
   e. 2 rubber-tipped clamps
   f. Alcoholic hibitane or betadine for skin preparation if infants more than 1500 g
   g. Aqueous chlorhexidine for infants less than 1500 g
   h. Scrub for doctor
   i. 1 mask
   j. 1 sterile gown
   k. 1 pair of sterile gloves.

Procedures

Preparation of Skin

1. The usual site for insertion for the intercostal catheter in the newborn chest is in the fourth intercostal space at the anterior axillary line.
2. The procedure is ideally carried out under sterile conditions with the operator gowned, gloved and masked.
3. The skin is prepared with alcoholic hibitane or betadine and the surrounding area draped with sterile towels. Use aqueous chlorhexidine if infant's weight less than 1500 g.

Insertion of Thoracostomy Tube

1. A small (approx. 0.5 cm) incision is made with a scalpel blade through the skin and subcutaneous tissue.
2. By blunt dissection with straight mosquito forceps through the intercostal muscle, the parietal pleura is opened **(Figs. 37.1A and B)**.
3. Insert trocar and cannula into the pleural cavity
4. The tube is advanced into the pleural cavity for 5 to 10 cm.
5. Withdraw the trocar partially so as to allow for clamping of the tube with rubber-tipped forceps prior to connecting to the drainage system.

Drainage with Continuous Negative Suction (Fig. 37.2)

1. The tube is immediately connected to tubing leading to suction apparatus. The clamp may then be removed.
2. Turn on suction at wail valve to the desired pressure (5 to 10 cm H_2O), regulate by adjusting fluid level in second drainage bottle.

Secure Thoracostomy Tube

1. A purse-string suture is placed around the tube through the surrounding skin and tied firmly once.
2. Both ends of the silk suture are then firmly wrapped around the tube 10 times and tied with a double knot.
3. The tube is then secured by "bridge" tape.

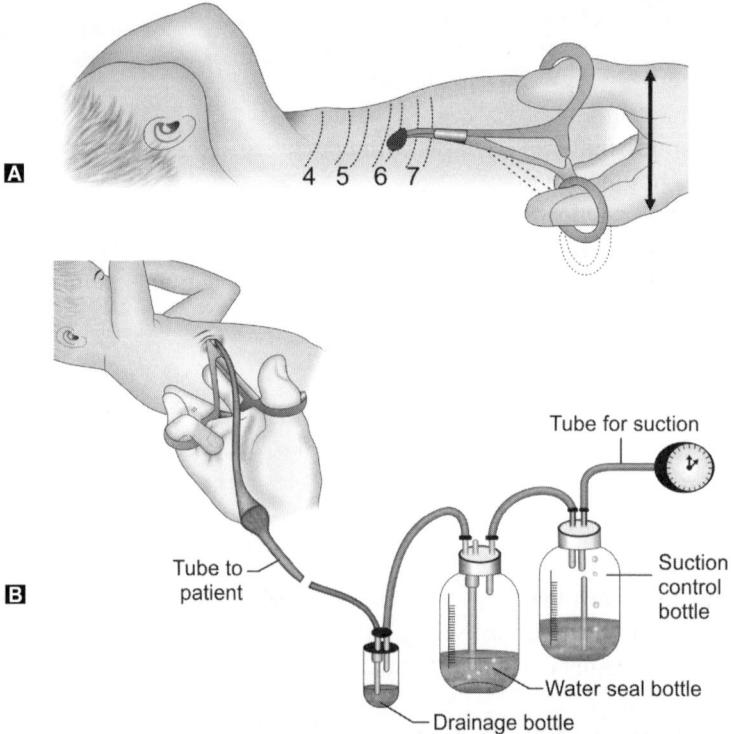

Figs. 37.1A and B: Showing insertion of thoracostomy tube.

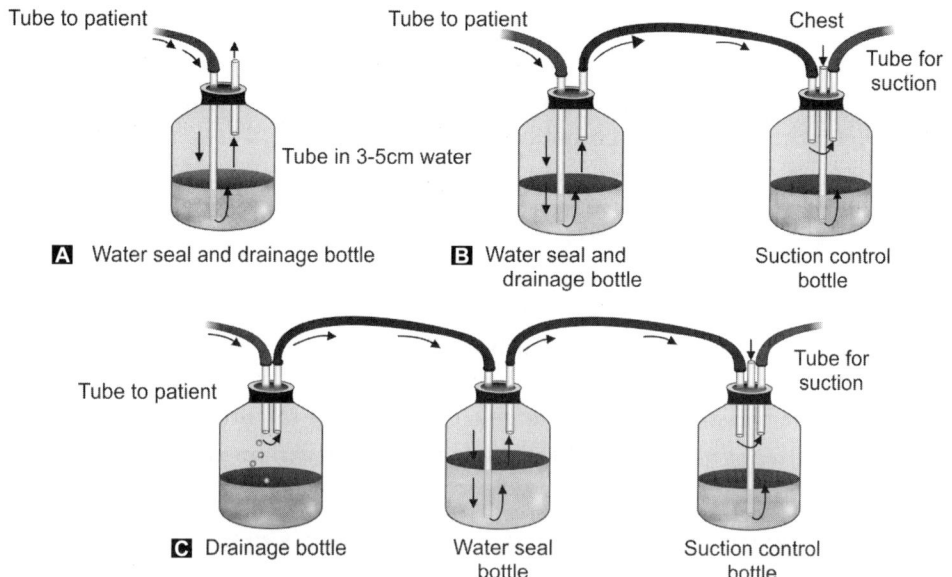

Figs. 37.2A to C: Water seal drainage bottles.

Check Position of Thoracostomy Tube
1. The position of the tube and resolution of the pneumothorax is checked by radiograph as soon as possible.

Precautions
1. Maintain a closed—drainage system, i.e. no leaks because pressure in the thoracic cavity is negative relative to the atmospheric pressure, therefore any break in system allows atmospheric, air to be sucked into the thoracic cavity preventing lung expansion or furthering lung collapse. Patient's tube should be submerged in at least 3 to 5 cm of fluid to prevent leaks.
2. Keep the container below the chest level to prevent fluid draining back to lungs.
3. Prevent blockages in tube by milking every hour or as required.
4. Ensure the fluid column is fluctuating because cessation of oscillation is indicative of a blocked tube or re-expansion of lung. If drainage and fluctuation is not resumed by milking, notify the doctor. A chest radiograph may be taken to verify re-expansion or if there is clinical deterioration suggestive of blocked tube, it may be irrigated or reinserted.
5. Measure drainage by reading of the container's markings 24 hourly or as needed (if excessive fluid is drained).
6. Clamp chest tube(s) close to chest wall with 2 clamps if there is a break in the closed circuit for any reason, there is a need to raise the container above chest level, or the container needs changing. Do not clamp for longer than 5 to 10 minutes.
7. Notify the doctors if:
   a. There is excessive fluid loss especially if fresh blood-stained fluid or plasma.
   b. There is increased bubbling from intercostal tube because tube may be blocked or a large leak may be present.
   c. Infant suddenly deteriorates.

Removal of Thoracostomy Tube

1. Cessation of continuous negative pressure suction can be considered if:
   a. Cessation of bubbling for 24 hours indicating air is no longer draining from the chest.
   b. No recurrence of the pneumothorax.
   c. Infant is not on assisted ventilation. Turn off the suction but leave the tube connected to the underwater seal system. Then, if a tension pneumothorax recurs, it can spontaneously decompress. Do not clamp the chest tube.
2. If there has been no bubbling from the chest for 24 hours, after stopping the suction arid no pneumothorax recurred on radiograph, clamping the tube can be considered.
3. If the condition remains stable for a further 24 hours, the tube can be removed.
4. Rapidly pull the tube out with one hand, in the other hand, have ready a sterile dressing to be applied as a pressure dressing. A large skin wound may require a suture for closure.
5. Follow the infant's vital signs closely and chest lung expansion with, a subsequent radiograph.

■ THE NURSE'S ROLE IN MANAGING UNPLANNED CHEST DRAIN EVENTS

1. **Accidental removal of chest drain child with air leak** (e.g. pneumothorax)
   - Cover site with occlusive dressing (yellow soft paraffin ointment and sterile gauze).
   - Notify medical and senior nursing staff immediately
   - Prepare for reinsertion of chest drain
   - Careful observation of child's respiratory and cardiovascular status
   - The staying suture if present and cover site with occlusive dressing (yellow soft paraffin ointment and sterile gauze)
   - If no staying suture, steri-strip wound and cover site with occlusive dressing
   - Notify medical and senior nursing staff immediately
   - Careful monitoring of child's respiratory status.
2. **Accidental disconnection/damage to drainage system child with air leak** (e.g. pneumothorax)
   - Clamp chest drain
     Emergency situation: It is generally contraindicated to clamp a chest drain with an air leak, however in this emergency the chest drain must be clamped, to prevent air being drawn into the chest, but for the shortest time possible.
   - Call for help
   - Use equipment from chest drain safety pack
   - Clean chest drainage system tubing approximately 10–15 cm below tubing disconnection site with Clinell swab
   - Using sterile scissors cut the tubing at the cleaned area
   - Insert sterile (appropriately sized) chest drain connector to the cut and clean tubing
   - Clean end of chest drain with Clinell swab. Reconnect chest drain to cleaned tubing and connector and remove clamp
   - Prepare new drainage system
   - Ensure connections are secure
   - Secure drainage container to the floor
   - Inform medical and senior nursing staff

- Clamp chest drain
- Place drain end on sterile drape
- Call for help
- Prepare new drainage system
- Clean drain end with Clinell swab
- Connect to drainage system, remove clamps
- Ensure connections are secure
- Secure drainage container to the floor
- Inform medical and senior nursing staff.
3. **Chest drain site infection/chest wall injury**
    - Regular assessment of chest drain site
    - In infection suspected—remove dressing
        - Obtain wound swab
        - Send to microbiology for culture and sensitivity
    - Apply dressing to chest drain site according to hospital wound chart or contact tissue.
    - Viability nurse for wound assessment
    - Document wound management plan, by completing wound chart
    - Re-assessment of wound as documented in wound chart
    - Utilize sterile technique when dressing/manipulating chest drain.
4. **Infection of chest drain tract**
    - Monitor chest drain losses for signs of infection
    - Obtain sample of chest drain loss
    - Sample collection procedure
    - Sample to be taken from drainage system tubing, not collecting chamber
    - Clean sample port with Clinell
    - Attach luer-lock syringe (e.g. 0.5 mL) to sample port
    - Manipulate chest drain system tubing to maneuver chest drain exudates towards sampling port
    - Aspirate sample into syringe
    - Insert aspirated chest drain exudates into universal container
    - Send to microbiology for culture and sensitivity and/or investigations requested by medical staff
    - Monitor child for signs of systemic sepsis.
5. **Chest drain tubing blockage**
    - Monitor chest drain losses at regular intervals
        - Post-cardiac surgery 15 minutes for 1st 6 hours, 30 minutes for following 6 hours, hourly
        - Pleural drains hourly or as required by child's clinical condition
    - Position chest drain tubing to prevent dependent loops and coiling by laying tubing across bed dropping vertically into drainage chamber
    - Monitor chest drain and tubing for clot formation and blockage
    - Position tubing over bed covers to allow constant observation
    (Blockage of chest drain can lead life-threatening complications:
    - Post-cardiac surgery: Unrecognized bleeding, cardiac tamponade
    - Pleural drains tension pneumothorax: Undrained pleural effusion leading to hemodynamic and respiratory compromise).

Inform medical and senior nursing staff of clot formation or blockage of chest drain and tubing.

Chapter 37: Thoracic Drainage for Tension Pneumothorax

POINTS TO NOTE
- Never lift drain above chest level.
- The unit and all tubing should be below patient's chest level to facilitate drainage.
- Tubing should have no kinks or obstructions that may inhibit drainage.
- Ensure all connections between chest tubes and drainage unit are tight and secure.
- Report should be made for any adverse events such as accidental disconnection or piece of tubing left in during removal of drain.

PRACTICE QUESTIONS
1. How will you manage a child with accidental removal of chest drain?
2. How will you manage a child with accidental disconnection/damage to drainage system with air leak?
3. How will you manage a child with chest drain tubing blockage?

MULTIPLE CHOICE QUESTIONS
1. Which of the following is a LATE sign of the development of a tension pneumothorax?
   a. Hypotension
   b. Tachycardia
   c. Tracheal deviation
   d. Dyspnea
2. While caring for a patient with a suspected pneumothorax, you note there are several areas on the patient's skin that appear to be "bulging" out. These "bulging" areas are located on the patient's neck, face, and abdomen. On palpation on these areas, you note they feel "crunchy". When charting your findings you would refer to these findings as:
   a. Subcutaneous paresthesia
   b. Pigment molle
   c. Subcutaneous emphysema
   d. Veisalgia
3. Which statement is CORRECT about a tension pneumothorax?
   a. This condition happens when an opening to the intrapleural space creates a two-way valve which causes pressure to build up in the space leading to shifting of the mediastinum.
   b. A tension pneumothorax is a medical emergency and is treated with needle decompression.
   c. Tracheal deviation is an early sign of a tension pneumothorax.
   d. An open pneumothorax is the only cause of a tension pneumothorax.

ANSWER KEY
1. c   2. c   3. b

Bibliography

1. Achar St. Text Book of Pediatrics,1st edition. Orient Longman publication; 1995.
2. Allibone L. Nursing management of chest drains. Nursing Standard. 2003;17(22):45-54.
3. American Academy of Paediatrics. Clinical Practice Guideline: Management of hyperbilirubinemia in the newborn Infant 35 weeks or more. Paediatrics. 2004;114:297-316.
4. American College of Ostetricians and Gynecologist (ACOG) Committee. Opinion Number 348: Umbilical Cord Blood Gas and Acid- Base Analysis. Obstetrics and Gynecology. 2006; 108(5):1319-22.
5. American Society of Health-System Pharmacists. How to use rectal suppositories properly, 2013.
6. Ball CG, Lord J, Laupland KB, et al. Chest tube complications: how well are we training our residents? Can J Surg. 2007;50:450-8.
7. Barber BK. Cultural, family, and personal contexts of parent-adolescent conflict. Journal of Marriage and the Family. 1994; 56: 375-86.
8. Bartelink IH, Rademaker CM, Schobben AF, van den Anker JN. Guidelines on paediatric dosing on the basis of developmental physiology and pharmacokinetic considerations. Clin Pharmacokinet. 2006; 45(11):1077
9. Bennett P, Smith C. Parents attitudinal and social influences on childhood vaccination. Health Educ Res. 1992;7: 341-8.
10. Bradford N, Edwards M, Chan R. Heparin versus 0.9% sodium chloride intermittent flushing for the prevention of occlusion in long term central venous catheters in infants and children: systematic review. International Journal of Nursing Studies. 2016; 59:51-59.
11. Bradshaw WT, Furdon SA. A Nurse's Guide to Early Detection of Umbilical Venous Catheter Complications in Infants. Advances in Neonatal Care. 2006; 6: 127-38.
12. Bray JH, Hetherington EM. Families in transition: Introduction and overview. Journal of Family Psychology. 1993;7:3-8.
13. Briggs D. Nursing care and management of patients with intraplueral drains. Nursing Standard. 2010;24(21):47-55.
14. Brockmeyer J, Simon T, Seery J, Johnson E, Armstrong P. Cerebral air embolism following removal of central venous catheter. Mil Med. 2009; 174(8):878-81.
15. Butler MG, Menitove JE. Umbilical cord blood banking: an update: J Assist Reprod Genet. 2011; 28(8): 669-76.
16. Canadian Paediatric Society. Oral rehydration therapy and early refeeding in the management of childhood gastroenteritis. Paediatr Child Health. 2006; 11(8):527-31.
17. Gregorio GV, Gonzales ML, Dans LF, Martinez EG. Polymer-based oral rehydration solution for treating acute watery diarrhoea. Cochrane Database Syst Rev 2016; 12:CD006519.
18. Institute for Safe Medical Practices. (n.d.). Administration of rectal suppositories or enemas.
19. Kevat AC, Bullen DV, Davis PG, Kamlin CO. A systematic review of novel technology for monitoring infant and newborn heart rate. Acta Paediatr. 2017;106(5):710-20.
20. Kozier B, et.al. Fundamental of nursing, 7th edition. India: Pearson Publication; 2005.pp.280-3.
21. Marlow DR. Textbook of Pediatrics Nursing, 6th edition. Elsevier publication.

22. Mascarenhas MR, Zemel B, Stallings VA. Nutritional assessment in pediatrics.Nutrition. 1998; 14:105-115.
23. Morrow B, Futter M, Argent A. Effect of endotracheal suction on lung dynamics in mechanically-ventilated paediatric patients. Aust J Physiother. 2006;52(2):121-6.
24. Navarrete C, Contreras M. Cord blood banking. A historical perspective. Br J Haematol. 2009;147: 236-45.
25. NSW Health GL 2007_001 Neonatal Exchange Transfusions in NSW: http//www.health.nsw.gov.au/policies/gl/2007/pdf/GL2007_001.pdf accessed 12th January 2011.
26. Pan SD, Zhu LL, Chen M, Xia P, Zhou Q. Weight-based dosing in medication use: what should we know? Patient Prefer Adherence. 2016;10:549-60.
27. Perlman JM, Risser R. Cardiopulmonary resuscitation in the delivery room. Associated clinical events. Arch Pediatr Adolesc Med. 1995;149:20-5.
28. Phillipos E, Solevåg AL, Pichler G, Aziz K, van Os S, O'Reilly M, et al. Heart Rate Assessment Immediately after Birth. Neonatology. 2016;109(2):130-8.
29. Quek S. Routine cord blood gas analysis: An overreaction? The Practising Midwife. 2004;7(10):20-3.
30. Sobczak A, Klepacka J, Amrom D, Żak I, Kruczek P, Kwinta P. Umbilical catheters as vectors for generalized bacterial infection in premature infants regardless of antibiotic use. Journal of Medical Microbiology. 2019;68(9):1306-13.
31. Society of Pediatric Nurses, American Nurses Association. Scope and standards of pediatric nursing practice. Washington, DC: Nurses book.org. 2003.
32. Thorp JA, Kildy GA, Yeomans ER, et al. Umbilical cord blood analysis at delivery. American Journal of Obstetrics and Gynecology.1996;175(3):517-22.
33. Tume LN, Copnell B. Endotracheal suctioning of the critically ill child. J Pediatr Intensive Care. 2015; 4(2): 56-63.
34. UWHealth. How to give your child a rectal suppository, 2014.
35. Viswanathan J, Desai AB (Eds). Achar's Textbook of Paediatrics, 3rd edition. Madras: Orientlongman. 1991:pp.1-16.
36. Wetzel R. Principles of monitoring/cardiopulmonary deviations. In: Yeh TS, Gioia FR, (Eds). Pediatric Critical are Clinical Review Series. Part 2. Fullerton, California: Society of Critical Care Medicine. 1990:87-103.
37. Wong's essentials of pediatric nursing, 7th edition. Elsevier Publication.
38. Woolley AP. Informed consent to immunization: the risks and benefits of individual autonomy. Calif Law Rev. 1977; 65:1286-314.
39. World Health Organization. Reduced osmolarity oral rehydration salts (ORS) formulation. UNICEF House, New York, NY; 2001. Available at: www.who.int/child-adolescent health/New_Publications/NEWS/Expert_consultation.htm (Accessed on January 18, 2006).
40. World Health Organization: Empowering parents and community: Efforts to Prevent Malnutrition Among Children, 36th scientific conference, 2021.

INDEX

Note: Page numbers followed by '*f*' figure; and '*t*' indicate table respectively.

A

Abdomen, radiograph of 251
Abdominal
    circumference 26, 30, 31
    restraint 130, 134
    veins 22
Acid-base and oxygenation monitoring 249
Acid-base blood gases 249
Acidifying solutions 102
Adrenaline 215
Air embolism 103, 234
    prevention and management 98
Airway
    clearance of 208
    open 208
Alcoholic chlorhexidine 249
Alkalinizing solution 102
Allergic reaction 103
Anemia, prevention and management 98
Angular scars 17
Angular stomatitis 17
Ankle dorsiflexion 23
Antecubital venous stick 238, 241
    complications 241
Antepartum factors 206
Anthropometric 26, 27
    measurements 1, 5, 16, 27
Antiseptic mouthwash 48
Apgar score 21, 21*t*
Arterial blood 197
Arterial blood pressure monitoring 249
Arterial catheter, insertion of 251
    umbilical 255
Arterial puncture 238, 242
    complications 243
    methods 242
Articles, preparation of 100
Aseptic none touch technique 184
Auto-disable syringes 52

B

Babinski reflex 20, 40*f*
Baby's clothing 67
Ballard scoring system 23
Bassinet procedure table 159
Betadine solution 53
Biochemical indices 18
Birth weight, caring low 64
Bitot's spot 17
Bladder catheterization 126
Blood, analyzing
Blood cultures 53
    preparation 53
    procedure 54
    purpose 53
    supplies and equipment 53
Blood decrease, levels in 197
Blood-drawing technique in 238, 239
    neonate, complications 240
Blood gas sampling 259
Blood gases 225, 229
Blood sample collection, assisting for 55*f*
Blood sugar 57
    level 60
Blood volume expanders 102
Body built 1
Body fluids 89
Bottle feeding 70, 72*f*
    equipment 72
    nursing alert 73
    procedure 72
    purpose 72
Bowel movement 51
Bowel pattern 16
Bradycardia 75
Breast tissue 22
Breastfeeding 64, 70, 71, 71*f*, 119
    procedure 71
    suction 65, 119
Bronchiectasis, severe 198
Bronze baby syndrome 150
Burns management 90

C

Calcium 235
Calculating weight, formula for 29
Canine 26
Caput succedaneum 20
Carbon dioxide, retention of 198
Carbon monoxide narcosis 203
Cardiopulmonary resuscitation 205
Cardio-respiratory monitoring 59
Cardiovascular and pulmonary examination 1
Caring ill children, component of 15
Catheter
    care 184
    choice of 254
    duration of 186

length of 187
removing 184, 189
selection 186
size 186
tip, location of 251, 254
Catheterization
factors to consider prior 185
in children 184
Cefotaxime 105
Cell damage 150
Central venous access devices 62
Central venous catheters 245
and long lines 245
dressing, procedure for changing 247
procedure 246
Central venous sites 246f
Cephalohematoma 20
Cheilosis 17
Chest compression 211f
technique of 210
finger method 210
thumb technique 211
two finger, and thumb technique 205
Chest drain 264
accidental disconnection of 264
accidental removal of 264
child with air leak 268
tract, infection of 269
tubing blockage 264, 269
Chest drainage systems 264
Chest wall injury 269
Child in incubator, care of 152
Child with air leak 264
Child's buttocks, holding 194f
Circulatory collapse 115
Clark's rule 79, 83
Clean-catch urine specimen 124, 126
Cold stress 234
Colostomies, types of 163
Colostomy 175f
double barrel 164
permanent 164
Colostomy care 162
and irrigation 162
Colostomy irrigation 162, 166, 167f
equipment 166
postoperative care 167
preliminary assessment 166
preparation of 167
procedure 167
types of 164
Communicable diseases 12
Compression, rate of 211
Conjunctival xerosis 17
Consanguineous marriage 1
Consent 93
Continuous monitoring, discontinuation of 62
Continuous negative suction 266

Continuous positive airway pressure 225, 227
Control panel 159
Cord blood pH 259
Counseling 66
Creatinine 18
Creatinine height index 18
Creativity 137
Crossed extension reflex 38, 39f, 46

D

Dehydration 89, 112
clinical assessment of 114
management of 89
mild 113, 114
moderate 113, 115
severe 114, 115
Deltoid site 85
IM injection 85f
Denver development
examination 43
screening test 36
Denver II test 42f
Dermatosis 17
Development, assessment of 37
Dextrose 234
Diarrheal disease 112
Dietary history 16
Discharging criteria 68
Documentation 177
possible complications 177
post-procedure care 177
preventing infection 178
Doll's eye 20
Dorsogluteal 79
Dorsogluteal site 87
IM injection 87f
Dosage calculations 105
Down syndrome 12
Drainage system child with air leak 268
Drawing blood 53
Dressing
and suture removal 179
purposes of 179
types of 179, 180
used, types of 179
Drug
administration 79
possible errors in 80
to children 79
dosage calculations 104
regimen 5
volume of 106
Dubowitz scoring scale 22, 22t

E

Elbow restraint 130, 132, 133f
equipment 132
procedure 133
purpose 132

Electrolyte imbalance 90
  management 90
Electrolyte requirement 91
Electrolyte solution 101
Embolism 249
Emesis basin 49
Endocrine system 17
Endotracheal intubation 213, 219*t*
  procedure of 214
Endotracheal tube
  insertion of 215*f*
  selecting size of 213
  size of 213
Endotracheal tube suction 217, 225, 229
  articles 218*f*
  equipment 229
  essential equipment 218
  general principles 229
  indications for 217
  nurses responsibilities 222
  potential complications of 219
  precautions with 218
  signs of excessive secretions 229
  technique 230
Enteral intake 60
Enterostomy care 172, 175
  equipment 176
  indications 176
  procedure 176
Equipment
  after care of 83
  and child, care of 88
  care of 102
  needed for procedure 126
  replacement of 73
Erythema toxicum 20
Exchange transfusion 79, 92
  equipment box 94
  formulae 93
  methods 95
Extracellular fluid 89
Extravasation 238
Extremity restraint 130, 133, 133*f*
  equipment 133
  procedure 133
Extrusion 20
Extubation 231
  equipment 231
  procedure 231
Eye care 149

F

Face mask 196
Face masks, types of 199
  non-rebreather 199
  partial rebreather 199
  simple 199
  venturi 199
Family assessment 9

Family health problems, describe 12
Family history 16
  areas of 10
Family tree 1
Feces, analyzing 46
Feeding 67, 117
  and weaning 118
  methods of 70
Fine motor 36, 37
Flow rate, calculation of 91
Fluid
  administration, infiltration of 236
  and electrolytes 91
  calculation 79, 88
  calculation of 91
  maintenance 57
  requirement, calculation of 91
  therapy, general guidelines for 150, 157, 160
Fluorescent tube lights 148
Fontanelle 26
  examination of 32
Fried's rule 84

G

Games 139
  in children 139*f*
Gastrointestinal effects 150
Gastrointestinal secretions 89
Gastrointestinal system 17
Gastrojejunal feeding 77
  precautions 77
Gastrojejunostomy feeding 70
Gastrostomy 170, 170*f*
Gastrostomy button 170, 171
Gastrostomy care 162, 169
Gastrostomy feeding 70, 76
  equipment 76
  procedure 76
  purpose 76
Gastrostomy tube 171
  feeding 76*f*
Gauze 180
Gavage feeding 70, 73, 74*f*
  equipment 74
  indications 74
  nursing alert 75
  procedure 74
  purpose 74
Genitalis 22
Gestational age 21
  of neonate, estimation of 21
Glabellar reflex 36, 38, 39*f*
Glucose 107
Glucose anhydrous 113
Grasp reflex 36, 38, 38*f*
Gross motor 36, 37
Grossed extension reflex 36
Guaiac fecal occult blood test 51

H

Habitual abortions 12
Hand hygiene 53, 193f, 193
Head
   circumference 26, 29, 30
   lag 23
   tilt-chin lift 208
   to foot assessment 3
Health information system 104
Heel puncture 238
   purpose 238
Heel to ear 23
Hematoma 238
Hemodynamic norms 57
Hepatomegaly 17
Heritable illness 9
Home fluids, recommended 112
Hood 159, 202
Humidification 152, 156
Humidity chamber 153
Humor and synovial 89
Hyaline membrane disease 21, 225
Hydrocolloid dressing 180
Hydrogel dressings 180
Hypercapnia 197, 259
Hyperglycemia 98
Hyperkalemia 90, 98
   management 90
Hypernatremia 90
   management 90
Hyperthermia 88
Hypertonic
   concentration 101
   dehydration 90
   solutions 89
Hypocalcemia 98
Hypoglycemia 20, 98, 234
Hypokalemia 90
   management 90
Hypothermia 98
   prevention and management 98
Hypotonic
   concentration 101
   solutions 89
Hypoventilation, reduced risk of 198
Hypoxia 197

I

Ibuprofen 106
Ideal suppository measures 191
Ileostomy 175, 175f
Immunization 121
   do's and don'ts 121, 121t
   empowering parents on 121
   record 61
   schedule 122, 123
Immunoglobulin infusion 92
Incubator 152, 153f, 154, 159, 202
   "T" piece circuit 196
   child care activities 157
   indications 154
   parts of 152
   temperature, setting of 154
Indicator light 152
Infant weighing scale 26, 28f
Infusion pump 234
Insensible water loss 150
Intellectual development 137
Interactional and relationship data 9
Intermittent indwelling 70
Intermittent mandatory ventilation 225, 227
Interviewing 9
   phases of 11
   principles of 11
   technique 11
Intracellular fluid 89
Intramuscular drug administration 84
Intramuscular injection sites 85
Intramuscular medications 79
Intrapartum asphyxia 259
Intrapartum factors 206
Intravenous therapy 234
   common IV additives 235
   common solutions 234
   equipment 235
   hints for prolonged 236
   indications for 234
   preparations 235
Intubation, technique of 213
Iron 17
Irradiation 148
Isoimmune hemolytic jaundice 92
Isolettes 154
Isotonic solutions 89
Isovolumetric method 96, 96f

J

Jacket restraint 130, 131f, 131
Jaundice 20, 148
Jaw thrust 208
Jejunostomy tube 171

K

Kangaroo mother care 64, 65f, 67f
   benefits of 65
   components of 65
   discontinuation of 68
   during sleep and resting 68
   monitoring during 67
   procedure 67
Kangaroo positioning 67
Katori feeding 70, 73f, 73
Kinetic stimulation 143
Klinefelter syndrome 12

L

Language 36, 37
   development 40

Laryngoscope, insertion of 214f
Length measurement 30f
Liquids, prepare 82
Low birth weight babies, fluid requirement for 149, 157, 160
Lubricate catheter 75

M

Magnesium 235
Malnutrition
 in children, prevention of 117
 risk of 15
Mask ventilation 210
Maternal syphilis 12
Measurement, techniques of 27
Mechanical ventilation 225, 227
Meconium 208
Medication, administrating 79, 82, 83
Medicine by mouth 81
Meningitis 48
Mental and emotional development 117
Metabolic acidosis 98, 197, 260
Metabolic needs 57
Metric units 104
Metronidazole 106
Mid-arm circumference 26, 31
 measurement 31f
Mile stones 36
 development 3
Milia 20
Mitts restraint 134
Mongolian spot 20
Monitoring equipment 93
Monitoring of babies 57
 management 61
 observations 58
Moro reflex 20, 36, 37, 38f
Mother's clothing 66
Mottled enamel 17
Mummy restraint 130, 131
 modified 132, 132f

N

Nalaxone hydrochloride 216
Nasal cannula
 equipment 200
 infant with 201f
 procedure 200
Nasal pongs 196, 227
Nasal trauma 227
Nasointestinal tube 171
Nebulizer 49
Necrotizing enterocolitis 21, 98
Neonatal intensive care unit 57
Neonatal osteomyelitis 238
Neonatal reflexes 71
Neonatal resuscitation, role of drug 215

Nerve damage 103
Nervous system 17
Neurological assessment 22
Neurological status, scoring of 23t
Neutral thermal environment 58, 152, 154
 by infant age 155
Newborn
 assessment 20
  immediate examination at birth 21
  purposes and precautions 20
 development of 37
 encephalopathy, moderate or severe 260
 fontanelles of 33f
 heel puncture of 239f
 reflexes of 20, 37
 screening test 61, 96
 total body water 88
Nipple level formation 22
Normal cord blood gas and pH 262
Nurses responsibilities 157, 160, 232
Nurses' roles in specimen collection 47
Nursing
 management 92, 94
 process 6
 responsibility 128
Nutrient solutions 101
Nutrition assessment 15
Nutritional deficiencies 17t
Nutritional parameters 15
Nutritional support
 long-term 170
 short-term 170
Nutritious foods 119

O

Optimum comfort, promotion of 191
Oral drug administration, infants 81f
Oral rehydration therapy 112
 preparation at home 115f
Organs, functional maturation of 36
Orotracheal intubation 213, 214
Osmotic dieresis 103
Ostomy care 162
Oxygen
 administration in children 196
 administration of 209
 high concentration 198
 hood 196
  infant in 202f
 inhalation, general instructions 202
 inlet 153
 masks, types of 199f
 need supplemental 197
 saturation 197
 tent 196, 201
 tent, infant in 201f
 therapy 197
  additional benefits of 197
  controlled 198

high concentration 198
indications for 197
long-term benefits of 197
low concentration 198
methods of 198
types of 198

P

Pain, clinical guideline 59
Paladi feeding 73
Paladin feeding 70
Palmar grasp 20
Panels 159
Paracetamol 106
Parkland formula 91
Pediatric drug calculation 104
Pediatric practice medication 104
Pediatric wards, isolette use in 58
Pedigree charts 1
Perinatal morbidity and mortality 21
Peritonitis 162
Permanent (secondary) teeth 33
Phlebotomy 52
Phosphate 235
Phototherapy 159
   care of child with 148
   complications of 150
   contraindications 149
   equipment 148
   indications 148
   nurses role 149
   set up of 149
   treatment of 150
   unit 148, 149f
Physical assessment 16
Physical growth parameters 27
Physical maturity 23
Physiological data 4
Pinnas 3
Plantar grasp 20
Plantar reflex 36, 39
Plasma proteins 18
Play
   associative 136, 141f, 141
   content of 138
   cooperative 136, 141f, 141
   development role of 138
   double barrel 136
   dramatic 139f
   during infancy 143
   functions of 137
   importance of 136
   magnifies 143, 144
   needle 146
   needs for different age groups 136
   onlooker 136, 140, 140f
   parallel 136, 140, 140f
   preschooler 144
   sense pleasure 136, 138, 138f
   skill 136, 138
   socioeffective 138
   solitary 141f
   therapeutic during bedside care 146
   types of 138, 139
   unoccupied 139f
Pleural and peritoneal fluids 89
Pleural drains tension pneumothorax 269
Plexiglas hood 153
Pneumonia 48
Pneumothorax, emergency relief of 265
Polycythemia 98
Popliteal angle 23
Positive pressure ventilation 205
   bag and mask 209
   technique of 209
Post-cardiac surgery 269
Potassium chloride 108, 113, 235
Pouches 162
   change of 165
   closed-ended 164
   open-ended 164
   types of 164
Premature infants 148
Premolars 26
Pre-school age children 81
Pressure dressing 179, 180
Preterm infants 152
Prior to test 44
Psychological support to mother 67
Psychosocial disorders 9
Pulmonary hypertension 198
Pulse oximetry 57
   monitoring 60
Push-pull method 95, 95f

R

Radial artery 242
   visualization for 242f
Radiant warmer 152, 159, 160
   care of child in 159
   parts of 159
Ratio calculation 108
Recap interview results 12
Recording genogram 10
Reflex, stepping 39f
Rehydration salts packet, oral 113f
Respiratory complications 260
Respiratory disease 198
   assessment of 59
Respiratory failure 197, 225
Respiratory rate 57, 59
Restraints 130
   hazards of 130, 134
   types of 131
Resuscitation
   equipment 93, 206
   indications 206
   initial steps of 207

preparation for 206
provision of 208
signs to evaluate for 207
TABC of 205, 207
Retinal damage 150
Retrolental fibroplasia 203
Rooting reflex 20, 36, 37, 37f

S

Safety measures 80
Scarf sign 23
School-age child 145
    athletic 145
    quite games and activities 145
    rules and rituals 145
    team play 145
Screening test, development 41
Self-adhesive dressing 179
Self-awareness 137
Sensorimotor development 137
Serum bilirubin level 148
Serum hepatitis 103
Servo control probe 152
Servo control system 159
Shaikir's tape 31
Shakins tape 26
Shock 226
    case of 244
    prevent and treat 99
    signs and symptoms of 197
Single random specimen 125
Skeletal system 17
Skin antisepsis 53
Skin fold thickness measurement 32f
Skin foldings 32
Skin necrosis 234
Skin-to-skin contact 64, 65
Sleep maximization 62
Sleep related disorders 198
Sloughing 234
Socialization 137, 139
Socioeffective play 136, 138f
Sodium bicarbonate 235
Sodium chloride 113, 234
Soft vinyl tube 77
Solitary play 136, 140
Solutions 105
Somatic proteins 18
Specimen, collection of 125
    concepts of 47
    importance of 47
    post-birth 260
Speech development of 41
Spoon feeding 70, 73f, 73
Sputum specimen collection 49
    preparation 49
    procedure 49

    purpose 49
    supplies and equipment 49
Square window 22
Stable internal environment 89
Stadiometer 26
Stepping reflex 36, 39
Sterile syringe 53, 100
Sterile tray 180
Stoma care 169
Stoma covers 162
    and caps 165
Stool specimen collection 50
    procedure 50
    purpose 50
    supplies and equipment 50
Storage area 159
Story telling 146
Streptococcus bacteria 48
Sucking reflex 20, 36, 37, 38f
Sunken anterior fontanelles 115
Suppositories
    complications 194
    contraindications 192
    equipment 192
    form packing, removing 194f
    indications 192
    insertion of 191
    pre-procedure guidelines 192
    procedure for insertion of 192
Surgical wounds 179
    care of 179
Sutures, removal of 179, 182
Swab 48
Swallowing reflex 37
Syringe pump 245

T

Tactile stimulation 208
Teaching mothers 118
Teeth eruption 26
Temperature 58
    indicator meter 152
    maintenance of 154
Temporal artery 242
    location of 243f
Temporary colostomy 163
Temporary teeth 26, 32
    eruption of 33
Tension pneumothorax 264, 265
Test tube method 124
    collecting urine 128
Therapeutic value 137
Thermometer 153
Thermoregulation 57, 152, 153
Thermostat knob 152
Thoracic drainage 264
Thoracostomy drainage 265

Thoracostomy tube 264
  check position of 267
  insertion of 266, 266f
  removal of 264, 268
  secure 266
Throat swab 46
Throat swab specimen collection 48
  procedure 48
  purpose 48
  supplies and equipment 48
Thrombocytopenia 98
Thrombosis 249, 251
Thyroid enlargement 17
Tissue infiltration 234
Toddler 81
Toddler oral drug administration 82f
Tongue depressor 48
Tonic neck reflex 36, 38, 39f
Tonsillitis 48
Tonsils 3
Total body water 89
Total parenteral nutrition 79, 99
  contraindications 99
  equipment 100
  indications 99
  instructions 100
Tourniquet 52, 100
Toy safety 142
  maintenance 142
  selection 142
  storage 143
  supervision 142
Transcellular fluid 89
Transtracheal oxygen delivery 202
Tray containing 100
Triceps skinfold 16
Tri-sodium citrate dihydrate 113
Tube feeding
  sites of 170
  types of 74
Tube, types of 171

U

Umbilical arterial catheterization 249, 254
  complications 251
  indications 249
  techniques 250
Umbilical artery 262
Umbilical catheter, preparation of 254
Umbilical cord blood collection 259
  and analysis 259
Umbilical cord pH 260
Umbilical vein 262
  catheterization 254
Umbilical venous catheter 255f, 257
  correct placement of 256f
Universal immunization program 121
Unsterile tray 181
Ureterostomies, types of 173

bilateral ureterostomy 173
double-barrel ureterostomy 173
single ureterostomy 173
transuretero-ureterostomy 173
Ureterostomy 172
  equipment and supplies 173
  indications 173
  purpose 173
  steps in procedure 173
Urethral catheterization
  aims of 184
  female 184, 185f, 188
  indications for 185
  male 184, 186f, 188
Urinalysis 124
Urinary catheterization 184
  general guidelines 187
Urinary drainage equipment 188
Urinary tract infections 124
Urine
  analysing 46
  in kidney 89
  screening 18
Urine specimen, collection 124
  female infant 127f
  male infant 126f
  methods of 128
Urine specimen, types of 125
Urostomy 169f
Urostomy care 162, 168
  equipment 169
  indications 168
  purposes 168

V

Vaccine 121, 122
  name of 2
Vastus lateralis 79, 86
Vastus lateralis injection site 86
  advantages of 86
  disadvantages 86
Venepuncture 46, 52
  equipment and supplies for 52
Venous catheter insertion, umbilical 255
Ventilation
  bradycardia in 231
  complications during 230
Ventilator care of
  child on 225
  infants on 228
Ventilator settings 230
Ventilator SIGHS 229
Ventilatory support, types of 227
Ventral suspension 23
Ventrogluteal site 79, 85
  IM injection 85f
Venture mask 196
Vernix caseosa 20
Vitamin C 17

Vitamin D 17
Volostomy in children 163*f*

W

Water play during bath 146
Water seal drainage bottles 267*f*
Weaning 117
   practices 118
   problems of 118
Weighting facility 153
Wet colostomy 164
Wet dressing 180
Whooping cough 48

World Health Organization 112
Wound dressing 179

X

Xerosis 17
Xiphoid process of sternum 75

Y

Young's rule 79, 83

Z

Zinc 17